Heart Failure with Preserved Ejection Fraction

Editors

MATTHEW C. KONERMAN
SCOTT L. HUMMEL

CARDIOLOGY CLINICS

www.cardiology.theclinics.com

November 2022 • Volume 40 • Number 4

ELSEVIER

1600 John F. Kennedy Boulevard • Suite 1800 • Philadelphia, Pennsylvania, 19103-2899

http://www.theclinics.com

CARDIOLOGY CLINICS Volume 40, Number 4
November 2022 ISSN 0733-8651, ISBN-13: 978-0-323-93981-2

Editor: Joanna Collett
Developmental Editor: Karen Justine Solomon

Cardiology Clinics (ISSN 0733-8651) is published quarterly by Elsevier Inc., 360 Park Avenue South, New York, NY 10010-1710. Months of issue are February, May, August, and November. Business and Editorial Offices: 1600 John F. Kennedy Blvd., Ste. 1800, Philadelphia, PA 19103-2899. Customer Service Office: 3251 Riverport Lane, Maryland Heights, MO 63043. Periodicals post-age paid at New York, NY and additional mailing offices. Subscription prices are $370.00 per year for US individuals, $948.00 per year for US institutions, $100.00 per year for US students and residents, $458.00 per year for Canadian individuals, $967.00 per year for Canadian institutions, $480.00 per year for international individuals, $967.00 per year for international institutions, $100.00 per year for Canadian students/residents and $220.00 per year for international students/residents. To receive student/resident rate, orders must be accompanied by name of affiliated institution, data of term, and the *signature* of program/residency coordinator on institution letterhead. Orders will be billed at individual rate until proof of status is received. Foreign air speed delivery is included in all *Clinics* subscription prices. All prices are subject to change without notice. **POSTMASTER:** Send address changes to *Cardiology Clinics*, Elsevier Health Sciences Division, Subscription Customer Service, 3251 Riverport Lane, Maryland Heights, MO 63043. **Customer Service: 1-800-654-2452 (U.S. and Canada); 314-447-8871 (outside U.S. and Canada). Fax: 314-447-8029. E-mail: journalscus-tomerservice-usa@elsevier.com (for print support); journalsonlinesupport-usa@elsevier.com (for online support).**

Reprints. For copies of 100 or more, of articles in this publication, please contact the Commercial Reprints Department, Elsevier Inc., 360 Park Avenue South, New York, NY 10010-1710. Tel.: 212-633-3874; Fax: 212-633-3820; E-mail: reprints@elsevier.com.

Cardiology Clinics is also published in Spanish by McGraw-Hill Interamericana Editores S. A., P.O. Box 5-237, 06500, Mexico D. F., Mexico; in Portuguese by Reichmann and Alfonso Editores Rio de Janeiro, Brazil; and in Greek by Dimitrios P. Lagos, 8 Pondon Street, GR115-28 Ilissia, Greece.

Cardiology Clinics is covered in *MEDLINE/PubMed (Index Medicus), Excerpta Medica, The Cumulative Index to Nursing and Allied Health Literature* (CINAHL).

Contributors

PACO E. BRAVO, MD
Assistant Professor of Medicine, Division of Cardiovascular Medicine, Department of Medicine, Division of Nuclear Medicine, Department of Radiology, Hospital of the University of Pennsylvania, Philadelphia, Pennsylvania, USA

SALVATORE CARBONE, PhD, MS, FHFSA
Assistant Professor, Department of Kinesiology and Health Sciences, College of Humanities and Sciences, VCU Pauley Heart Center, Division of Cardiology, Department of Internal Medicine, Virginia Commonwealth University, Richmond, Virginia, USA

JULIO A. CHIRINOS, MD, PhD
Assistant Professor of Medicine, Division of Cardiovascular Medicine, Department of Medicine, Hospital of the University of Pennsylvania, Perelman School of Medicine, University of Pennsylvania, Philadelphia, Pennsylvania, USA

ADAM D. DEVORE, MD, MHS
Division of Cardiology, Duke University School of Medicine, Duke Clinical Research Institute, Durham, North Carolina, USA

MARAT FUDIM, MD, MHS
Division of Cardiology, Department of Medicine, Duke University, Duke Clinical Research Institute, Durham, North Carolina, USA

PARAG GOYAL, MD, MSc
Associate Professor of Medicine, Etingen Family Clinical Scholar of Medicine, Director, Weill Cornell Medicine HFpEF Program, Department of Medicine, Weill Cornell Medicine, New York, New York, USA

GILLIAN GRAFTON, DO
Division of Cardiovascular Medicine, Department of Internal Medicine, Henry Ford Hospital, Detroit, Michigan, USA

TOMONARI HARADA, MD, PhD
Department of Cardiovascular Medicine, Gunma University Graduate School of Medicine, Maebashi, Gunma, Japan

STEVEN HSU, MD
Division of Cardiology, Department of Medicine, Johns Hopkins University, Baltimore, Maryland, USA

SCOTT L. HUMMEL, MD, MS, FACC, FHFSA
Associate Professor of Internal Medicine, Division of Cardiovascular Medicine, University of Michigan Frankel Cardiovascular Center, Cardiology Section Chief, Department of Medicine, University of Michigan, Ann Arbor Veterans Affairs Health System, Ann Arbor, Michigan, USA

HIDEKI ISHII, MD, PhD
Department of Cardiovascular Medicine, Gunma University Graduate School of Medicine, Maebashi, Gunma, Japan

C. CHARLES JAIN, MD
Clinical Fellow, Assistant Professor of Medicine, Cardiovascular Medicine, Mayo Clinic, Rochester, Minnesota, USA

KAZUKI KAGAMI, MD
Department of Cardiovascular Medicine, Gunma University Graduate School of Medicine, Maebashi, Gunma, Japan; Division of Cardiovascular Medicine, National Defense Medical College, Tokorozawa, Saitama, Japan

DANIELLE L. KIRKMAN, PhD, MS, RCEP
Assistant Professor, Department of Kinesiology and Health Sciences, College of Humanities and Sciences, VCU Pauley Heart Center, Division of Cardiology, Department of Internal Medicine, Virginia Commonwealth University, Richmond, Virginia, USA

DALANE W. KITZMAN, MD
Kermit Glenn Phillips II Chair in Cardiovascular Medicine Professor, Department of Internal Medicine, Sections on Cardiovascular Disease and Geriatrics, Wake Forest School of Medicine, Winston-Salem, North Carolina, USA

MATTHEW C. KONERMAN, MD, MSc, FACC
Assistant Professor of Internal Medicine, Ambulatory Care Clinical Chief, Division of Cardiovascular Medicine, Department of Medicine, University of Michigan, University of Michigan Frankel Cardiovascular Center, Cardiology Section Chief, Ann Arbor, Michigan, USA

ALLISON P. LEVIN, MD
Department of Medicine, Harvard Medical School, Massachusetts General Hospital, Boston, Massachusetts, USA

DYLAN MARSHALL, MD
Cardiovascular Medicine Fellow, Department
of Medicine, Weill Cornell Medicine, New York,
New York, USA

MATHEW S. MAURER, MD
Cardiac Amyloidosis Program, Columbia
University Irving Medical Center, NewYork-
Presbyterian Hospital, New York, New York,
USA

VICTOR M. MOLES, MD
Clinical Assistant Professor, Division of
Cardiovascular Medicine, Department of
Internal Medicine, University of Michigan, Ann
Arbor, Michigan, USA

MASARU OBOKATA, MD, PhD
Department of Cardiovascular Medicine,
Gunma University Graduate School
of Medicine, Maebashi, Gunma,
Japan

KAZUNORI OMOTE, MD, PhD
Department of Cardiovascular Medicine, Mayo
Clinic, Rochester, Minnesota, USA

ANTHONY E. PETERS, MD, MS
Division of Cardiology, Duke University School
of Medicine, Duke Clinical Research Institute,
Durham, North Carolina, USA

YOGESH N.V. REDDY, MD, MSc
Senior Associate Consultant, Assistant
Professor of Medicine, Cardiovascular Medicine,
Mayo Clinic, Rochester, Minnesota, USA

CARLOS M. RODRIGUEZ, MD
Cardiac Amyloidosis Program, Columbia
University Irving Medical Center, NewYork-
Presbyterian Hospital, New York, New York,
USA

HUSAM M. SALAH, MD
Department of Medicine, University of
Arkansas for Medical Sciences, Little Rock,
Arkansas, USA

DIA A. SMILEY, DO
Cardiac Amyloidosis Program, Columbia
University Irving Medical Center, NewYork-
Presbyterian Hospital, New York, New York,
USA

MAHESH K. VIDULA, MD
Assistant Professor of Medicine, Division of
Cardiovascular Medicine, Department of
Medicine, Hospital of the University of
Pennsylvania, Philadelphia, Pennsylvania, USA

OMAR ZAINUL, BS, MD
Candidate, Weill Cornell Medical College, New
York, New York, USA

Contents

Heart failure with preserved ejection fraction (HFpEF) is common and increasing in prevalence. Despite this, HFpEF is challenging to diagnose due in part to its shared clinical features with other comorbid conditions. HFpEF is now understood as a systemic syndrome, often driven by pro-inflammatory comorbidities, rather than solely a cardiac disease. This review summarizes the epidemiology, diagnostic criteria, and pathophysiology of HFpEF and proposes a clinical approach for patients suspected of having or diagnosed with HFpEF.

Pathophysiological heterogeneity is considered the primary reason for the limited effective treatment options for patients with heart failure with preserved ejection fraction (HFpEF). Recent studies have focused on HFpEF phenotyping that categorizes patients as pathophysiologically homogeneous groups to develop personalized treatment strategies. This approach relies on comorbidities, cardiac structure and function, central hemodynamics at rest and during exercise, or machine learning techniques. Although some phenotypes have been successfully identified, efforts are still ongoing. This review summarizes the current understanding of phenotyping approaches in patients with HFpEF, highlighting its pathophysiology and potential treatment strategies.

As echocardiography is universally performed in the evaluation of suspected heart failure with preserved ejection fraction (HFpEF), a number of structural and functional characteristics relevant to both the diagnosis and phenotyping of HFpEF can be elucidated. Exclusion of alternate causes of heart failure is a critical first step performed principally by echocardiography. Once HFpEF is confirmed, echocardiography may provide insight into pathophysiology and phenotyping by quantifying atrial mechanics, pericardial restraint, degree of pulmonary hypertension, and atrial valvular regurgitation. Although current echo-Doppler assessment of filling pressures is insensitive to diagnose HFpEF, there are emerging technologies such as left atrial (LA) strain that hold promise for noninvasive diagnosis.

Heart failure with preserved ejection fraction (HFpEF) is highly prevalent, affecting approximately half of all patients with HF. The diagnosis of HFpEF can be notoriously challenging in clinical practice, given the many overlapping etiologies of dyspnea or reduced exercise tolerance in patients at risk for HFpEF. Multimodality imaging has an important role in establishing the diagnosis of HFpEF and the presence of elevated left ventricular filling pressures, identifying specific etiologies of HFpEF that can benefit from approved therapies, and discerning distinct phenogroups or mechanistic abnormalities that may inform the development of novel therapeutics.

Heart failure (HF) with preserved ejection fraction (HFpEF) is characterized by an inability of the heart to perfuse the body without pathologic increases in filling pressure at rest or during exertion. Right heart catheterization provides direct assessment for HF, providing the most robust and direct method to evaluate the central hemodynamic abnormalities, and serves as the gold standard to confirm or refute the presence of HFpEF. This article reviews current understanding of the best practices in the performance and interpretation of hemodynamic assessment, relates important pathophysiologic concepts to clinical care, and discusses current and evidence-based applications of hemodynamics in HFpEF.

The management of heart failure with preserved ejection fraction (HFpEF) is rapidly evolving. The pharmacologic treatment of patients with HFpEF includes symptom management with diuretics and optimization of comorbidities, including hypertension, obesity, diabetes mellitus, and atrial fibrillation. Specific therapies, including angiotensin II receptor blockers, mineralocorticoid receptor antagonists, angiotensin receptor–neprilysin inhibitors, and sodium–glucose cotransporter-2 inhibitors, are well tolerated and can reduce the risk of HF hospitalization, particularly in those on the lower end of the HFpEF left ventricular ejection fraction spectrum. Ongoing trials should continue to inform optimal therapy in this evolving field.

Patients with heart failure with preserved ejection fraction (HFpEF) suffer from a high rate of cardiometabolic comorbidities with limited pharmaceutical therapies proven to improve clinical outcomes and cardiorespiratory fitness (CRF). Nonpharmacologic therapies, such as exercise training and dietary interventions, are promising strategies for this population. The aim of this narrative review is to present a summary of the literature published to date and future directions related to the efficacy of nonpharmacologic, lifestyle-related therapies in HFpEF, with a focus on exercise training and dietary interventions.

Heart failure with preserved ejection fraction (HFpEF) is a heterogeneous syndrome with few options for effective pharmacologic therapies. Numerous device-based approaches to HFpEF therapy have emerged, which aim to treat the clinical and pathophysiologic features common to the varied causes of this syndrome. This review summarizes the current landscape of device therapy in HFpEF with a focus on structural interventions, such as left-to-right atrial shunts; cardiac contractility modulation; autonomic modulation, such as baroreflex activation therapy and splanchnic nerve modulation; and respiratory modulation, such as phrenic nerve stimulation.

Because heart failure with preserved ejection fraction (HFpEF) is closely linked to aging processes and disproportionately affects older adults, consideration of geriatric domains is paramount to ensure high-quality care to older adults with HFpEF. Multimorbidity, polypharmacy, cognitive impairment, depressive symptoms, frailty, falls, and social isolation each have important implications on quality of life and clinical events including hospitalization and mortality. There are multiple strategies to screen for these conditions. This narrative review underscores the importance of screening for multiple geriatric conditions, integrating these conditions into decision making, and addressing these conditions when caring for older adults with HFpEF.

Heart failure with preserved ejection fraction (HFpEF) is a common medical condition associated with increased morbidity and mortality. Through different mechanisms, including passive left-sided congestion and/or vasculopathy, patients with HFpEF can develop pulmonary hypertension (PH). This association -PH-HFpEF- is linked with worsening symptomatology and long-term outcomes. Although pulmonary vasodilators have been effective in treating patients with a pulmonary vasculopathy, such as pulmonary arterial hypertension (PAH), these results have not been replicated in those with PH-HFpEF. There is an unmet need to develop effective medical therapy for this challenging population. In this article, we focus on understanding the definition, epidemiology, diagnosis, clinical implications, and treatment for PH in the setting of HFpEF.

Heart failure with preserved ejection fraction (HFpEF) is a heterogeneous syndrome, and cardiac amyloidosis (CA) is one of the causes of HFpEF, that has established and emerging treatment options. However, it remains an underdiagnosed and often overlooked cause of HFpEF. The importance of early diagnosis cannot be emphasized enough, as emerging therapies are more effective early in the course of the disease. Further, because of the unique physiologic and hemodynamic features of CA, patients poorly tolerate traditional heart failure medications and experience worse outcomes compared with other causes of HFpEF. With the aging of the population, transthyretin (ATTR) CA, once thought to be a rare disease, will become the most common type of systemic amyloidosis. ATTR-CA is increasingly recognized due to enhanced clinical awareness; advances in diagnostic imaging that have led to a diagnostic approach that does not require a biopsy, as well as the recent introduction of novel disease-modifying treatments. ATTR-CA causes restrictive and infiltrative cardiomyopathy that results in heart failure, atrial and ventricular arrhythmias, and conduction disease, and is associated with significant morbidity and mortality. Our goal in this review is to provide an overview of the historical, epidemiologic, diagnostic, and therapeutic evolution of ATTR-CA, and to emphasize the importance of early suspicion and detection of HFpEF.

CARDIOLOGY CLINICS

SERIES OF RELATED INTEREST

Heart Failure Clinics
Available at: https://www.heartfailure.theclinics.com/
Interventional Cardiology Clinics
Available at: https://www.interventional.theclinics.com/
Cardiac Electrophysiology Clinics
Available at: https://www.cardiacep.theclinics.com/

Preface

Heart Failure with Preserved Ejection Fraction: The Future Is Now

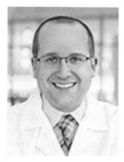
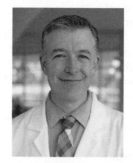

Matthew C. Konerman, MD, MSc   Scott L. Hummel, MD, MS

Editors

The epidemic of heart failure with preserved ejection fraction (HFpEF) has compelled both of us since the start of our training. There are few greater unmet needs in medicine today. Millions of patients with HFpEF have quality of life on par with severe cancer or disabling rheumatoid arthritis and suffer frequent hospitalizations and shortened lifespan. Until recently, this large and growing problem appeared unsolvable, and even incremental improvements were difficult to achieve.

The past 10 to 15 years have brought crucial understanding of how HFpEF develops and progresses. The terminology shift from "diastolic heart failure" to HFpEF is not merely semantics[1]; beyond diastolic dysfunction, HFpEF involves a multidimensional failure of cardiovascular reserve. Comorbid conditions, such as hypertension, diabetes mellitus, and obesity, are not only common in HFpEF but also likely directly contribute to its pathophysiology. A related and important recent insight is that HFpEF is not just a cardiovascular disease but also a systemic syndrome with multiorgan manifestations.[2]

Based on these advances, a broadly applicable evidence base for treating HFpEF is beginning to emerge. Successful recent clinical trials have improved participant selection criteria and have studied treatments with pleotropic effects, such as SGLT-2 inhibitors and exercise. However, much more work is needed, particularly in developing strategies that can sustainably improve quality of life. One major challenge is the heterogeneity of HFpEF. Precision phenotyping at multiple levels, including genetic, molecular, hemodynamic, and systems biology/whole person, may be needed to effectively target therapies. In this issue of *Cardiology Clinics*, we are privileged to share insights from experts in the field on diagnosing, phenotyping, and treating HFpEF.

As a primer for later articles, Anderson and Konerman give an overview of HFpEF

Cardiol Clin 40 (2022) xiii–xiv
https://doi.org/10.1016/j.ccl.2022.07.002
0733-8651/22/© 2022 Published by Elsevier Inc.

epidemiology, pathophysiology, and diagnosis along with a suggested approach to initial evaluation. Obokata and colleagues outline how to assess and manage key phenotypes of HFpEF. Jain and Reddy provide an outstanding review of echocardiography, and Vidula and colleagues summarize how multimodality imaging can uncover the underlying mechanisms and etiologies of HFpEF. Borlaug and team illustrate the critical importance of hemodynamic assessment in diagnosis and hemodynamic phenotyping. The next section reveals the exciting and rapidly changing landscape of HFpEF treatment. Peters and Devore offer a thorough review of pharmacologic clinical trials; Carbone and Kirkman expertly outline the importance of diet and exercise, and Fudim and colleagues assess novel device-based therapies for HFpEF. The last section of the issue provides in-depth information on three important facets of HFpEF diagnosis and management. Zainul and team's article clearly demonstrates the importance of geriatric domains; Moles and Grafton review pulmonary hypertension in HFpEF, and Smiley and colleagues provide an essential and comprehensive article on transthyretin cardiac amyloidosis.

We believe that the future is bright for researchers, clinicians, and most importantly, our patients with or at risk of HFpEF. We hope that you find the articles in this issue of *Cardiology Clinics* as informative, exciting, and relevant as we have.

Matthew C. Konerman, MD, MS, FACC
Division of Cardiovascular Medicine
University of Michigan Frankel Cardiovascular Center
1500 East Medical Center Drive, SPC 5853
Ann Arbor, MI, 48109, USA

Scott L. Hummel, MD, MS, FACC, FHFSA
University of Michigan Frankel Cardiovascular Center
1500 East Medical Center Drive, SPC 5853
Ann Arbor, MI, 48109, USA

Ann Arbor Veterans Affairs Health System
2215 Fuller Road
Ann Arbor, MI, 48105, USA

E-mail addresses:
mkonerma@med.umich.edu (M.C. Konerman)
scothumm@med.umich.edu (S.L. Hummel)

REFERENCES

1. Maurer MS, Hummel SL. Heart failure with preserved ejection fraction: what's in a name? J Am Coll Cardiol 2021;58(3):275–7.
2. Shah SJ, Borlaug BA, Kitzman DW, et al. Research priorities for heart failure with preserved ejection fraction. Circulation 2020;141(12):1001–26.

Epidemiology, Diagnosis, Pathophysiology, and Initial Approach to Heart Failure with Preserved Ejection Fraction

Theresa Anderson, MD[a],*, Scott L. Hummel, MD, MS[b,c],
Matthew C. Konerman, MD, MSc[b]

KEYWORDS

- Heart failure with preserved ejection fraction • HFpEF diagnosis • HFpEF pathophysiology
- HFpEF comorbid conditions

KEY POINTS

- The diagnosis of heart failure with preserved ejection fraction (HFpEF) involves clinical signs and symptoms with an EF > 50% plus objective evidence of elevated left ventricular filling pressures.
- Recently published scores using clinical and echocardiographic data can be used to determine the probability of an HFpEF diagnosis in patients with unexplained dyspnea.
- HFpEF is heavily influenced by pro-inflammatory comorbid conditions causing endothelial dysfunction, collagen dysregulation, and myocyte hypertrophy.
- HFpEF is a heterogenous syndrome of impaired cardiac reserve function.
- Treatment of both cardiac manifestations and noncardiac comorbid conditions is essential for the management of HFpEF.

EPIDEMIOLOGY

Heart failure affects an estimated 26 million individuals globally with an average of 3.6 million diagnosed annually worldwide.[1] In the United States, heart failure affects 5.7 million individuals and is the leading cause of hospitalization.[1] Heart failure with preserved ejection fraction (HFpEF) has increased in prevalence over the past 3 decades,[2,3] and is associated with poor quality of life, high hospitalization rates, and increased mortality.[3–5] Outcomes have improved in heart failure with reduced ejection fraction (HFrEF) because of the increased use of evidence-based medications and devices. However, few evidence-based therapies have been established for HFpEF. A significant proportion of patients with HFpEF die of cardiovascular (CV) related causes (eg, sudden death, worsening heart failure, and myocardial infarction).[4] Patients with HFpEF are often older and commonly have multiple comorbid conditions such as obesity, hypertension, diabetes mellitus (DM), renal disease, and pulmonary disease that contribute to high rates of non-CV morbidity and mortality.[2,6,7]

HFpEF is the most common form of heart failure in older adults,[8] in part due to the increased prevalence of key risk factors with aging. Despite this, HFpEF has been called the "ultimate form of premature cardiac aging" since aging is associated with several HFpEF pathophysiologic mechanisms.[9] These mechanisms include the following: increased left

[a] University of Michigan, Internal Medicine Residency Department, 1500 East Medical Center Drive, Ann Arbor, MI 48109, USA; [b] University of Michigan Frankel Cardiovascular Center, 1500 East Medical Center Dr., SPC 5853, Ann Arbor, MI 48109, USA; [c] Charles S. Kettles VA Medical Center, 2215 Fuller Road, Ann Arbor, MI 48105, USA
* Corresponding author.
E-mail address: tandersn@med.umich.edu

Cardiol Clin 40 (2022) 397–413
https://doi.org/10.1016/j.ccl.2022.07.001
0733-8651/22/Published by Elsevier Inc.

Table 1
Diagnostic criteria for heart failure with reduced, mildly reduced (HFmrEF), and preserved ejection fraction

	Clinical	Imaging/Diagnostic Labs
HFrEF	Signs and symptoms	EF < 40%
HFmrEF	Signs and symptoms	EF 41%–49% plus evidence of elevated filling pressures (baseline or provoked)
HFpEF	Signs and symptoms	EF > 50% plus evidence of elevated filling pressures (baseline or provoked—ie, elevated brain natriuretic peptide, noninvasive, and invasive hemodynamic measurements)

ventricular diastolic stiffness, impaired left ventricular diastolic relaxation, increased arterial stiffness, chronotropic incompetence, blunted cardiac output reserve with exercise, and endothelial dysfunction.[10–13] Mechanistic pathways for these changes include increased oxidative stress, systemic microvascular inflammation, cellular senescence, and interstitial fibrosis as well as changes in mitochondrial function.[14]

Women have a twofold higher prevalence of HFpEF compared with men and HFpEF is the most common form of heart failure for women worldwide.[15–18] Some analyses suggest that this may be the result of increased age since women have a longer life expectancy than men.[16] For example, in a pooled analysis of over 28,000 patients from four community-based cohorts, men were not at lower risk of developing HFpEF compared with women after controlling for age and other risk factors.[19] Cohort studies differ on whether men or women have poorer outcomes once HFpEF develops.[20,21] Further research is needed to develop a greater understanding of sex-related differences with HFpEF pathophysiology and outcomes.

CLINICAL PRESENTATION AND DIAGNOSTIC CRITERIA

Heart failure is a clinical syndrome characterized by symptoms (eg, dyspnea, fatigue, orthopnea, and paroxysmal nocturnal dyspnea) and clinical signs (eg, peripheral edema, lung rales, and jugular venous distention) along with evidence of cardiac structural or functional abnormalities. Symptoms of HFpEF can be similar to other CV conditions (eg, coronary artery disease [CAD] and atrial fibrillation) and non-CV conditions (eg, obesity, venous insufficiency, chronic obstructive pulmonary disease, sleep-disordered breathing, thyroid dysfunction, and anemia). As a result, efforts should be made to assess the contribution of comorbid conditions and evaluate for alternative diagnoses.

Heart failure classification requires an assessment of left ventricular ejection fraction (LVEF) with imaging, which is most commonly performed via echocardiography. Although heart failure classification schemes and terms have changed over time, the American Heart Association (AHA), American College of Cardiology (ACC), and Heart Failure Society of America recently updated the diagnostic criteria for heart failure, replacing the prior 2013 guidelines (**Table 1**). The diagnosis of HFpEF involves both LVEF > 50% and evidence of increased filling pressures by invasive studies or noninvasive hemodynamic measurements (ie, echocardiogram) as described by (see Omote and colleagues, "Hemodynamic Assessment in Heart Failure with Preserved Ejection Fraction," in this issue) and (see Jain and colleagues, Approach to Echocardiography in Heart Failure with Preserved Ejection Fraction," in this issue).[22]

EVALUATION FOR ALTERNATIVE DIAGNOSES

Clinical symptoms and structural cardiac changes seemingly diagnostic for HFpEF may also present in other syndromes. It is imperative to rule out alternative etiologies for signs and symptoms such as dyspnea, edema, and jugular venous distention. For example, left ventricular hypertrophy (LVH) and diastolic dysfunction (DD) may develop as a sequela of infiltrative disease (amyloidosis, sarcoidosis), longstanding uncontrolled hypertension, or with fixed valvular lesions (ie, aortic stenosis). Constrictive pericardial disease can lead to elevated intracardiac filling pressures and jugular venous distention. Nephropathy, chronic kidney disease (CKD), and cirrhosis phenotypically can present with rapidly progressive edema and volume overload. Anemia and chronic obstructive pulmonary disease often display exertional dyspnea.

Furthermore, many of these conditions are commonly found in patients with HFpEF and need to be optimized to improve their quality of life.

ADDRESSING MISCONCEPTIONS ABOUT HEART FAILURE WITH PRESERVED EJECTION FRACTION DIAGNOSIS

Misconception #1: Diastolic Dysfunction is Needed for Heart Failure with Preserved Ejection Fraction Diagnosis

Left ventricular DD is common in HFpEF, and prognosis worsens in parallel with the severity of DD in both community cohorts and among patients with diagnosed HFpEF.[10,23] However, it is crucial to note that (1) not all individuals with DD have or will develop HFpEF and (2) not all patients with HFpEF have DD. Among 935 participants in the Treatment of Preserved Cardiac Function Heart Failure With an Aldosterone Antagonist Trial (TOPCAT) study, DD was present in only 66%.[24] Similarly, in the Candesartan in Heart failure: Assessment of Reduction in Mortality and morbidity (CHARM)-Preserved trial, 67% of patients with HFpEF had DD, with fewer than one-half of these having moderate to severe DD.

Other abnormalities on echocardiography can aid in the diagnosis of HFpEF, and are extensively reviewed by (see Jain and colleagues, Approach to Echocardiography in Heart Failure with Preserved Ejection Fraction," in this issue). Briefly, in addition to DD LVH and left atrial enlargement (LAE) are often present.[24,25] Individuals with HFpEF often have multiple risk factors for the development of LVH including hypertension, obesity, obstructive sleep apnea, and older age. Furthermore, cardiac myocytes may still hypertrophy in the absence of overt LVH.[26,27] However, patients with HFpEF more commonly have a reduced isovolumetric relaxation time and increased E/E' ratio on echocardiography compared with patients with LVH that do not have heart failure.[24,25] The presence of LVH has been associated with increased morbidity and mortality in patients with HFpEF.[26] Left ventricular DD leads to a pressure overloaded state that contributes to the development of LAE. The severity of LAE may also serve as a marker for DD of the heart and has been associated with adverse outcomes both in the community and among individuals with HFpEF.[24–26,28,29]

Misconception #2: "Normal" Natriuretic Peptide Levels Rule Out a Heart Failure with Preserved Ejection Fraction Diagnosis

Natriuretic peptides are commonly used to aid in the diagnosis of heart failure in patients with dyspnea, and elevated levels are associated with increased risk for heart failure readmissions and mortality among patients with HFpEF.[30,31] However, a normal B-natriuretic peptide (BNP) does not exclude the diagnosis of HFpEF. In a study evaluating 159 symptomatic patients diagnosed with HFpEF by an elevated pulmonary capillary wedge pressure (>25 mm Hg) at right heart catheterization, 29% had a BNP of less than 100.[32] Mechanisms explaining this feature with HFpEF relate to wall tension and obesity. BNP rises with greater wall tension; however, individuals with HFpEF, especially if LVH is present and the LV is non-dilated, experience a reduced wall tension despite being in heart failure. In addition, obesity contributes to lower BNP levels as visceral fat increases the clearance of natriuretic peptides. Other factors that have been associated with reduced levels of natriuretic peptide levels in HFpEF include genetics, insulin resistance, androgens, and African ancestry.[33]

AN OVERVIEW OF HEART FAILURE WITH PRESERVED EJECTION FRACTION PATHOPHYSIOLOGY: FOUR MAJOR THEMES

The following themes can serve as a foundation for understanding HFpEF pathophysiology. However, HFpEF is a heterogeneous syndrome comprised of various pathophysiologic mechanisms (many of which are still being eluicdated) and impacted by a patient's comorbid conditions. Some patients may demonstrate only a few of the features outlined in the section below, while others may present with all of the features listed. Keeping this in mind when assessing a patient is critical for the diagnosis and management of HFpEF.

Theme #1: Heart Failure with Preserved Ejection Fraction is Characterized by Impaired Cardiac Reserve in Multiple Domains

The cardinal manifestation of HFpEF is exercise intolerance. Healthy CV function with exercise requires appropriate diastolic function (increased filling), systolic function (increased contractility), chronotropy (increased heart rate), and vascular function (reduced vascular resistance).

Left ventricular diastolic dysfunction

The left ventricle depends on efficient diastolic function for adequate filling of the ventricle and off-loading of the left atrium within the cardiac cycle. Diastolic function of the ventricle is influenced by both active relaxation of the LV, also known as LV pressure decay, and the intrinsic stiffness of the myocardium.[9,34] Approximately two-thirds of patients with HFpEF have DD due to one or both of these mechanisms.[9] Prior studies have shown prolonged LV pressure decay during isovolumetric relaxation in HFpEF leading to higher LV filling pressures over time. Potential contributing mechanisms to this impairment in relaxation time may be related to intracellular calcium levels. Cardiac relaxation depends on a reduced level of intracellular calcium, allowing for myofilament dissociation. In HFpEF, myocyte intracellular calcium levels are elevated reflecting impairment in the removal of calcium, which may affect myocardial relaxation.[9,35]

Although DD may be present at rest in HFpEF, as shown in **Fig. 2**, the effects of DD may be accentuated with exercise.[36] As the cardiac cycle shortens during exercise due to an elevation in heart rate, the ventricle needs to relax more rapidly to create an intraventricular gradient to pull blood rapidly into the ventricle.[9] Prior invasive cardiac studies have evaluated the pressure–volume (PV) relationship of individuals with HFpEF during exercise and have found a leftward shift in the PV curve, indicating that the LV is operating with higher pressures at any given volume (**Fig. 1**).[37] Therefore, patients with HFpEF may experience increased LV filling pressures with exercise that have been shown to result from inadequate relaxation and increased LV stiffness.[38]

In addition to impaired LV relaxation, increased LV stiffness contributes to DD and elevated filling pressures.[9,34,35,39] This depends on collagen quality (type I vs type III), collagen quantity in the extracellular matrix, and titin stiffness. In the setting of a systemic pro-inflammatory state with increasing LV filling pressures, fibrillar collagen deposition is augmented and favors stiffer type I collagen leading to diffuse cardiac fibrosis. Collagen surrounds cardiomyocyte fascicles. As collagen is dysregulated in HFpEF, studies have suggested that this may cause ventricular dyssynchrony.[40] Studies

have also shown mechanical dyssynchrony in both diastole and systole, and its magnitude was related to the extent of DD.[41]

Titin, a large bidirectional spring-like protein, is a key contributor to the passive stiffness of the left ventricle and has two isoforms: a short and stiffer N2B, and a longer flexible N2BA. In animal models of HFpEF, the stiffer N2B form predominantes.[35] In addition, systemic inflammation associated with common comorbidities (ie, diabetes, obesity, and hypertension (HTN)) causes hypophosphorylation of titin, which further increases the passive stiffness of the left ventricular (LV).

Overall, DD in HFpEF is driven by complex interactions between delayed LV pressure decay, increased collagen deposition, contractile dyssynchrony, and titin hypophosphorylation.[42] DD results in higher LV end-diastolic filling pressures.[43] This leads to pulmonary congestion causing symptoms of dyspnea[44] and exercise intolerance[45] as well as increased risk of hospitalization[46] and death, even if pressures are normal at rest.[10,23,47] Furthermore, increased LV filling pressures contribute to left atrial dilation, atrial arrhythmias, pulmonary hypertension, and right ventricular remodeling and dysfunction that are observed in HFpEF and contribute to significant morbidity and mortality. Aggressive treatment to reduce filling pressures has been associated with reduced hospitalizations and symptom burden for HFpEF.[48]

Systolic dysfunction, chronotropic incompetence, and vascular stiffening

Although patients with HFpEF by definition have a preserved EF, LV systolic dysfunction can also contribute to impaired CV reserve.[9] Several studies by Borlaug and colleagues have demonstrated that patients with HFpEF are less able to augment their cardiac index with exercise because of blunted increases in heart rate, contractility, and vasodilatation.[36,49–51] This results partly from an inability to increase LV and right ventricular (RV) systolic function with exercise. For example, patients with HFpEF show higher end-systolic LV volume with no significant difference in end-diastolic volume compared with patients without HFpEF.[36,49] This not only reduces forward stroke volume, but also affects early diastolic filling.[9,36]

An inability to reduce vascular resistance with exercise is one reason that patients with HFpEF are unable to increase stroke volume with exercise.[52,53] Reddy and colleagues[52] evaluated 98 patients with HFpEF and 22 patients with hypertension without HFpEF using cardiopulmonary exercise testing, right heart catheterization, and invasive blood pressure (BP) monitoring. During

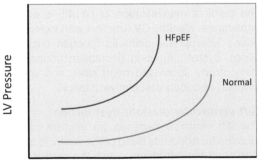

Fig. 1. Diastolic dysfunction in the HFpEF. Given increased stiffness and reduced left ventricular pressure decay, the heart resides at higher filling pressures as depicted by the red line displaying patients with HFpEF.

exercise, patients with HFpEF displayed reduced total arterial compliance, increased arterial resistance, and higher effective arterial elastance despite similar BP at baseline. In other words, attenuated reductions in systemic vascular resistance were observed in patients with HFpEF that were associated with higher LV filling pressures and decreased cardiac output reserve. Similar changes in the pulmonary vasculature have been observed to affect RV systolic function in HFpEF,[36] which will be described later in this article. With exercise, patients with HFpEF demonstrate impaired pulmonary vasodilatation, less reduction in pulmonary vascular resistance, and greater reduction in pulmonary artery compliance when compared with controls.

Abnormal vascular stiffening in HFpEF is likely because of comorbid conditions such as hypertension, older age, and obesity, which have been shown to increase arterial stiffness.[42,52,54–57] In addition, as discussed above, an imbalance in nitric oxide (NO) and reactive oxygen species (ROS) occurs in HFpEF on a systemic level and this has been suspected to contribute to arterial stiffening. The abnormal ventricular–vascular coupling contributes to decreased exercise capacity in patients with HFpEF.[51,52,58,59]

Even though HFpEF is defined by a normal EF at rest, several studies demonstrate that patients with HFpEF often have abnormal systolic function using other measures such as strain imaging.[36,60–64] In an analysis from the Treatment of Preserved Cardiac Function Heart Failure with an Aldosterone Antagonist (TOPCAT) trial, Shah and colleagues[62] showed that 52% of patients with HFpEF have impaired longitudinal strain, which was associated with a significantly increased risk of the composite outcome of CV death, heart failure hospitalization, and aborted cardiac arrest. Reduced global longitudinal stain has been observed in patients with HFpEF and is associated with abnormal diastolic function and reduced exercise capacity.[65] Coronary microvascular dysfunction (CMD) may contribute to impaired LV systolic function in HFpEF that has been hypothesized to worsen with exercise-induced ischemia.[42,66,67] In short, impaired systolic function may further contribute to decreased cardiac output reserve in patients with HFpEF.[36,64]

Lastly, chronotropic incompetence also contributes to impaired cardiac reserve in HFpEF as it contributes to decreased cardiac output with exercise.[36,49,50] This has been shown in studies by Borlaug and colleagues using exercise hemodynamic data. Based on the data from patients without heart failure, some have hypothesized that systemic inflammation and endothelial dysfunction contribute to chronotropic incompetence in HFpEF though further studies are needed to establish this.[68,69] Chronotropic incompetence may also be related to impairments in autonomic tone that are also characterized by impaired heart rate recovery with exercise, which may also contribute to adverse outcomes.[9,70,71]

Theme #2: Heart Failure with Preserved Ejection Fraction is a Systemic Syndrome of Decreased Physiologic Reserve

Although cardiac dysfunction is necessary to diagnose HFpEF, many patients present with a systemic syndrome that may involve changes to the pulmonary vasculature, renal function, and even metabolism. For example, skeletal muscle dysfunction is common in patients with HFpEF.

Several studies have shown that abnormal skeletal muscle function contributes to decreased exercise tolerance in patients with HFpEF.[72] These studies have used cardiopulmonary stress testing with or without invasive hemodynamic monitoring to demonstrate that a substantial percentage of patients with HFpEF have decreased peripheral oxygen extraction characterized by a lack of widening of the arteriovenous oxygen difference.[58,73] Abnormal skeletal muscle oxygen extraction is the result of both peripheral microvascular dysfunction because of systemic inflammation and structural changes to the skeletal muscle.[68,74–76] In a study of muscle biopsy specimens, patients with HFpEF have abnormal skeletal muscle displaying a shift in muscle fiber type distribution and a reduced capillary-to-fiber ratio, both of which contribute to exercise intolerance.[77] MRI has shown increased intermuscular fat to skeletal muscle ratios in lower extremity muscle in patients with HFpEF, which predicted decreased exercise capacity.[78] Furthermore, cardiac and skeletal muscle mitochondrial function is abnormal in HFpEF.[79] Skeletal muscle oxidative capacity, mitochondrial content, and mitochondrial fusion have all been shown to be abnormal.[80] Analyses have concluded that improved skeletal muscle oxygen extraction could have a greater impact on exercise capacity in HFpEF than any hemodynamic variable.[81] Importantly, exercise training has been shown to improve peripheral oxygen extraction and exercise capacity.[82]

Patients with HFpEF commonly have significant frailty, or the decreased resilience to handle physiologic stressors, which is an evolving risk factor for outcomes in patients with HFpEF. One study assessing frailty and physical performance in older patients with HFpEF found that lower extremity function independently predicted hospitalization burden.[83] In addition, in a large clinical trial assessing HFpEF, 94% of subjects were considered frail and found to have a greater mortality risk with an increasing frailty burden.[84] Frailty significantly affects the quality of life in patients with HFpEF and its presence may interact with the management of other comorbid conditions and play a role in patient-centered care. The approach to care for geriatric patients with HFpEF, including those with frailty, has been reviewed by Goyal and colleagues.

Theme #3: Heart Failure with Preserved Ejection Fraction is an Inflammatory Syndrome Caused by Common Comorbidities

Extracardiac comorbid conditions are common in HFpEF, and they play a critical role in disease pathophysiology. Specific comorbidities such as obesity have been implicated in multiple pathophysiologic changes. As discussed in detail by (see Kagami and colleagues, "Key Phenotypes of Heart Failure with Preserved Ejection Fraction Pathophysiologic Mechanisms and Potential Treatment Strategies," in this issue) comorbid conditions play a role in phenotyping patients with HFpEF. Here, we will introduce a paradigm that likely contributes to disease pathophysiology in many patients with HFpEF. This paradigm

describes how several comorbid conditions contribute to the onset and progression of HFpEF. Specific comorbid conditions will be discussed individually later in this article.

Prior paradigms suggested for HFpEF focused on increased afterload (myocardial wall stress) from hypertension resulting in LVH and DD. However, recent research has proposed a new paradigm focused on myocardial inflammation.[85] Noncardiac comorbidities such as obesity, diabetes, and hypertension are very common in patients with HFpEF, and these comorbidities are the impetus for a systemic pro-inflammatory state. The "systemic microvascular paradigm" of HFpEF (**Fig. 2**) suggests metabolic comorbidities drive endothelial inflammation in the coronary microvasculature, which leads to LV remodeling and cardiac dysfunction.[86,87] This inflammation involves cytokines such as interleukin-6 (IL-6), soluble interleukin-1 receptor like 1, C-reactive protein, and tumor necrosis factor alpha (TNF-α).[88–90] These factors influence the cardiac endothelium in two distinct ways.[91] First, the endothelium begins to develop ROS which interact with NO, limiting its availability to function within cardiomyocytes. The combination of reduced NO bioavailability and an increased burden of oxidative stress results in a reduced vasodilatory capacity of the coronary endothelium leading to impaired

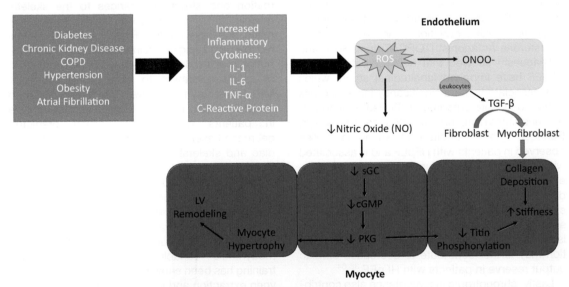

Fig. 2. The Systemic Microvascular Paradigm of HFPEF depicting the interplay between comorbid conditions increasing inflammatory cytokines and their influence on myocardial remodeling through dysregulation of reactive oxygen species (ROS), titin alteration, myocyte hypertrophy and collagen deposition. COPD: Chronic obstructive pulmonary disease, IL-1: Interleukin 1, IL-6: Interleukin 6, TNF-α: tumor necrosis factor alpha, TGF-β: tissue growth factor beta, sGC: guanylate cyclase, cGMP: cyclic guanosine 3′,5′-monophosphate, PKG: protein kinase G, LV: left ventricular. (*Adapted from* Paulus WJ, Tschöpe C. A novel paradigm for heart failure with preserved ejection fraction: comorbidities drive myocardial dysfunction and remodeling through coronary microvascular endothelial inflammation. J Am Coll Cardiol. 2013 Jul 23;62(4):263-71.)

coronary flow and myocardial perfusion.[35] In addition, reduced NO bioavailability also decreases protein kinase G (PKG) activity, which typically functions as a "brake" for limiting myocyte hypertrophy. With lower NO levels and lower PKG activity, cardiac myocytes hypertrophy leads to LV remodeling. Low PKG activity also reduces phosphorylation of the cytoskeleton titin, increasing myocardial stiffness.[92–97]

Inflammatory cytokines such as TNF-α and IL-6 also influence the endothelium to recruit monocytes. These monocytes release transforming growth factor beta (TGF-β) to stimulate the production of myofibroblasts to secrete collagen. Collagen found in the extracellular matrix of the heart consists of Type I (stiff) and Type III (flexible) collagen fibers. One histologic study of HFpEF myocardium revealed increased collagen volume and a greater expression of type I collagen, reflecting a dysregulation in this pathway.[39,86,98] In this way, collagen deposition and fibrosis differs in HFpEF compared with HFrEF. In HFrEF, direct myocardial injury leads to apoptosis and fibrosis, which can be focal when it results from myocardial ischemia and infarction. This is contrasted with HFpEF in which fibrosis is not mediated by apoptosis nor is it localized. Rather, coronary microvascular endothelial inflammation leads to diffuse fibrosis and stiffening of the myocardium.[35]

The mechanisms described that result from systemic inflammation contribute to the unique pathophysiology of HFpEF. As myocytes hypertrophy and stiffen, these histologic changes lead to LVH and DD. Although the above focuses on the effect of systemic inflammation on the myocardium, systemic inflammation affects other organ systems such as the kidneys, pulmonary vasculature, and skeletal muscle as discussed elsewhere.[68,99]

Theme #4: Optimal Treatment of Heart Failure with Preserved Ejection Fraction Requires Comprehensive Management of Both Cardiac and Noncardiac Diseases

As emphasized above, patients with HFpEF have several comorbid conditions that are risk factors for the disease, impact HFpEF pathophysiology, and contribute to symptoms and functional capacity, which is illustrated in **Fig. 3**. Just as much as these patients require excellent cardiac care, they require comprehensive primary care of these issues. Here, we highlight a few of the most important comorbid conditions, although these and other conditions will be discussed in more detail in the sections that follow.

Risk factors and comorbid conditions

Hypertension Although HFpEF is a heterogenous disease of multiple phenotypes, hypertension is present in the vast majority. In a recent major clinical trial of patients with HFpEF, 95% carried a diagnosis of hypertension[100] with 55% having systolic BP at screening more than 130 mm Hg. Resistant hypertension was present in 32% of patients with HFpEF in another major trial.[101] Hypertension has been implicated as contributing to a systemic pro-inflammatory state that promotes HFpEF development.[86] It is known to increase afterload on the left ventricle, increasing pro-hypertrophic signaling leading to LVH and DD, two morphologic changes associated with HFpEF.[11] Hypertension also increases arterial stiffness, impairs ventricular–vascular coupling, and worsens endothelial

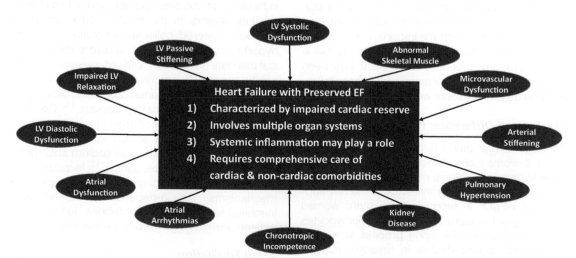

Fig. 3. HFpEF is a systemic syndrome characterized by impaired cardiac reserve but involving multiple organ systems. It requires comprehensive care of cardiac and noncardiac comorbidities. Many pathophysiologic mechanisms contribute to the disease with some represented above.

function.[9,12] Moreover, it is a major risk factor for CV events, which are common in HFpEF.[4] Importantly, treatment of hypertension has been linked to improvement in DD and LVH.[102] In a recent study, patients with HFpEF with a systolic BP of 120 to 129 mm Hg were shown to have the lowest risk of CV death and HF hospitalization.[103] This finding is consistent with ACC/AHA guidelines recommending a goal systolic BP of less than 130 mm Hg in patients with HFpEF.[104] Please note while patients with hypertension may share common changes in myocardial structure and function with HFpEF, these abnormalities are usually more advanced in HFpEF and patients with HFpEF display additional unique pathophysiologic mechanisms.[56]

Obesity and Physical Activity

Obesity is very common in HFpEF (60%–80%) and has been established as a risk factor for disease development.[68,105,106] In a large study of over 50,000 patients, Pandey and colleagues[107] demonstrated that a body mass index (BMI) greater than 25 kg/m^2 is associated with an increased risk of HFpEF. In the same study, low levels of physical activity assessed as metabolic equivalent (MET)-min/wk were not associated with increased HFpEF risk; however, increased levels of activity were associated with a reduced risk of HFpEF. In relatively healthy seniors, physical activity has been associated with improved left ventricular compliance and distensibility.[108] In another study of almost 20,000 patients, cardiorespiratory fitness was shown to explain a significant portion of the risk of HFpEF associated with an elevated BMI.[109] These studies highlight the relationship between these important risk factors. In the next article, the distinct pathophysiologic mechanisms contributing to HFpEF that have been linked to obesity will be reviewed. Many have emphasized the importance of obesity as a modifiable risk factor, not only given its role in pathophysiology, but also because it has been linked to adverse CV outcomes such a hospitalization and death in patients with HFpEF.[110,111]

Sex-Related Difference: Prevalence in Women

Although further study is needed to fully understand if women are at increased risk of HFpEF, several pathophysiologic mechanisms or risk factors may have a greater influence in the development of HFpEF in women. From birth, women have roughly the same number of cardiomyocytes as men; however, the aging process in women has an attenuated decline in myocyte number compared with men with less eccentric remodeling and a greater amount of concentric hypertrophy. Women also have smaller LV chambers and stroke volume comparatively with a higher reliance on chronotropic competence to maintain cardiac output during exertion.[112] One study found a greater association of vascular and ventricular stiffness even in the absence of CV disease for women, which may potentially place women at a greater risk for the development of HFpEF.[12]

Estrogen deficiency, specifically in the postmenopausal stage, can influence left ventricular remodeling, which may be different from that seen in men.[113] With a decline in estrogen, postulated theories contributing to the development of HFpEF for women include activation of the renin–angiotensin–aldosterone system, which may contribute to increased collagen synthesis and the development of DD.[112]

Diabetes Mellitus

Approximately 20% to 45% of individuals with HFpEF suffer from DM and this condition is associated with increased morbidity and long-term mortality.[56,68] As discussed above, it has been hypothesized to contribute to a systemic, proinflammatory state associated with oxidative stress and microvascular dysfunction that promotes the development of HFpEF.[86,114,115] In a study of endomyocardial biopsy samples from heart failure patients, a diagnosis of DM was associated with higher left ventricular diastolic stiffness attributed to increased cardiomyocyte resting tension.[116] DM has also been associated with greater age-associated increases in left ventricular wall thickness. Hyperglycemia and insulin resistance also increase free-fatty acid usage in cardiac myocytes, which produces toxic lipid metabolites and dysregulation of ROS.[117,118] As discussed above, imbalance in oxygen species and inflammation are key players in the microvascular paradigm leading to altered collagen deposition, myocyte hypertrophy, and increased cardiac stiffness. Clinical trial data have shown DM reduces exercise capacity, worsen vascular congestion causing elevated filling pressures, and are associated with increased inflammatory markers.[117] Congestion and volume overload may in part be related to the upregulation of sodium–glucose cotransporter type 2, which increases sodium absorption and reduces diuretic response.[117] In addition to worsening HFpEF through the above-mentioned mechanisms, insulin-dependent diabetes was identified as a risk factor for sudden death among patients from a major HFpEF clinical trial.[4]

Atrial Fibrillation

Structural changes and the pathophysiology associated with atrial dysfunction in HFpEF has been reviewed by (see Obokata et al., "Key Phenotypes of Heart Failure with Preserved Ejection Fraction Pathophysiologic Mechanisms and Potential Treatment Strategies," in this issue) Briefly, in HFpEF, the heart becomes dependent on increased left atrial pressure for LV filling because of LV DD and impairment in early diastolic suction particularly with exercise. Increased left atrial pressure leads to LAE, left atrial dysfunction, and atrial fibrillation. Left atrial dysfunction is common in HFpEF and associated with increased pulmonary vascular resistance, RV dysfunction, heart failure hospitalization, and increased mortality.[119–123] Patients with HFpEF display higher left atrial pressures and increased left atrial stiffness compared with patients with HFrEF.[124] In a study of 308 patients with HFpEF, left atrial dysfunction identified with strain imaging was associated with increased pulmonary artery systolic pressure, increased pulmonary vascular resistance, decreased cardiac output, and decreased peak oxygen consumption on cardiopulmonary exercise testing. In addition, abnormal left atrial reservoir strain was independently associated with the composite outcome of CV hospitalization or death.

As a result of increased left atrial pressure and left atrial dysfunction, atrial fibrillation is a common comorbidity found in heart failure and approximately two-thirds of patients with HFpEF will develop this condition.[120] Conversely, the presence of atrial fibrillation increases the risk of incident HFpEF.[123] Patients with HFpEF who have atrial fibrillation have worse systolic function, diastolic function, pulmonary artery pressure, and right ventricular function as well as decreased exercise capacity and an increased risk for death.[9,120,125–127] Further discussion regarding the role of atrial fibrillation in HFpEF pathophysiology is also included in Chapter 2.

Coronary Artery Disease and Dyslipidemia

Myocardial ischemia can lead to the development of biventricular dysfunction, and it is well known that infarction induces inflammation in the myocardium. CAD is prevalent in HFpEF with one study finding that 91% of hospitalized patients with HFpEF have some form of either CAD or CMD, which was associated with more adverse events including death or hospitalization from CV causes or heart failure.[128] CAD is associated with an increased risk of sudden death in HFpEF.[129] Data suggest revascularization may improve outcomes in HFpEF though data from randomized trials are lacking.[130] The roles of both CAD and CMD in HFpEF pathophysiology will be discussed in detail in Chapter 2.

Chronic Kidney Disease

CKD has been shown to be associated with CV disease (arrhythmias, HFrEF, HFpEF, coronary disease, and so forth), and 50% of all patients with advanced CKD also have some form of CV disease.[131] Patients with advanced CKD (stage IV or V) have an increased cardiovascular disease (CVD) mortality rate approximating 40% to 50% of all deaths, in contrast to a CVD mortality rate of ~26% in patients with normal kidney function.[131] When considering the relationship between CKD and HFpEF, individuals who have worsening kidney function are more likely to have HFpEF when compared with those without renal dysfunction.[132] In the Prevention of Renal and Vascular End-stage Disease (PREVEND) trial, albuminuria and elevated cystatin C secretion increased the risk for developing HFpEF.[133,134]

CKD produces a pro-inflammatory state with neurohormonal changes and dysregulation of the renin–angiotensin–aldosterone system (RAAS), sympathetic hyperactivity, and increased ROS and uremic toxins, which together increase fibrosis, alter myocardial remodeling, and contribute to arterial stiffening.[131,135] In addition, as kidney function declines, the ability to adequately maintain fluid and salt homeostasis is derailed leading to volume overload. This may explain data supporting diuretic therapy in preventing HFpEF incidence and improving outcomes in HFpEF. In ALLHAT (Antihypertensive and Lipid-Lowering Treatment to Prevent Heart Attack Trial), the diuretic chlorthalidone significantly reduced the incidence of new-onset HFpEF and HFpEF hospitalizations compared with non-diuretic antihypertensives.[136] In the TOPCAT (Treatment of Preserved Cardiac Function Heart Failure with an Aldosterone Antagonist) trial, spironolactone reduced heart failure hospitalizations in patients with HFpEF. Overall, CKD is a complex disorder with a clear impact on HFpEF pathophysiology and prognosis.

SUGGESTED INITIAL DIAGNOSTIC AND THERAPEUTIC APPROACH TO HEART FAILURE WITH PRESERVED EJECTION FRACTION
Initial Diagnostic Assessment

Some patients with heart failure symptoms and an EF $\geq$ 50% will clearly meet the criteria for HFpEF based on history, physical examination, echocardiography, biomarker data, and invasive hemodynamics if available. Many other patients may not meet all criteria for HFpEF; for example, patients may have risk factors for the disease though may have a natriuretic peptide level in the normal range or lack findings on echocardiography suggestive of HFpEF. Even in patients meeting diagnostic criteria, symptoms may also be related to other conditions such as anemia, obesity, lung disease, sleep apnea, and deconditioning, which complicates the diagnosis of HFpEF. When clinically appropriate, laboratory studies, pulmonary function tests, ventilation–perfusion imaging, chest imaging, polysomnography, and cardiopulmonary exercise testing should be considered to evaluate for noncardiac contributors to symptoms.

Predictive models to estimate the probability of HFpEF have recently been developed and are recommended in cases where the diagnosis remains unclear. In patients with undifferentiated dyspnea who have had an echocardiogram, the H_2FPEF score was created by Reddy and colleagues.[137] The H_2FPEF score was developed in a quaternary care referral population, with HFpEF confirmed by invasive hemodynamics, but has since been validated in clinical trial and community populations. The H_2FPEF model incorporates age, comorbidities, and readily available echocardiographic parameters (**Table 2**) into an integer point scoring system. The resulting scores may then be used to estimate the probability that HFpEF is present: low (score 0–1, <25% probability), intermediate (score 2–5), and high probability (score 6–9, >90% probability). The Heart Failure Association of the European Society of Cardiology has developed the HFA-PEFF model, a similar point-scoring system to estimate HFpEF probability as low, intermediate, or high.[138] As the HFA-PEFF score incorporates volumetric measurements from echocardiography that are sometimes challenging to obtain in patients with obesity, the H_2FPEF model may be more broadly applicable.

Hemodynamic assessment to diagnose heart failure with preserved ejection fraction

In patients with intermediate probability of HFpEF based on scoring systems or where the diagnosis otherwise remains in question (eg, high probability of HFpEF but with comorbid conditions that could also explain symptoms), the recommended next step is invasive hemodynamic assessment as reviewed extensively by (see Omote and colleagues, "Hemodynamic Assessment in Heart Failure with Preserved Ejection Fraction," in this issue). Elevated resting left ventricular filling pressures (as measured directly via left heart catheterization or estimated with a pulmonary capillary wedge pressure on right heart catheterization) provide direct confirmation of HFpEF. However, normal pressures at rest should not exclude the diagnosis. HFpEF typically presents as exercise intolerance characterized by dyspnea and fatigue with exertion. Therefore, exercise right heart catheterization may be necessary to reveal the hemodynamic abnormalities to explain these symptoms.[139–141] For example, in a study of 55 patients with unexplained dyspnea on exertion, yet normal natriuretic peptide levels and resting hemodynamics, 58% had an increased PCWP with exercise of greater than 25 mm Hg.[139] Normal left-sided filling pressures during symptom-limited exercise right heart catheterization should prompt further evaluation for alternative etiologies.

Treatment approach to heart failure with preserved ejection fraction

Once HFpEF is diagnosed, the treatment approach begins with the consideration of other cardiac and noncardiac conditions that may be contributing to symptoms or have specific evidence-based management. As discussed by (see Vidula and colleagues, "The Role of Multimodality Imaging in

Table 2
H_2FPEF score for assessing probability of heart failure with preserved ejection fraction in patients with unexplained dyspnea

			H_2FPEF Score			
		H_2	**F**	**P**	**E**	**F**
Clinical variable	Heavy	Hypertensive	Atrial fibrillation	Pulmonary hypertension	Elder	Filling pressures
Criteria	BMI > 30 kg/m²	>2 antihypertensives	Paroxysmal or Persistent	Doppler PASP > 35 mm Hg	Age >60	E/E' >9
Points	2	1	3	1	1	1
Total possible score: 9						
0–1 points: <25% probability; 6+ points: >90% probability						

Abbreviations: BMI, body mass index; E/E', early mitral inflow velocity/mitral annular early diastolic velocity; PASP, pulmonary artery systolic pressure (assessed via echocardiogram with Doppler).

the Evaluation of Heart Failure with Preserved Ejection Fraction," in this issue) special attention should be given to ruling out obstructive CAD, as many HFpEF risk factors are also risk factors for CAD. Similarly, as discussed by Reddy and colleagues, echocardiography should be carefully reviewed as valvular disease, pulmonary hypertension, pericardial syndromes, and right ventricular dysfunction are common mimickers of HFpEF. In addition, a high index of suspicion should be maintained for infiltrative cardiomyopathies, especially cardiac amyloidosis as reviewed by (see Smiley and colleagues, "Transthyretin Cardiac Amyloidosis An Evolution in Diagnosis and Management of an "Old" Disease," in this issue). Delayed gadolinium enhancement or other abnormalities on cardiac MRI may provide important clues to nonstandard etiologies and mimickers of HFpEF, such as sarcoidosis, amyloidosis, hypertrophic cardiomyopathy, Fabry's disease, and others.

In parallel with evaluating HFpEF etiology, the next step in the therapeutic approach is to lower cardiac filling pressures and achieve BP control, since uncontrolled hypertension contributes to worsening symptoms and progression of HFpEF. Patients should track daily weights and vital signs, and regular laboratory monitoring is needed in patients undergoing active diuresis. Given the steep pressure–volume curves observed in HFpEF, euvolemia may be difficult to achieve. In some cases, right heart catheterization to assess volume status or pulmonary artery pressure sensor placement may be needed, especially in cases of cardiorenal syndrome. As discussed by (see Peters and colleagues, "Pharmacologic Therapy for Heart Failure with Preserved Ejection Fraction," in this issue) spironolactone can augment diuresis, particularly if its use can replace potassium supplementation for a patient and can be effective if hypertension is treatment-resistant. SGLT-2 inhibitors may also be used to augment diuresis, particularly considering recent clinical trial data demonstrating beneficial outcomes for patients with HFpEF.

Once euvolemia and BP control are achieved, a phenotype-specific approach may guide treatment given the heterogeneity of pathophysiologic mechanisms in HFpEF.[142,143] As detailed by (see Kagami and colleagues, "Key Phenotypes of Heart Failure with Preserved Ejection Fraction Pathophysiologic Mechanisms and Potential Treatment Strategies," in this issue) and (see Moles and colleagues, "Pulmonary Hypertension in Heart Failure with Preserved Ejection Fraction," in this issue) identifying phenotypes such as obesity- or exercise-induced HFpEF and pathophysiologic mechanisms such as CMD, left ventricular systolic dysfunction, left atrial dysfunction, or pulmonary

vascular disease with or without right ventricular dysfunction can be critical to developing the best treatment plan for a patient.

Throughout the whole therapeutic evaluation for any patient with HFpEF, common comorbid conditions such as CAD, DM, obstructive sleep apnea, obesity, hypertension, and CKD must be optimally managed. As reviewed by (see Carbone and Kirkman, "Nonpharmacological Strategies in Heart Failure with Preserved Ejection Fraction," in this issue) non-pharmacologic interventions focusing on diet and exercise are important as they have established benefits in HFpEF and address many of the comorbid conditions listed above. As emphasized by (see Goyal and colleagues, "Geriatric Domains in Patients with Heart Failure with Preserved Ejection Fraction," in this issue) in medically complex older adults, depression, poor social support, frailty, cognitive impairment, polypharmacy, and other geriatric domains may complicate the implementation of or response to treatment. Ideally, patients should be considered for clinical trials of phenotype-specific pharmacologic and device therapies that hold promise for changing disease trajectory. During this whole process, patient education is crucial to establish a foundation for understanding this complex syndrome and the multidisciplinary interventions needed to improve quality of life and clinical outcomes.

SUMMARY

HFpEF is common, increasing in prevalence, and associated with poor quality of life and clinical outcomes. Impaired CV reserve function is often present in multiple domains, and this heterogeneity complicates assessment and management. HFpEF is now understood as a systemic syndrome with multi-organ involvement, often driven by microvascular dysfunction associated with pro-inflammatory comorbidities. Recently developed predictive algorithms can help diagnose HFpEF, and results of initial testing can direct additional evaluation for underlying etiology. Effective management of HFpEF requires a holistic consideration of both cardiac and noncardiac domains. Emerging methods of disease phenotyping may lead to more precisely targeted therapies for this major public health threat.

CLINICS CARE POINTS

- The diagnosis of HFpEF requires an EF > 50% and evidence of elevated filling pressures at rest or provoked.

- The diagnosis of HFpEF does not require diastolic dysfunction on echocardiography or elevated natriuretic peptide levels.
- HFpEF is a heterogenous disease that can include multiple abnormalities in cardiac function.
- HFpEF is a systemic disease that can involve multiple organ systems.
- Treatment of comorbid conditions is imperative to prevent HFpEF progression and optimize quality of life.

DISCLOSURE

Dr. Hummel is supported by the National Institutes of Health (R01-AG062582, R01-HL139813) and the Department of Veterans Affairs (RDC-2017-1066). Otherwise regarding this publication and contents written, all authors have nothing to disclose.

REFERENCES

1. Ambrosy AP, Fonarow GC, Butler J, et al. The global health and economic burden of hospitalizations for heart failure. J Am Coll Cardiol 2014;63(12): 1123–33.
2. Owan TE, Jacobsen SJ, Redfield MM. Trends in prevalence and outcome of heart failure with preserved ejection fraction. N Engl J Med 2006;9: 251–9.
3. Savarese G, Lund LH. Global public health burden of heart failure. Card Fail Rev 2017;03(01):7.
4. Vaduganathan M, Patel RB, Michel A, et al. Mode of death in heart failure with preserved ejection fraction. J Am Coll Cardiol 2017;69(5):556–69.
5. Fonarow GC, Abraham WT, Albert NM, et al. Association between performance measures and clinical outcomes for patients hospitalized with heart failure. JAMA 2007;297(1):61.
6. Steinberg BA, Zhao X, Heidenreich PA, et al. Trends in patients hospitalized with heart failure and preserved left ventricular ejection fraction: prevalence, therapies, and outcomes. Circulation 2012;126(1):65–75.
7. Henkel DM, Redfield MM, Weston SA, et al. Death in heart failure: a community perspective. Circ Heart Fail 2008;1(2):91–7.
8. Lin Y, Fu S, Yao Y, et al. Heart failure with preserved ejection fraction based on aging and comorbidities. J Transl Med 2021;19(1):291.
9. Borlaug BA. The pathophysiology of heart failure with preserved ejection fraction. Nat Rev Cardiol 2014;11(9):507–15.
10. Redfield MM, Jacobsen SJ, Burnett JC, et al. Burden of systolic and diastolic ventricular dysfunction in the community appreciating the scope of the heart failure epidemic. ACC Curr J Rev 2003;12(3):50–1.
11. Gevaert AB, Boen JRA, Segers VF, et al. Heart failure with preserved ejection fraction: a review of cardiac and noncardiac pathophysiology. Front Physiol 2019;10:638.
12. Redfield MM, Jacobsen SJ, Borlaug BA, et al. Age- and gender-related ventricular-vascular stiffening: a community-based study. Circulation 2005; 112(15):2254–62.
13. Shah AM, Claggett B, Kitzman D, et al. Contemporary assessment of left ventricular diastolic function in older adults: the atherosclerosis risk in communities study. Circulation 2017;135(5): 426–39.
14. Pandey A, Shah SJ, Butler J, et al. Exercise intolerance in older adults with heart failure with preserved ejection fraction. J Am Coll Cardiol 2021; 78(11):1166–87.
15. Tadic M, Cuspidi C, Plein S, et al. Sex and heart failure with preserved ejection fraction: from pathophysiology to clinical studies. J Clin Med 2019;8(6): 792. https://doi.org/10.3390/jcm8060792.
16. Dunlay SM, Roger VL, Weston SA, et al. Longitudinal changes in ejection fraction in heart failure patients with preserved and reduced ejection fraction. Circ Heart Fail 2012;5(6):720–6.
17. Masoudi FA, Havranek EP, Smith G, et al. Gender, age, and heart failure with preserved left ventricular systolic function. J Am Coll Cardiol 2003;41(2):217–23.
18. Brouwers FP, de Boer RA, van der Harst P, et al. Incidence and epidemiology of new onset heart failure with preserved vs. reduced ejection fraction in a community-based cohort: 11-year follow-up of PREVEND. Eur Heart J 2013;34(19):1424–31.
19. Ho JE, Enserro D, Brouwers FP, et al. Predicting heart failure with preserved and reduced ejection fraction: the international collaboration on heart failure subtypes. Circ Heart Fail 2016;9(6). https://doi.org/10.1161/CIRCHEARTFAILURE.115.003116.
20. Sharma K, Mok Y, Kwak L, et al. Predictors of mortality by sex and race in heart failure with preserved ejection fraction: ARIC Community Surveillance Study. JAHA 2020;9(19). https://doi.org/10.1161/JAHA.119.014669.
21. Sotomi Y, Hikoso S, Nakatani D, et al. Sex differences in heart failure with preserved ejection fraction. JAHA 2021;10(5). https://doi.org/10.1161/JAHA.120.018574.
22. Heidenreich PA, Bozkurt B, Aguilar D, et al. 2022 AHA/ACC/HFSA guideline for the management of heart failure. J Am Coll Cardiol 2022;79(17): e263–421.
23. Persson H, Lonn E, Edner M, et al. Diastolic dysfunction in heart failure with preserved systolic function: need for objective evidence. J Am Coll Cardiol 2007;49(6):687–94.

24. Shah AM, Shah SJ, Anand IS, et al. Cardiac structure and function in heart failure with preserved ejection fraction: baseline findings from the echocardiographic study of the treatment of preserved cardiac function heart failure with an aldosterone antagonist trial. Circ Heart Fail 2014;7(1):104–15.

25. Melenovsky V, Borlaug BA, Rosen B, et al. Cardiovascular features of heart failure with preserved ejection fraction versus nonfailing hypertensive left ventricular hypertrophy in the urban baltimore community. J Am Coll Cardiol 2007;49(2):198–207.

26. Zile MR, Gottdiener JS, Hetzel SJ, et al. Prevalence and significance of alterations in cardiac structure and function in patients with heart failure and a preserved ejection fraction. Circulation 2011;124(23):2491–501.

27. Nayor M, Cooper LL, Enserro DM, et al. Left ventricular diastolic dysfunction in the community: impact of diagnostic criteria on the burden, correlates, and prognosis. JAHA 2018;7(11).

28. Pritchett AM, Mahoney DW, Jacobsen SJ, et al. Diastolic dysfunction and left atrial volume. J Am Coll Cardiol 2005;45(1):87–92.

29. Shin S, Claggett B, Inciardi RM, et al. Prognostic value of minimal left atrial volume in heart failure with preserved ejection fraction. JAHA 2021;10(15):e019545.

30. Fonarow GC, Peacock WF, Phillips CO, et al. Admission B-type natriuretic peptide levels and in-hospital mortality in acute decompensated heart Failure. J Am Coll Cardiol 2007;49(19):1943–50.

31. Verbrugge FH, Omote K, Reddy YNV, et al. Heart failure with preserved ejection fraction in patients with normal natriuretic peptide levels is associated with increased morbidity and mortality. Eur Heart J 2022. https://doi.org/10.1093/eurheartj/ehab911. ehab911.

32. Anjan VY, Loftus TM, Burke MA, et al. Prevalence, clinical phenotype, and outcomes associated with normal b-type natriuretic peptide levels in heart failure with preserved ejection fraction. The Am J Cardiol 2012;110(6):870–6.

33. Shah SJ. BNP: biomarker not perfect in heart failure with preserved ejection fraction. Eur Heart J 2022; 43(20):1952–4.

34. Zile MR, Baicu CF, Gaasch WH. Diastolic heart failure — abnormalities in active relaxation and passive stiffness of the left ventricle. N Engl J Med 2004;350(19):1953–9. https://doi.org/10.1056/NEJMoa032566.

35. Simmonds SJ, Cuijpers I, Heymans S, et al. Cellular and molecular differences between HFpEF and HFrEF: a step ahead in an improved pathological understanding. Cells 2020;9(1):242.

36. Borlaug BA, Kane GC, Melenovsky V, et al. Abnormal right ventricular-pulmonary artery coupling with exercise in heart failure with preserved ejection fraction. Eur Heart J 2016;37(43):3293–302.

37. Wachter R, Schmidt-Schweda S, Westermann D, et al. Blunted frequency-dependent upregulation of cardiac output is related to impaired relaxation in diastolic heart failure. Eur Heart J 2009;30(24):3027–36.

38. Borlaug BA, Jaber WA, Ommen SR, et al. Diastolic relaxation and compliance reserve during dynamic exercise in heart failure with preserved ejection fraction. Heart 2011;97(12):964–9.

39. Westermann D, Lindner D, Kasner M, et al. Cardiac inflammation contributes to changes in the extracellular matrix in patients with heart failure and normal ejection fraction. Circ Heart Fail 2011;4(1):44–52.

40. Baicu CF, Stroud JD, Livesay VA, et al. Changes in extracellular collagen matrix alter myocardial systolic performance. Am J Physiology-Heart Circulatory Physiol 2003;284(1):H122–32.

41. Yu CM, Zhang Q, Yip GWK, et al. Diastolic and systolic asynchrony in patients with diastolic heart failure. J Am Coll Cardiol 2007;49(1):97–105.

42. Obokata M, Reddy YNV, Borlaug BA. Diastolic dysfunction and heart failure with preserved ejection fraction. JACC: Cardiovasc Imaging 2020; 13(1):245–57.

43. Ohara T, Niebel CL, Stewart KC, et al. Loss of adrenergic augmentation of diastolic intra-lv pressure difference in patients with diastolic dysfunction. JACC: Cardiovasc Imaging 2012; 5(9):861–70.

44. Obokata M, Olson TP, Reddy YNV, et al. Haemodynamics, dyspnoea, and pulmonary reserve in heart failure with preserved ejection fraction. Eur Heart J 2018;39(30):2810–21.

45. Reddy YNV, Olson TP, Obokata M, et al. Hemodynamic Correlates and diagnostic role of cardiopulmonary exercise testing in heart failure with preserved ejection fraction. JACC: Heart Fail 2018;6(8):665–75.

46. Adamson PB, Abraham WT, Bourge RC, et al. Wireless pulmonary artery pressure monitoring guides management to reduce decompensation in heart failure with preserved ejection fraction. Circ Heart Fail 2014;7(6):935–44.

47. Dorfs S, Zeh W, Hochholzer W, et al. Pulmonary capillary wedge pressure during exercise and long-term mortality in patients with suspected heart failure with preserved ejection fraction. Eur Heart J 2014;35(44):3103–12.

48. Abraham WT, Adamson PB, Bourge RC, et al. Wireless pulmonary artery haemodynamic monitoring in chronic heart failure: a randomised controlled trial. The Lancet 2011;377(9766):658–66.

49. Borlaug BA, Olson TP, Lam CSP, et al. Global cardiovascular reserve dysfunction in heart failure

with preserved ejection fraction. J Am Coll Cardiol 2010;56(11):845–54.

50. Borlaug BA, Melenovsky V, Russell SD, et al. Impaired chronotropic and vasodilator reserves limit exercise capacity in patients with heart failure and a preserved ejection fraction. Circulation 2006; 114(20):2138–47.

51. Abudiab MM, Redfield MM, Melenovsky V, et al. Cardiac output response to exercise in relation to metabolic demand in heart failure with preserved ejection fraction. Eur J Heart Fail 2013;15(7):776–85.

52. Reddy YNV, Andersen MJ, Obokata M, et al. Arterial stiffening with exercise in patients with heart failure and preserved ejection fraction. J Am Coll Cardiol 2017;70(2):136–48.

53. Ennezat PV, Lefetz Y, Maréchaux S, et al. Left ventricular abnormal response during dynamic exercise in patients with heart failure and preserved left ventricular ejection fraction at rest. J Card Fail 2008;14(6):475–80.

54. Lee HY, Oh BH. Aging and arterial stiffness. Circ J 2010;74(11):2257–62.

55. Safar ME, Czernichow S, Blacher J. Obesity, arterial stiffness, and cardiovascular risk. JASN 2006; 17(4 suppl 2):S109–11.

56. Mohammed SF, Borlaug BA, Roger VL, et al. Comorbidity and ventricular and vascular structure and function in heart failure with preserved ejection fraction: a community-based study. Circ Heart Fail 2012;5(6):710–9.

57. Fernandes-Silva MM, Shah AM, Claggett B, et al. Adiposity, body composition and ventricular-arterial stiffness in the elderly: the Atherosclerosis Risk in Communities Study: adiposity and ventricular-arterial stiffness. Eur J Heart Fail 2018; 20(8):1191–201.

58. Haykowsky MJ, Brubaker PH, John JM, et al. Determinants of exercise intolerance in elderly heart failure patients with preserved ejection fraction. J Am Coll Cardiol 2011;58(3):265–74.

59. Kitzman DW, Herrington DM, Brubaker PH, et al. Carotid arterial stiffness and its relationship to exercise intolerance in older patients with heart failure and preserved ejection fraction. Hypertension 2013;61(1):112–9.

60. Kraigher-Krainer E, Shah AM, Gupta DK, et al. Impaired systolic function by strain imaging in heart failure with preserved ejection fraction. J Am Coll Cardiol 2014;63(5):447–56.

61. Park JJ, Park JB, Park JH, et al. Global longitudinal strain to predict mortality in patients with acute heart failure. J Am Coll Cardiol 2018;71(18):1947–57.

62. Shah AM, Claggett B, Sweitzer NK, et al. Prognostic importance of impaired systolic function in heart failure with preserved ejection fraction and the impact of spironolactone. Circulation 2015; 132(5):402–14.

63. Borlaug BA, Lam CSP, Roger VL, et al. Contractility and ventricular systolic stiffening in hypertensive heart disease. J Am Coll Cardiol 2009;54(5): 410–8.

64. Tan YT, Wenzelburger F, Lee E, et al. The pathophysiology of heart failure with normal ejection fraction. J Am Coll Cardiol 2009; 54(1):36–46.

65. Hasselberg NE, Haugaa KH, Sarvari SI, et al. Left ventricular global longitudinal strain is associated with exercise capacity in failing hearts with preserved and reduced ejection fraction. Eur Heart J - Cardiovasc Imaging 2015;16(2):217–24.

66. Shah SJ, Lam CSP, Svedlund S, et al. Prevalence and correlates of coronary microvascular dysfunction in heart failure with preserved ejection fraction: PROMIS-HFpEF. Eur Heart J 2018; 39(37):3439–50.

67. Obokata M, Reddy YNV, Melenovsky V, et al. Myocardial injury and cardiac reserve in patients with heart failure and preserved ejection fraction. J Am Coll Cardiol 2018;72(1):29–40.

68. Shah SJ, Kitzman DW, Borlaug BA, et al. Phenotype-specific treatment of heart failure with preserved ejection fraction: a multiorgan roadmap. Circulation 2016;134(1):73–90.

69. Huang PH. Comparison of endothelial vasodilator function, inflammatory markers, and N-terminal pro-brain natriuretic peptide in patients with or without chronotropic incompetence to exercise test. Heart 2006;92(5):609–14.

70. Phan TT, Shivu GN, Abozguia K, et al. Impaired heart rate recovery and chronotropic incompetence in patients with heart failure with preserved ejection fraction. Circ Heart Fail 2010; 3(1):29–34.

71. Cole CR, Blackstone EH, Pashkow FJ, Snader CE, Lauer MS. Heart-rate recovery immediately after exercise as a predictor of mortality. Heart 1999; 341(18):1351–7.

72. Haykowsky MJ, Brubaker PH, Morgan TM, et al. Impaired aerobic capacity and physical functional performance in older heart failure patients with preserved ejection fraction: role of lean body mass. The Journals Gerontol Ser A: Biol Sci Med Sci 2013;68(8):968–75.

73. Dhakal BP, Malhotra R, Murphy RM, et al. Mechanisms of Exercise Intolerance in Heart Failure With Preserved Ejection Fraction: the role of abnormal peripheral oxygen extraction. Circ Heart Fail 2015;8(2):286–94. https://doi.org/10.1161/CIRCHEARTFAILURE.114.001825. Epub 2014 Oct 24. PMID: 25344549; PMCID: PMC5771713.

74. Lee JF, Barrett-O'Keefe Z, Nelson AD, et al. Impaired skeletal muscle vasodilation during

exercise in heart failure with preserved ejection fraction. Int J Cardiol 2016;211:14–21.

75. Tucker WJ, Haykowsky MJ, Seo Y, et al. Impaired exercise tolerance in heart failure: role of skeletal muscle morphology and function. Curr Heart Fail Rep 2018;15(6):323–31.

76. Zizola C, Schulze PC. Metabolic and structural impairment of skeletal muscle in heart failure. Heart Fail Rev 2013;18(5):623–30.

77. Kitzman DW, Nicklas B, Kraus WE, et al. Skeletal muscle abnormalities and exercise intolerance in older patients with heart failure and preserved ejection fraction. Am J Physiology-Heart Circulatory Physiol 2014;306(9):H1364–70.

78. Haykowsky MJ, Kouba EJ, Brubaker PH, et al. Skeletal muscle composition and its relation to exercise intolerance in older patients with heart failure and preserved ejection fraction. The Am J Cardiol 2014;113(7):1211–6.

79. Kumar AA, Kelly DP, Chirinos JA. Mitochondrial dysfunction in heart failure with preserved ejection fraction. Circulation 2019;139(11):1435–50.

80. Molina AJA, Bharadwaj MS, Van Horn C, et al. Skeletal muscle mitochondrial content, oxidative capacity, and mfn2 expression are reduced in older patients with heart failure and preserved ejection fraction and are related to exercise intolerance. JACC: Heart Fail 2016;4(8):636–45.

81. Houstis NE, Eisman AS, Pappagianopoulos PP, et al. Exercise intolerance in heart failure with preserved ejection fraction: diagnosing and ranking its causes using personalized O$_2$ pathway analysis. Circulation 2018;137(2):148–61.

82. Haykowsky MJ, Brubaker PH, Stewart KP, et al. Effect of endurance training on the determinants of peak exercise oxygen consumption in elderly patients with stable compensated heart failure and preserved ejection fraction. J Am Coll Cardiol 2012;60(2):120–8.

83. Hornsby WE, Sareini MA, Golbus JR, et al. Lower extremity function is independently associated with hospitalization burden in heart failure with preserved ejection fraction. J Card Fail 2019;25(1):2–9.

84. Sanders NA, Supiano MA, Lewis EF, et al. The frailty syndrome and outcomes in the TOPCAT trial: frailty in HFpEF. Eur J Heart Fail 2018;20(11):1570–7.

85. Mishra S, Kass DA. Cellular and molecular pathobiology of heart failure with preserved ejection fraction. Nat Rev Cardiol 2021;18(6):400–23.

86. Paulus WJ, Tschöpe C. A novel paradigm for heart failure with preserved ejection fraction. J Am Coll Cardiol 2013;62(4):263–71.

87. Franssen C, Chen S, Unger A, et al. Myocardial microvascular inflammatory endothelial activation in heart failure with preserved ejection fraction. JACC: Heart Fail 2016;4(4):312–24.

88. Cheng JM, Akkerhuis KM, Battes LC, et al. Biomarkers of heart failure with normal ejection fraction: a systematic review. Eur J Heart Fail 2013;15(12):1350–62.

89. Sanders-van Wijk S, van Empel V, Davarzani N, et al. Circulating biomarkers of distinct pathophysiological pathways in heart failure with preserved vs. reduced left ventricular ejection fraction: biomarkers in heart failure with preserved vs. reduced EF. Eur J Heart Fail 2015;17(10):1006–14.

90. D'Elia E, Vaduganathan M, Gori M, et al. Role of biomarkers in cardiac structure phenotyping in heart failure with preserved ejection fraction: critical appraisal and practical use: role of biomarkers in cardiac structure phenotyping in HFpEF. Eur J Heart Fail 2015;17(12):1231–9.

91. Kalogeropoulos A, Georgiopoulou V, Psaty BM, et al. Inflammatory markers and incident heart failure risk in older adults. J Am Coll Cardiol 2010;55(19):2129–37.

92. van Heerebeek L, Hamdani N, Falcão-Pires I, et al. Low myocardial protein kinase G activity in heart failure with preserved ejection fraction. Circulation 2012;126(7):830–9.

93. Linke WA, Hamdani N. Gigantic business: titin properties and function through thick and thin. Circ Res 2014;114(6):1052–68.

94. Zile MR, Baicu CF, Ikonomidis J S, et al. Myocardial stiffness in patients with heart failure and a preserved ejection fraction: contributions of collagen and titin. Circulation 2015;131(14):1247–59.

95. Borbély A, van der Velden J, Papp Z, et al. Cardiomyocyte stiffness in diastolic heart failure. Circulation 2005;111(6):774–81.

96. van Heerebeek L, Franssen CPM, Hamdani N, et al. Molecular and cellular basis for diastolic dysfunction. Curr Heart Fail Rep 2012;9(4):293–302.

97. Krüger M, Kötter S, Grützner A, et al. Protein Kinase G modulates human myocardial passive stiffness by phosphorylation of the titin springs. Circ Res 2009;104(1):87–94.

98. Kasner M, Westermann D, Lopez B, et al. Diastolic tissue Doppler indexes correlate with the degree of collagen expression and cross-linking in heart failure and normal ejection fraction. J Am Coll Cardiol 2011;57(8):977–85.

99. Cowley AW, Abe M, Mori T, et al. Reactive oxygen species as important determinants of medullary flow, sodium excretion, and hypertension. Am J Physiology-Renal Physiol 2015;308(3):F179–97.

100. Solomon SD, McMurray JJV, Anand IS, et al. Angiotensin–Neprilysin inhibition in heart failure with preserved ejection fraction. N Engl J Med 2019;381(17):1609–20.

101. Tsujimoto T, Kajio H. Spironolactone use and improved outcomes in patients with heart failure with preserved ejection fraction with resistant hypertension. JAHA 2020;9(23).

102. Tam MC, Lee R, Cascino TM, et al. Current perspectives on systemic hypertension in heart failure with preserved ejection fraction. Curr Hypertens Rep 2017;19(2):12.

103. Selvaraj S, Claggett BL, Böhm M, et al. Systolic blood pressure in heart failure with preserved ejection fraction treated with sacubitril/valsartan. J Am Coll Cardiol 2020;75(14):1644–56.

104. Yancy CW, Jessup M, Bozkurt B, et al. 2017 ACC/AHA/HFSA focused update of the 2013 ACCF/AHA guideline for the management of heart failure: a report of the American College of Cardiology/American Heart Association Task Force on Clinical practice Guidelines and the Heart Failure Society of America. Circulation 2017;136(6). https://doi.org/10.1161/CIR.0000000000000509.

105. Savji N, Meijers WC, Bartz TM, et al. The association of obesity and cardiometabolic Traits with incident HFpEF and HFrEF. JACC: Heart Fail 2018;6(8):701–9.

106. Borlaug BA. Evaluation and management of heart failure with preserved ejection fraction. Nat Rev Cardiol 2020;17(9):559–73.

107. Pandey A, LaMonte M, Klein L, et al. Relationship between physical activity, body mass index, and risk of heart failure. J Am Coll Cardiol 2017;69(9):1129–42.

108. Bhella PS, Hastings JL, Fujimoto N, et al. Impact of lifelong exercise "dose" on left ventricular compliance and distensibility. J Am Coll Cardiol 2014;64(12):1257–66.

109. Pandey A, Cornwell WK, Willis B, et al. Body mass index and cardiorespiratory fitness in mid-life and risk of heart failure hospitalization in older age. JACC: Heart Fail 2017;5(5):367–74.

110. Tsujimoto T, Kajio H. Abdominal obesity is associated with an increased risk of all-cause mortality in patients with HFpEF. J Am Coll Cardiol 2017;70(22):2739–49.

111. Haass M, Kitzman DW, Anand IS, et al. Body mass index and adverse cardiovascular outcomes in heart failure patients with preserved ejection fraction: results from the irbesartan in heart failure with preserved ejection fraction (I-PRESERVE) Trial. Circ Heart Fail 2011;4(3):324–31.

112. Beale AL, Meyer P, Marwick TH, et al. Sex differences in cardiovascular pathophysiology: why women are overrepresented in heart failure with preserved ejection fraction. Circulation 2018;138(2):198–205.

113. Merz AA, Cheng S. Sex differences in cardiovascular ageing. Heart 2016;102(11):825–31.

114. Tabit CE, Chung WB, Hamburg NM, et al. Endothelial dysfunction in diabetes mellitus: molecular mechanisms and clinical implications. Rev Endocr Metab Disord 2010;11(1):61–74.

115. Cheng S, Xanthakis V, Sullivan LM, et al. Correlates of echocardiographic indices of cardiac remodeling over the adult life course: longitudinal observations from the framingham heart study. Circulation 2010;122(6):570–8.

116. van Heerebeek L, Hamdani N, Handoko ML, et al. Diastolic stiffness of the failing diabetic heart: importance of fibrosis, advanced glycation end products, and myocyte resting tension. Circulation 2008;117(1):43–51.

117. McHugh K, DeVore AD, Wu J, et al. Heart failure with preserved ejection fraction and diabetes. J Am Coll Cardiol 2019;73(5):602–11.

118. Dei Cas A, Khan SS, Butler J, et al. Impact of diabetes on epidemiology, treatment, and outcomes of patients with heart failure. JACC: Heart Fail 2015;3(2):136–45.

119. Omote K, Borlaug BA. Left atrial myopathy in heart failure with preserved ejection fraction. Circ J 2021. https://doi.org/10.1253/circj.CJ-21-0795. CJ-21-0795.

120. Zakeri R, Chamberlain AM, Roger VL, et al. Temporal relationship and prognostic significance of atrial fibrillation in heart failure patients with preserved ejection fraction: a community-based study. Circulation 2013;128(10):1085–93.

121. Santos ABS, Kraigher-Krainer E, Gupta DK, et al. Impaired left atrial function in heart failure with preserved ejection fraction: impaired left atrial function in HFpEF. Eur J Heart Fail 2014;16(10):1096–103.

122. Santos ABS, Roca GQ, Claggett B, et al. Prognostic relevance of left atrial dysfunction in heart failure with preserved ejection fraction. Circ Heart Fail 2016;9(4):e002763.

123. Santhanakrishnan R, Wang N, Larson MG, et al. Atrial fibrillation begets heart failure and vice versa: temporal associations and differences in preserved versus reduced ejection fraction. Circulation 2016;133(5):484–92.

124. Melenovsky V, Hwang SJ, Redfield MM, et al. Left atrial remodeling and function in advanced heart failure with preserved or reduced ejection fraction. Circ Heart Fail 2015;8(2):295–303.

125. Melenovsky V, Hwang SJ, Lin G, et al. Right heart dysfunction in heart failure with preserved ejection fraction. Eur Heart J 2014;35(48):3452–62.

126. Mohammed SF, Hussain I, AbouEzzeddine OF, et al. Right ventricular function in heart failure with preserved ejection fraction: a community-based study. Circulation 2014;130(25):2310–20.

127. Obokata M, Reddy YNV, Melenovsky V, et al. Deterioration in right ventricular structure and function

over time in patients with heart failure and preserved ejection fraction. Eur Heart J 2019;40(8):689–97.

128. Rush CJ, Berry C, Oldroyd KG, et al. Prevalence of coronary artery disease and coronary microvascular dysfunction in patients with heart failure with preserved ejection fraction. JAMA Cardiol 2021; 6(10):1130.

129. Rusinaru D, Houpe D, Szymanski C, et al. Coronary artery disease and 10-year outcome after hospital admission for heart failure with preserved and with reduced ejection fraction. Eur J Heart Fail 2014;16(9):967–76.

130. Hwang SJ, Melenovsky V, Borlaug BA. Implications of coronary artery disease in heart failure with preserved ejection fraction. J Am Coll Cardiol 2014; 63(25):2817–27.

131. Jankowski J, Floege J, Fliser D, et al. Cardiovascular disease in chronic kidney disease: pathophysiological insights and therapeutic options. Circulation 2021;143(11):1157–72.

132. Mavrakanas TA, Khattak A, Wang W, et al. Association of chronic kidney disease with preserved ejection fraction heart failure is independent of baseline cardiac function. Kidney Blood Press Res 2019;44(5):1247–58.

133. Smink PA, Lambers Heerspink HJ, Gansevoort RT, et al. Traditional risk factors, and incident cardiovascular disease: the PREVEND (prevention of renal and vascular Endstage disease) study. Am J Kidney Dis 2012;60(5):804–11.

134. Fang JC. Heart failure with preserved ejection fraction: a kidney disorder? Circulation 2016;134(6): 435–7.

135. van de Wouw J, Broekhuizen M, Sorop O, et al. Chronic kidney disease as a risk factor for heart failure with preserved ejection fraction: a focus on microcirculatory factors and therapeutic targets. Front Physiol 2019;10:1108.

136. Davis BR, Kostis JB, Simpson LM, et al. Heart failure with preserved and reduced left ventricular ejection fraction in the antihypertensive and lipid-lowering treatment to prevent heart attack trial. Circulation 2008;118(22):2259–67.

137. Reddy YNV, Carter RE, Obokata M, et al. A simple, evidence-based approach to help guide diagnosis of heart failure with preserved ejection fraction. Circulation 2018;138(9):861–70.

138. Pieske B, Tschöpe C, de Boer RA, et al. How to diagnose heart failure with preserved ejection fraction: the HFA–PEFF diagnostic algorithm: a consensus recommendation from the Heart Failure Association (HFA) of the European Society of Cardiology (ESC). Eur Heart J 2019;40(40):3297–317.

139. Borlaug BA, Nishimura RA, Sorajja P, et al. Exercise hemodynamics enhance diagnosis of early heart failure with preserved ejection fraction. Circ Heart Fail 2010;3(5):588–95.

140. Gorter TM, Obokata M, Reddy YNV, et al. Exercise unmasks distinct pathophysiologic features in heart failure with preserved ejection fraction and pulmonary vascular disease. Eur Heart J 2018; 39(30):2825–35.

141. Obokata M, Kane GC, Reddy YNV, et al. Role of diastolic stress testing in the evaluation for heart failure with preserved ejection fraction: a simultaneous invasive-echocardiographic study. Circulation 2017;135(9):825–38.

142. Senni M, Paulus WJ, Gavazzi A, et al. New strategies for heart failure with preserved ejection fraction: the importance of targeted therapies for heart failure phenotypes. Eur Heart J 2014;35(40): 2797–815.

143. Shah SJ, Borlaug BA, Kitzman DW, et al. Research priorities for heart failure with preserved ejection fraction: National Heart, Lung, and Blood Institute Working Group Summary. Circulation 2020; 141(12):1001–26.

Key Phenotypes of Heart Failure with Preserved Ejection Fraction
Pathophysiologic Mechanisms and Potential Treatment Strategies

Kazuki Kagami, MD[a,b], Tomonari Harada, MD, PhD[a], Hideki Ishii, MD, PhD[a], Masaru Obokata, MD, PhD[a],*

KEYWORDS

- Heart failure with preserved ejection fraction • Heterogeneity • Phenotyping
- Personalized treatment

KEY POINTS

- Treatments for patients with heart failure with preserved ejection fraction (HFpEF) are limited, largely owing to the pathophysiologic heterogeneity of the underlying mechanisms.
- Phenotyping patients with HFpEF into pathophysiologically homogeneous groups may allow for personalized treatment.
- Phenotyping approaches based on comorbidities, cardiac structure and function, resting and exercise hemodynamics, and machine-learning techniques have been proposed.
- Further studies are warranted to develop optimal approaches for the HFpEF phenotyping.
- Ultimately, the efficacy of phenotype-specific treatment strategies should be tested in randomized clinical trials.

INTRODUCTION

Heart failure (HF) is a growing health-care problem worldwide, with an increasing prevalence, high mortality and hospitalization rates, and high medical costs.[1] Approximately 64.3 million people worldwide had HF in 2017[2] and the prevalence is expected to increase further in the coming years due to population aging and the increasing burden of comorbidities.[3] Currently, more than half of the patients with HF have preserved ejection fraction (HFpEF).[4] In contrast to HF with reduced ejection fraction , large clinical trials have shown few effective treatments to reduce mortality and HF hospitalization in patients with HFpEF.[4–7] Given its increasing prevalence and limited therapeutic options, HFpEF is a substantial and growing public health problem.

HFpEF is increasingly recognized as a pathophysiologically heterogeneous syndrome.[4,8] Rather than left ventricular (LV) diastolic dysfunction alone, patients with HFpEF display multiple cardiac and noncardiac abnormalities, including LV systolic dysfunction, left atrial (LA) dysfunction and remodeling, altered pulmonary gas change, pulmonary vascular remodeling, pulmonary hypertension (PH) and right ventricular (RV) dysfunction, and peripheral abnormalities.[4,9–15] The extent to which each of these abnormalities affects individual patients substantially varies.[8] To make matters more complex, key clinical phenotypes, such as obesity, coronary artery disease (CAD), and pulmonary vascular disease, may cause distinct pathophysiologic changes in the cardiovascular system.[12,16–18] This pathophysiologic heterogeneity has been considered

[a] Department of Cardiovascular Medicine, Gunma University Graduate School of Medicine, 3-39-22 Showa-machi, Maebashi, Gunma 371-8511, Japan; [b] Division of Cardiovascular Medicine, National Defense Medical College, 3-2 Namiki, Tokorozawa, Saitama 359-8513, Japan
* Corresponding author.
E-mail address: obokata.masaru@gunma-u.ac.jp

Cardiol Clin 40 (2022) 415–429
https://doi.org/10.1016/j.ccl.2022.06.001
0733-8651/22/© 2022 Elsevier Inc. All rights reserved.

the leading cause of the failure of clinical trials to identify effective treatments for HFpEF and motivated us to phenotype patients based on pathophysiological features to develop personalized treatments.[19] In this review, we summarize the current understanding of HFpEF phenotyping, focusing on its pathophysiology and potential treatment strategies for major phenotypes.

HFpEF Phenotyping: How Should This be Achieved?

To date, substantial efforts have been made to better characterize and group patients into distinct phenotypes. Although no consensus exists on how HFpEF phenotyping should be achieved, there are key approaches for classification, including comorbidity-based methods,[12,16–18] biomarker profiling-based methods,[17,20] cardiovascular imaging-based methods (echocardiography, cardiac magnetic resonance [CMR], or comuputed tomography) to detect pathophysiological mechanisms,[8,14,21–26] and exercise hemodynamic signatures-based methods.[27] Machine learning or data-driven precision medicine approaches have also emerged.[28–30] Regardless of the phenotyping methods, candidate phenotypes will require potential treatment strategies that are better tailored to the underlying abnormality, and it is ultimately necessary to verify the efficiency of the treatment for the specific phenotype identified.

Phenotyping Based on Comorbidities

Obesity-related HFpEF

The prevalence of obesity has been increasing at an alarming rate in most Western countries, especially in the United States, where one-third of adults are currently obese (31% of men and 35% of women).[31] This prevalence is projected to increase further, and one in two American adults will become obese by 2030.[32] Recent studies have reported an even higher prevalence of obesity (~75%) in patients with HFpEF.[4,7,16,33] Obesity and increased fat accumulation have multiple adverse effects on the cardiovascular system, including hemodynamic, inflammatory, metabolic, neurohormonal, and mechanical effects (including obstructive sleep apnea), as well as lipotoxicity and systemic and coronary microvascular dysfunction (CMD).[16,34–39] Given its high prevalence and pathophysiological significance, obesity is recognized as the most important phenotype of the HFpEF syndrome.[8,34]

Patients with obesity-related HFpEF have multiple pathophysiological characteristics that differentiate them from other phenotypes of HFpEF.

The most important feature of obesity-related HFpEF may be increased plasma volume and fluid retention, which has been reported to be 40% greater in grade $\geq$ 2 obesity-related HFpEF than in nonobesity-related HFpEF.[16] Volume expansion contributes to chamber remodeling and hemodynamic perturbations (high biventricular filling pressures) at rest and during exercise in obesity-related HFpEF.[16,35] Intriguingly, the increase in chamber volumes and excess epicardial adipose tissue may enhance pericardial restraint and ventricular interdependence, contributing to a more severe elevation in left-side filling pressures, reduced exercise capacity, and poorer clinical outcomes[16,40–42] (Fig. 1).

Rather than general adiposity, growing evidence has demonstrated the pathophysiological importance of regional adipose tissue distribution in patients with HFpEF.[39,43] Increased visceral adiposity is associated with low-grade systemic inflammation through the upregulation of proinflammatory adipokines (tumor necrosis factor-α, interleukin-6 [IL-6], IL-8, and resistin) and downregulation of anti-inflammatory adipokines (e.g., adiponectin and omentin-1).[44–46] Recent studies have reported that visceral adipose tissue (VAT) is greater in patients with HFpEF than in controls without HF.[38,39] In addition to inflammatory effects, women with HFpEF with excess VAT displayed marked elevation in pulmonary capillary wedge pressure (PCWP) during exercise, suggesting a potential role for hemodynamic derangements.[38] Importantly, increased VAT is associated with reduced exercise capacity and poorer clinical outcomes.[39,43,47]

The presence of obesity is important in the diagnostic evaluation of HFpEF. Despite elevated PCWP, obesity is associated with substantially lower natriuretic peptide levels, which may be related to enhanced clearance in adipose tissue, alteration in sex hormones, increased neprilysin activity, or reduced chamber distending pressure due to heightened pericardial restraint.[16,48,49] Regardless of the mechanism, this leads to underestimation of the severity of hemodynamic congestion and thus under-recognition of HFpEF in obese patients.[50,51] Natriuretic peptides may not accurately reflect changes in congestion following treatment to reduce adipose tissue distribution, such as sodium-glucose cotransporter 2 (SGLT2) inhibitors, caloric restriction, or bariatric surgery.[7] Neurohormonal markers including C-terminal pro-endothelin-1 and mid-regional pro-adrenomedullin may be less dependent on body mass for estimating congestion.[50]

Based on pathophysiological mechanisms, obesity-related HFpEF is potentially targeted by

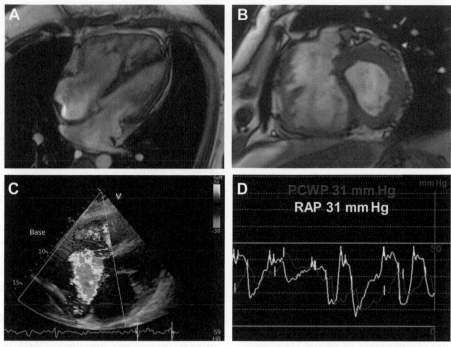

Fig. 1. A representative case of obesity-related heart failure with preserved ejection fraction. A 60-year-old man was referred to our echocardiography laboratory for evaluation of progressive exertional dyspnea and peripheral edema. He was morbidly obese with a body mass index of 55.1 kg/m². (*A, B*) Cardiac magnetic resonance imaging showing RV dilation with a flattened interventricular septum, suggesting heightened ventricular interdependence. (*C*) Right heart chamber dilation associated with functional moderate-to-severe TR. (*D*) Right heart catheterization showing severely elevated right atrial (RA) pressure with ventricularized waveforms, possibly due to significant TR (yellow). Pulmonary capillary wedge pressure was also elevated to a similar degree as the RA pressure (*red*), indicative of heightened ventricular interaction and pericardial restraint.

reducing adiposity (reducing overall body mass or regional adiposity, such as visceral or epicardial adipose tissue), volume expansion, and inflammation. Some therapies may exert multiple beneficial effects on these pathways. In a landmark randomized study by Kitzman and colleagues,[52] body weight decreased by aerobic exercise training or caloric restriction (−3 kg and −7 kg, respectively), leading to improvements in exercise capacity (peak oxygen consumption), quality of life, and symptoms of dyspnea in patients with obesity and HFpEF (mean body mass index 39.3 kg/m²). Caloric restriction also leads to a reduction in visceral and abdominal subcutaneous fat, with a decrease in high-sensitivity C-reactive protein levels.[52] Pharmacotherapies, such as orlistat, lorcaserin, naltrexone–bupropion, liraglutide, and phentermine–topiramate, are an option as an adjunct to lifestyle modification in overweight or obese patients to reduce body weight.[53] A recent meta-analysis demonstrated that phentermine–topiramate and semaglutide, which are glucagon-like peptide 1 (GLP-1) receptor agonists, maybe the most effective in reducing body weight (percent body weight change of −8.0% and

−5.6%, respectively).[53] Experimental studies have shown that GLP-1 receptor agonists ameliorate LV diastolic dysfunction, although clinical studies of GLP-1 receptor agonists in patients with HFpEF are lacking.[54] SGLT2 inhibitors are emerging drugs that may exert multiple beneficial effects in obese patients with HFpEF. These inhibitors reduce overall body mass and visceral and epicardial fat mass and ameliorate adipocyte hypertrophy and inflammation, cardiac fibrosis, and plasma volume expansion.[55,56] These effects may explain the reduced risk of cardiovascular death or HF hospitalization with empagliflozin in patients with HFpEF in the Empagliflozin Outcome Trial in Patients with Chronic Heart Failure with Preserved Ejection Fraction (EMPEROR-Preserved) trial.[7] Obesity is associated with increased neprilysin activity, which promotes the degradation of natriuretic peptides,[49] suggesting that sacubitrilvalsartan (angiotensin II receptor blocker and neprilysin inhibitor) has particular benefits in the obesity-related HFpEF phenotype.[57,58] In contrast to the modest contribution of behavioral (<5 kg) or pharmacological interventions to weight loss (5 kg–10 kg), bariatric surgery effects a substantial and sustained reduction in body weight (25 kg–75 kg).[59] Bariatric surgery is associated with improvements in LV systolic and diastolic function and lowers the risk of new-onset HF[60–62] although further prospective randomized trials in obesity-related HFpEF are needed. Given the possible existence of the obesity paradox, there may be concerns regarding aggressive therapeutic weight loss in patients with HFpEF.[47] However, abdominal obesity and morbid obesity may be better targets for HFpEF therapy.[43,47]

CAD and CMD in HFpEF

CAD is common in patients with HFpEF (~68%).[18,63–65] This may be explained by the shared risk factors between CAD and HFpEF, but there are potential mechanistic links: myocardial ischemia may worsen LV diastolic dysfunction, and increases in LV filling pressures secondary to LV diastolic dysfunction may reduce diastolic coronary perfusion and myocardial O_2 supply, causing myocardial ischemia.[17,66] The presence of CAD in patients with HFpEF is associated with the deterioration of global LV systolic function and increased risks of all-cause mortality and sudden death compared with those without CAD.[18,63–65] In addition to the high prevalence and prognostic significance, it is of note that CAD is modifiable or treatable. Thus, the identification of CAD is important in the evaluation of HFpEF[66] and can be achieved using coronary angiography or coronary computed tomography. Noninvasive ischemic stress testing with echocardiography or nuclear imaging may be less accurate, with higher rates of false-negative and false-positive results.[18]

Accumulating evidence demonstrates that a substantial proportion of patients with HFpEF have CMD.[63,67,68] It has been proposed that coronary microvascular inflammation that develops from proinflammatory cardiac and metabolic comorbidities (hypertension, diabetes, obesity, metabolic syndrome, smoking, chronic kidney disease, and lung disease) leads to CMD and coronary microvascular rarefaction.[69] Identification of CMD may be challenging based on clinical characteristics and comorbidities[67] and relies on the gold standard of invasive coronary physiology testing or noninvasive approaches using biomarkers (troponin), Doppler echocardiography, myocardial position emission tomography, or CMR.[67,70,71] CMD in patients with HFpEF can be caused by endothelium-dependent mechanisms (imbalance between endothelium-derived relaxing factors and vasoconstrictors), endothelium-independent mechanisms (e.g., impaired vascular myocyte tone), or a combination of both.[67] CMD is now recognized as an important factor in the pathophysiology of HFpEF. The severity of CMD is associated with more severe myocardial fibrosis, poorer LV diastolic function and RV function, higher LV filling pressures at rest and during exercise, and reduced exercise capacity.[70,72,73] Of note, increasing data suggest that CMD is associated with adverse outcomes in patients with HFpEF.[63,67,68]

Revascularization is associated with the restoration of LV systolic function and lower mortality rates in patients with HFpEF and CAD.[18] However, in a post hoc analysis of the International Study of Comparative Health Effectiveness with Medical and Invasive Approaches (ISCHEMIA) trial, no clinical benefit was observed in patients with HFpEF (EF>45%) assigned to initial coronary revascularization compared with those with conservative medical therapy, although the number of participants was small ($n = 177$).[74] Further large-scale randomized trials are warranted to determine the efficacy of revascularization for the HFpEF ischemic phenotype. Unfortunately, there are no proven therapies targeting CMD in HFpEF patients.

Phenotyping Based on Pathophysiology

LV systolic dysfunction phenotype

By definition, patients with HFpEF have preserved EF; however, it is now clear that LV systolic function is often abnormal. LV systolic function can be evaluated using tissue Doppler or deformation imaging on echocardiography or CMR imaging.[75–77] Subtle impairment in LV systolic dysfunction at rest becomes apparent during exercise in patients with HFpEF and is associated with depressed cardiac output reserve and reduced exercise capacity.[78] The mechanism causing the limitations in systolic function and reserve is unclear but may be related to CMD, which contributes to subendocardial ischemia and myocardial supply–demand mismatch.[41] This may be supported by the fact that patients with HFpEF with ischemic heart disease demonstrate a marked decrease in EF over time.[79] Importantly, subtle impairments in LV systolic function, systolic reserve limitation, and decline in EF are all associated with poorer clinical outcomes in patients with HFpEF.[79–81]

In the Prospective Comparison of ARNI with ARB Global Outcomes in HF with Preserved Ejection Fraction (PARAGON-HF) trial, sacubitril-valsartan did not reduce the rates of the primary composite outcomes of HF hospitalization and cardiovascular death compared with valsartan alone in patients with HFpEF (EF $\geq$ 45%).[6] Prespecified subgroup analysis demonstrated a possible benefit of sacubitril-valsartan treatment among patients with an EF below the median value (EF ≤ 57%). In the pooled analysis of the PARAGON-HF and PARADIGM-HF trials, patients with EF below the normal range appeared to benefit from sacubitril-valsartan treatment compared with a renin–angiotensin–aldosterone system inhibitor alone, which was observed with spironolactone treatment in the Treatment of Preserved Cardiac Function Heart Failure With an Aldosterone Antagonist (TOPCAT) trial.[82,83] Current guidelines from ACC/AHA/HFSA recommend the use of mineralocorticoid receptor antagonists and sacubitril-valsartan in selected patients with HFpEF, particularly those with an EF below normal.[84] A recent study demonstrated that β-blocker use is associated with a reduced risk of all-cause mortality in patients with lower global longitudinal strain (GLS, <14%) regardless of EF, but not in those with preserved GLS (≥14%).[85] These data suggest that patients with HFpEF with LV systolic dysfunction may represent a phenotype in which neurohormonal activation is enhanced, and as such, neurohormonal blockers may be effective. Further prospective trials are required to confirm the benefits of neurohormonal blockers to this HFpEF phenotype.

LA dysfunction phenotype

The LA is a cardiac chamber that maintains cardiac performance by modulating LV filling through its reservoir, conduit, and booster pump functions. In the early stages of LV diastolic dysfunction and HFpEF, the relative contributions of LA function to LV filling increases. However, as LV diastolic dysfunction progresses, LA function progressively worsens with increasing LA remodeling and often atrial fibrillation (AF).[10,24] Hence, LA dysfunction and remodeling are common in HFpEF patients.[86] LA dysfunction and remodeling in tandem with increasing AF burden in HFpEF are associated with LA stiffening. In this condition, elevation in LA pressure can develop disproportionately to LV filling pressure in some patients (so-called LA myopathy).[10,24] The elevation in LA pressure becomes dramatic during exercise, with increased blood flow from the pulmonary veins to the LA, contributing to reduced ventilation efficiency, more severe pulmonary vascular disease and pulmonary artery (PA)-RV coupling, impaired cardiac output reserve, and reduced exercise capacity (Fig. 2).[10,24,87] Notably, LA dysfunction and remodeling in HFpEF are associated with an increased risk of adverse outcomes.[24] Given the pathophysiological and prognostic importance of

LA dysfunction, assessment of LA function, rather than simply remodeling and dilation, is increasingly recognized as important to develop optimal therapeutic approaches for this syndrome. Although LA volume index is a widely used indicator of LA remodeling reflecting the chronic effects of LV filling pressure, it is insufficient to assess the severity of LA dysfunction.[21] Recent studies have demonstrated the potential for LA deformation imaging using speckle tracking echocardiography to evaluate LA function in patients with HFpEF (see Fig. 2).[10,86] LA function can also be evaluated using CMR-derived strain imaging.[77]

LA dysfunction and remodeling in patients with HFpEF could be targeted by three fundamental approaches: reduction of LA or LV filling pressures; modification to LA structural and electrical remodeling with neurohormonal inhibitors; and maintenance of sinus rhythm. LA unloading through an interatrial shunt device could mitigate LA dysfunction and remodeling in HFpEF.[88] In a small randomized trial, interatrial shunt device implantation reduced PCWP during exercise by 3 mm Hg at the 1-month follow up in patients with HFpEF (EF ≥ 40%),[89] and patients with preserved LA compliance at baseline showed a greater reduction in LA volume following the procedure.[90] However, in the REDUCE LAP-HF II pivotal randomized trial, placement of an atrial shunt device did not reduce the primary hierarchical composite outcome of cardiovascular death or nonfatal ischemic stroke, total HF events, and change in Kansas City Cardiomyopathy Questionnaire overall summary score in patients with HFpEF (EF ≥ 40%).[27] Other device-based therapies targeting LA unloading are currently underway.[91]

Neurohormonal antagonists could be useful by directly targeting myocardial structure and function in the LA. In the Prospective Comparison of ARNI with ARB on Management of Heart Failure with Preserved Ejection Fraction (PARAMOUNT) trial, sacubitril-valsartan treatment resulted in a greater reduction in the LA volume index in HFpEF, with decreases in N-terminal pro-B-type natriuretic peptide levels, than valsartan alone.[92] This may be related to the beneficial therapeutic effects of neprilysin inhibition on endogenous natriuretic peptide activation, especially atrial natriuretic peptide. However, the PARAGON-HF trial comparing sacubitril-valsartan with valsartan did not show improved clinical outcomes in patients with HFpEF, as mentioned above.[6] Large clinical trials assessing the efficacy of angiotensin-converting enzyme inhibitors and angiotensin II receptor blockers in HFpEF have also shown neutral results.[4]

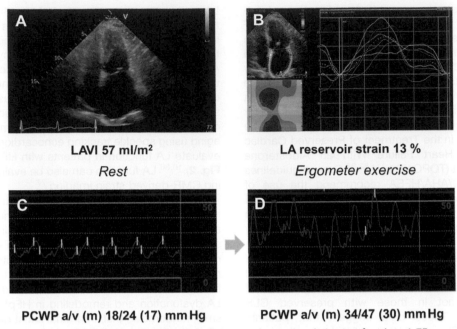

LAVI 57 ml/m²
Rest

LA reservoir strain 13 %
Ergometer exercise

PCWP a/v (m) 18/24 (17) mm Hg

PCWP a/v (m) 34/47 (30) mm Hg

Fig. 2. A representative case of LA myopathy heart failure with preserved ejection fraction. A 75-year-old woman with a history of repeated catheter ablation for AF was evaluated for exertional dyspnea. Despite maintaining the sinus rhythm, her dyspnea progressively worsened. (*A, B*) Echocardiography showing LA dilation and LA dysfunction, as evidenced by low LA reservoir strain. (*C, D*) Right heart catheterization revealed relatively large v-waves of PCWP waveforms at rest (24 mm Hg), which dramatically increased to 47 mm Hg during ergometer exercise, indicating severely reduced LA compliance.

Catheter ablation may be an effective treatment for restoring sinus rhythm and mitigating the adverse consequences of AF in patients with HFpEF and AF.[93] A previous study has shown that catheter ablation reduces the hospitalization rate for HF in patients with HFpEF.[94] In a subanalysis from the Catheter Ablation vs Antiarrhythmic Drug Therapy for Atrial Fibrillation (CABANA) trial, catheter ablation treatment was associated with lower rates of the primary composite endpoint of all-cause mortality, disabling stroke, serious bleeding, or cardiac arrest (hazard ratio [HR] 0.64, 95% confidence intervals [CI], 0.41–0.99) and all-cause mortality (HR 0.57, 95% CI 0.33–0.96) compared with drug therapy alone in patients with stable HF and AF, of which 79% had an EF ≥ 50%.[95] Prospective trials testing the efficacy of catheter ablation in patients with HFpEF are warranted.

PH, pulmonary vascular disease, and right heart dysfunction

PH is common in patients with HFpEF (~75%) and is strongly associated with poor prognosis.[75,96] PH in HFpEF is primarily caused by passive backward transmission of elevated LV filling pressures, but chronic and sustained increases in LV filling and pulmonary venous pressures lead to pulmonary vascular remodeling.[97] Recent histological data

examining patients with HFpEF demonstrated pulmonary vascular remodeling in the veins, small vessels, and arteries, and severity was associated with elevated pulmonary vascular resistance.[98] In addition to interstitial edema secondary to elevated pulmonary venous pressure, pulmonary vascular remodeling in HFpEF may reduce alveolar–capillary membrane gas conductance and thus the diffusion capacity for carbon monoxide (DLCO), which is associated with mortality.[99,100] Patients with pulmonary vascular disease have limitations in RV systolic function and reserve, more severe right heart congestion, enhanced ventricular interaction, and reduced exercise tolerance (**Fig. 3**).[12] Importantly, this phenotype is associated with poorer clinical outcomes than isolated post-capillary PH.[101]

Reduction of downstream left-sided filling pressures lowers the post-capillary component of PH. In the (CardioMEMS Heart Sensor Allows Monitoring of Pressure to Improve Outcomes in NYHA Class III Heart Failure Patients (CHAMPION) trial, a significant reduction in hospitalization rates was observed in patients with HFpEF by primarily adjusting diuretics to maintain the control of remotely monitored PA pressures.[102] The interatrial shunt device is designed to lower LA pressure during exercise through a left-to-right shunt. In addition

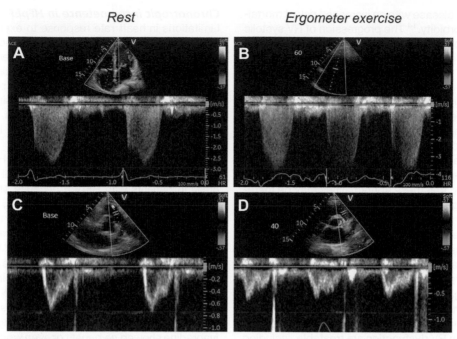

Fig. 3. A representative case of heart failure with preserved ejection fraction with pulmonary vascular disease. Diastolic stress echocardiography was performed on a 69-year-old man with progressive exertional dyspnea. (*A*, *C*) At rest, Doppler echocardiography showed normal peak TR velocity (2.6 m/s), but estimated pulmonary vascular resistance (mean PA pressure/cardiac output) was elevated due to low cardiac output (cardiac index 1.9 L/min/m²). There was a mid-systolic notch in the RV outflow Doppler, suggesting the presence of pulmonary vascular disease. (*B*, *D*) During supine bicycle exercise, TR velocity increased to 3.5 m/s with an elevation in E/e′ ratio from 7.3 to 17.1. The ventricular septum was flattened in the short-axis view, suggesting heightened ventricular interdependence. Of note, mid-systolic notch became more remarkable in the RV outflow Dopper with a reduction in velocity-time integral from 12.5 cm to 10.3 cm. This was associated with worsening RV systolic function, evidenced by the reduction in peak systolic tissue velocity of the tricuspid annulus from 10.4 m/s at rest to 10.1 m/s.

to LA unloading, this device can improve pulmonary vascular resistance, PA compliance, and PA elastance, possibly through enhanced recruitment and distension of the pulmonary circulation, indicative of salutary effects on both the post- and precapillary components of PH.[103] However, more understanding of these issues will be critical, since in the recent REDUCE-LAP HF II trial, interatrial shunting appeared harmful in patients with elevated pulmonary vascular resistance during exercise.[27]

Clinical trials testing the efficacy of pharmacological therapies targeting the nitric oxide–cyclic guanosine monophosphate (NO-sCG-cGMP) pathway in HFpEF have demonstrated largely neutral results.[104] In a single-center study, 1-year treatment with sildenafil, a phosphodiesterase 5 inhibitor, improved PA hemodynamics (decreased PA pressure and pulmonary vascular resistance), lung function (increased DLCO), and RV systolic function in HFpEF patients with evidence of right-sided HF.[104] However, a larger multicenter trial showed that sildenafil did not improve exercise capacity (peak VO$_2$ and 6-min walk distance) or quality of

life in unselected HFpEF patients.[105] A recent single-center study also showed that treatment with sildenafil did not improve PA hemodynamics or exercise capacity (peak VO$_2$) in HFpEF patients with predominantly isolated post-capillary PH.[106] To date, other candidate agents targeting NO-sCG-cGMP have been evaluated for the treatment of HFpEF. Acute treatment with inorganic nitrite has been shown to reduce left-sided filling pressure at rest and during exercise.[107] In multicenter randomized trials testing the efficacy of isosorbide mononitrate or inorganic nitrite on physical activity levels, however, no clinical benefit was observed.[108,109] A recent clinical trial on vericiguat, an sGC stimulator, has shown neutral results.[110]

RV systolic dysfunction in HFpEF results from PH but may also be caused by load-independent factors, such as myocardial ischemia, AF, tricuspid regurgitation (TR), obesity, and neurohormonal activation.[41,111] HFpEF syndrome initially presents with isolated LV diastolic dysfunction; however, RV systolic dysfunction can develop over time.[14] Hence, RV dysfunction may represent a more advanced disease with an increased risk of mortality and morbidity.[14] The progression of RV systolic dysfunction is associated with global right heart remodeling and dilation, which extends not only to the RV but also to the right atrium (RA).[14] AF may be a major driver of RA dilation and dysfunction even in the absence of PH and RV dilation.[112] RA enlargement and subsequent tricuspid annular dilation may worsen functional TR (**Fig. 4**).[26] Of note, RA dilation and dysfunction and TR severity are each associated with poorer clinical outcomes independent of RV dysfunction and PH in HFpEF, suggesting that these abnormalities may be therapeutic targets rather than merely reflecting disease progression.[25,112,113]

Treatment of right heart dysfunction and remodeling is challenging. Given that afterload mismatch is clearly an important contributor to RV dysfunction, therapies that lower pulmonary pressure may mitigate or prevent the progression of right heart remodeling and dysfunction.[104] Some of the load-independent risk factors identified for developing RV dysfunction are treatable, including AF, CAD, and obesity.[14] Therapies targeting these modifiable risks, such as restoring sinus rhythm, coronary revascularization, or weight loss, may prevent right heart remodeling and dysfunction.[18] Diuretics are the most commonly used treatment for relieving symptoms of right HF in patients with significant functional impairment. Novel transcatheter tricuspid valve interventions have demonstrated promising results in recent trials with better survival and reduced hospitalization rate for HF compared with standard medical treatments.[114] This intervention may be effective in patients with HFpEF with significant TR, especially in those with atrial functional TR owing to the absence of PH.[26]

Chronotropic incompetence in HFpEF

Limitations in heart rate response to exercise (i.e., chronotropic incompetence) are common in patients with HFpEF.[15] The potential mechanisms remain unclear but may be related to sinus node dysfunction, autonomic dysfunction, or premature cessation of exercise before maximal sinus node activation due to exertional dyspnea and fatigue.[115,116] Importantly, chronotropic incompetence is associated with reduced exercise capacity and poorer clinical outcomes in HFpEF.[117] Of note, β-blockers are frequently prescribed (up to 80%) in patients with HFpEF because of the high prevalence of comorbidities such as AF, systemic hypertension, and CAD, and possibly on the premise that heart rate lowering may enhance diastolic filling time and exercise capacity.[6,118–120] However, there are concerns that β-blockers may worsen chronotropic response during exercise in HFpEF, contributing to limitations in cardiac output reserve and exercise capacity. Prior clinical trials reported that pharmacological heart rate lowering through ivabradine showed no benefit or even worsened exercise capacity in HFpEF (6-min walk distance, peak oxygen consumption).[121,122]

Recent studies have demonstrated the potential benefit of β-blocker withdrawal in patients with HFpEF, in which exercise capacity improved after β-blocker cessation.[123,124] These data suggest that β-blocker cessation may be an option for patients with HFpEF and chronotropic incompetence. The pacing-induced heart rate increase has been reported to be associated with lower LV filling pressures and improvements in quality of life and functional capacity in patients with HFpEF.[125] Therefore, pacemaker-based therapies are currently being tested in patients with HFpEF (NCT0214351 and NCT04546555).[126]

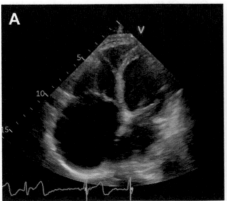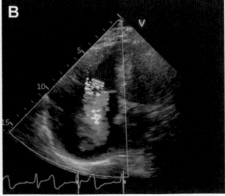

Fig. 4. A representative case of atrial function TR in heart failure with preserved ejection fraction (HFpEF). (*A*) Echocardiography demonstrated severe RA dilation in an 86-year-old man with HFpEF and long-standing AF. (*B*) RA dilation was associated with tricuspid annular enlargement and subsequent severe TR.

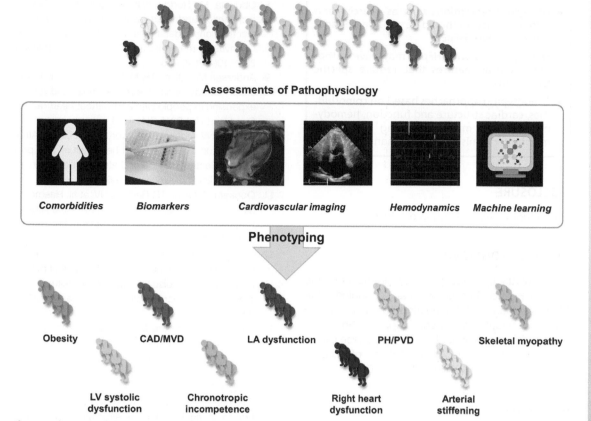

Fig. 5. Schematic illustration for HFpEF phenotyping. CAD/MVD, coronary artery disease/microvascular dysfunction, LA, left atrial, PH/PVD, pulmonary hypertension/pulmonary vascular disease.

Phenotyping Based on Machine Learning

The role of artificial intelligence (AI) is now expanding to the field of HFpEF. Recently, AI has been applied to identify novel HFpEF phenotypes. A machine learning-based clustering approach using multidimensional data, including clinical variables, physical characteristics, laboratory data, electrocardiogram parameters, and echocardiographic parameters, identified three distinct phenogroups that markedly differed in clinical characteristics, cardiac structure and function, and clinical outcomes.[28] Recent studies using data from the TOP-CAT trial also demonstrated the utility of machine learning-based phenotyping in patients with HFpEF.[29,127] Interestingly, a phenogroup that had the poorest outcomes but had a potential benefit from spironolactone treatment has been identified.[127] The machine learning approach has the potential to identify new phenotypes that cannot be defined by ordinary means. However, it may be difficult to understand the pathophysiologic implications of the identified phenotypes. A recent National Heart, Lung, and Blood Institute Working Group Summary document advocated for predictive systems biology and computational modeling,[128] and such physiology-informed phenotyping has strong potential.[129,130]

SUMMARY AND FUTURE DIRECTIONS

Failure of large clinical trials to identify effective treatments in patients with HFpEF is largely related to pathophysiological heterogeneity. Detailed characterization and classification of patients based on comorbidities, underlying pathophysiology, or novel machine learning technology may allow personalized treatment to overcome heterogeneity (**Fig. 5**). Further studies are warranted to establish the optimal approaches for HFpEF phenotyping. Ultimately, the efficacy of phenotype-specific treatment strategies should be tested in future randomized clinical trials.

CLINICS CARE POINTS

- Diuretics are the first-line therapy for congestion.

- Lifestyle interventions such as exercise and caloric restriction should be considered especially for obese HFpEF.
- Some patients with HFpEF may have pathophysiological features that require specific treatments.
- Phenotyping approaches based on comorbidities, cardiac structure and function, hemodynamics, and machine-learning techniques may hold promise for better management.

DISCLOSURE

The authors have nothing to disclose.

ACKNOWLEDGMENTS

Dr. Obokata received research grants from the Fukuda Foundation for Medical Technology, the Mochida Memorial Foundation for Medical and Pharmaceutical Research, Nippon Shinyaku, Takeda Science Foundation, the Japanese Circulation Society, the Japanese College of Cardiology, and JSPS KAKENHI (21K1607800).

REFERENCES

1. Savarese G, Becher PM, Lund LH, et al. Global burden of heart failure: a comprehensive and updated review of epidemiology. Cardiovasc Res 2022. https://doi.org/10.1093/cvr/cvac013.
2. GBD 2017 Disease and Injury Incidence and Prevalence Collaborators. Global, regional, and national incidence, prevalence, and years lived with disability for 354 diseases and injuries for 195 countries and territories, 1990-2017: a systematic analysis for the Global Burden of Disease Study 2017. Lancet 2018;392(10159):1789–858.
3. Dunlay SM, Roger VL, Redfield MM. Epidemiology of heart failure with preserved ejection fraction. Nat Rev Cardiol 2017;14(10):591–602.
4. Borlaug BA. Evaluation and management of heart failure with preserved ejection fraction. Nat Rev Cardiol 2020;17(9):559–73.
5. Mentz RJ, Kelly JP, Von Lueder TG, et al. Noncardiac comorbidities in heart failure with reduced versus preserved ejection fraction. J Am Coll Cardiol 2014;64(21):2281–93.
6. Solomon SD, McMurray JJV, Anand IS, et al. Angiotensin–neprilysin inhibition in heart failure with preserved ejection fraction. N Engl J Med 2019; 381(17):1609–20.
7. Anker SD, Butler J, Filippatos G, et al. Empagliflozin in heart failure with a preserved ejection fraction. N Engl J Med 2021;385(16):1451–61.
8. Obokata M, Reddy YNV, Borlaug BA. Diastolic dysfunction and heart failure with preserved ejection fraction: understanding mechanisms by using noninvasive methods. JACC Cardiovasc Imaging 2020;13(1 Pt 2):245–57.
9. Andersen MJ, Olson TP, Melenovsky V, et al. Differential hemodynamic effects of exercise and volume expansion in people with and without heart failure. Circ Heart Fail 2015;8(1):41–8.
10. Reddy YNV, Obokata M, Verbrugge FH, et al. Atrial dysfunction in patients with heart failure with preserved ejection fraction and atrial fibrillation. J Am Coll Cardiol 2020;76(9):1051–64.
11. Obokata M, Olson TP, Reddy YNV, et al. Haemodynamics, dyspnoea, and pulmonary reserve in heart failure with preserved ejection fraction. Eur Heart J 2018;39(30):2810–21.
12. Gorter T, Obokata M, Reddy Y, et al. Exercise unmasks distinct pathophysiologic features of pulmonary vascular disease in heart failure with preserved ejection fraction. Eur Heart J 2018; 39(30):2825–35.
13. Kagami K, Takemura M, Yoshida K, et al. Pulmonary Vascular alterations on ct imaging and outcomes in heart failure with preserved ejection fraction : a preliminary data. J Card Fail 2021; 27(9):1031–3.
14. Obokata M, Reddy YNV, Melenovsky V, et al. Deterioration in right ventricular structure and function over time in patients with heart failure and preserved ejection fraction. Eur Heart J 2019;40(8):689–98.
15. Haykowsky MJ, Brubaker PH, John JM, et al. Determinants of exercise intolerance in elderly heart failure patients with preserved ejection fraction. J Am Coll Cardiol 2011;58(3):265–74.
16. Obokata M, Reddy YNV, Pislaru SV, et al. Evidence supporting the existence of a distinct obese phenotype of heart failure with preserved ejection fraction. Circulation 2017;136(1):6–19.
17. Obokata M, Reddy YNV, Melenovsky V, et al. Myocardial injury and cardiac reserve in patients with heart failure and preserved ejection fraction. J Am Coll Cardiol 2018;72(1):29–40.
18. Hwang SJ, Melenovsky V, Borlaug BA. Implications of coronary artery disease in heart failure with preserved ejection fraction. J Am Coll Cardiol 2014; 63(25 PART A):2817–27.
19. Cunningham JW, Claggett BL, O'Meara E, et al. Effect of sacubitril/valsartan on biomarkers of extracellular matrix regulation in patients with HFpEF. J Am Coll Cardiol 2020;76(5):503–14.
20. Obokata M, Kane GC, Reddy YNV, et al. The neurohormonal basis of pulmonary hypertension in heart failure with preserved ejection fraction. Eur Heart J 2019;40(45):3707–17.
21. Obokata M, Reddy YNV. The role of echocardiography in heart failure with preserved ejection fraction:

what do we want from imaging? Heart Failure Clin 2019;15(2):241–56.

22. Harada T, Kagami K, Kato T, et al. Echocardiography in the diagnostic evaluation and phenotyping of heart failure with preserved ejection fraction. J Cardiol 2022;79(6):679–90.

23. Tamargo M, Obokata M, Reddy YNV, et al. Functional mitral regurgitation and left atrial myopathy in heart failure with preserved ejection fraction. Eur J Heart Fail 2020;22(3):489–98.

24. Melenovsky V, Hwang SJ, Redfield MM, et al. Left atrial remodeling and function in advanced heart failure with preserved or reduced ejection fraction. Circ Heart Fail 2015;8(2):295–303.

25. Harada T, Obokata M, Omote K, et al. Independent and incremental prognostic value of semiquantitative measures of tricuspid regurgitation severity in heart failure with preserved ejection fraction. Eur Heart J Cardiovasc Imaging 2020. https://doi.org/10.1093/ehjci/jeaa264.

26. Harada T, Obokata M, Omote K, et al. Functional tricuspid regurgitation and right atrial remodeling in heart failure with preserved ejection fraction. Am J Cardiol 2022;162:129–35.

27. Shah SJ, Borlaug BA, Chung ES, et al. Atrial shunt device for heart failure with preserved and mildly reduced ejection fraction (REDUCE LAP-HF II): a randomised, multicentre, blinded, sham-controlled trial. Lancet 2022;399(10330):1130–40.

28. Shah SJ, Katz DH, Selvaraj S, et al. Phenomapping for novel classification of heart failure with preserved ejection fraction. Circulation 2015;131(3):269–79.

29. Segar MW, Patel KV, Ayers C, et al. Phenomapping of patients with heart failure with preserved ejection fraction using machine learning-based unsupervised cluster analysis. Eur J Heart Fail 2020;22(1):148–58.

30. Cohen JB, Schrauben SJ, Zhao L, et al. Clinical phenogroups in heart failure with preserved ejection fraction. JACC Heart Fail 2020;8(3):172–84.

31. Article O. Health effects of overweight and obesity in 195 countries over 25 Years. N Engl J Med 2017;377(1):13–27.

32. Ward ZJ, Bleich SN, Cradock AL, et al. Projected U.S. state-level prevalence of adult obesity and severe obesity. N Engl J Med 2019;381(25):2440–50.

33. Reddy YNV, Rikhi A, Obokata M, et al. Quality of life in heart failure with preserved ejection fraction: importance of obesity, functionalcapacity, and physical inactivity. Eur J Heart Fail 2020;22(6):1009–18. https://doi.org/10.1002/ejhf.1788.

34. Harada T, Obokata M. Obesity-related heart failure with preserved ejection fraction. Heart Failure Clin 2020;16(3):357–68.

35. Sorimachi H, Burkhoff D, Verbrugge FH, et al. Obesity, venous capacitance, and venous compliance in heart failure with preserved ejection fraction. Eur J Heart Fail 2021;23(10):1648–58.

36. Reddy YNV, Obokata M, Testani JM, et al. Adverse renal response to decongestion in the obese phenotype of heart failure with preserved ejection fraction: renal response of hospitalized obese HFpEF. J Card Fail 2020;26(2):101–7.

37. Harada T, Sunaga H, Sorimachi H, et al. Pathophysiological role of fatty acid-binding protein 4 in Asian patients with heart failure and preserved ejection fraction. ESC Heart Fail 2020;7(6):4256–66.

38. Sorimachi H, Obokata M, Takahashi N, et al. Pathophysiologic importance of visceral adipose tissue in women with heart failure and preserved ejection fraction. Eur Heart J 2021;42(16):1595–605.

39. Haykowsky MJ, Nicklas BJ, Brubaker PH, et al. Regional adipose distribution and its relationship to exercise intolerance in older obese patients who have heart failure with preserved ejection fraction. JACC Heart Fail 2018;6(8):640–9.

40. Koepp KE, Obokata M, Reddy YNV, et al. Hemodynamic and functional impact of epicardial adipose tissue in heart failure with preserved ejection fraction. JACC Heart Fail 2020;8(8):657–66.

41. Churchill TW, Li SX, Curreri L, et al. Evaluation of 2 existing diagnostic scores for heart failure with preserved ejection fraction against a comprehensively phenotyped cohort. Circulation 2021;143(3):289–91.

42. Pugliese NR, Paneni F, Mazzola M, et al. Impact of epicardial adipose tissue on cardiovascular haemodynamics, metabolic profile, and prognosis in heart failure. Eur J Heart Fail 2021;23(11):1858–71.

43. Tsujimoto T, Kajio H. Abdominal obesity is associated with an increased risk of all-cause mortality in patients with HFpEF. J Am Coll Cardiol 2017;70(22):2739–49.

44. Fontana L, Eagon JC, Trujillo ME, et al. Visceral fat adipokine secretion is associated with systemic inflammation in obese humans. Diabetes 2007;56(4):1010–3.

45. Reddy YNV, Lewis GD, Shah SJ, et al. Characterization of the obese phenotype of heart failure with preserved ejection fraction: a RELAX trial ancillary study. Mayo Clin Proc 2019;94(7):1199–209.

46. Shah SJ, Kitzman DW, Borlaug BA, et al. Phenotype-specific treatment of heart failure with preserved ejection fraction. Circulation 2016;134(1):73–90.

47. Chandramouli C, Ting W, Id T, et al. Association of obesity with heart failure outcomes in 11 Asian regions : a cohort study. PLos Med 2019;16(9):e1002916.

48. Chang AY, Abdullah SM, Jain T, et al. Associations among androgens, estrogens, and natriuretic

peptides in young women. observations from the dallas heart study. J Am Coll Cardiol 2007;49(1):109–16.

49. Standeven KF, Hess K, Carter AM, et al. Neprilysin, obesity and the metabolic syndrome. Int J Obes 2011;35(8):1031–40.

50. Obokata M, Reddy YNV, Melenovsky V, et al. Uncoupling between intravascular and distending pressures leads to underestimation of circulatory congestion in obesity. Eur J Heart Fail 2022;24(2):353–61.

51. Myhre PL, Vaduganathan M, Claggett BL, et al. Association of natriuretic peptides with cardiovascular prognosis in heart failure with preserved ejection fraction: secondary analysis of the TOPCAT randomized clinical trial. JAMA Cardiol 2018;02115:1–6.

52. Kitzman DW, Brubaker P, Morgan T, et al. Effect of caloric restriction or aerobic exercise training on peak oxygen consumption and quality of life in obese older patients with heart failure with preserved ejection fraction: a randomized clinical trial. JAMA 2016;315(1):36–46.

53. Shi Q, Wang Y, Hao Q, et al. Pharmacotherapy for adults with overweight and obesity: a systematic review and network meta-analysis of randomised controlled trials. Lancet 2022;399(10321):259–69.

54. Nguyen TD, Shingu Y, Amorim PA, et al. GLP-1 improves diastolic function and survival in heart failure with preserved ejection fraction. J Cardiovasc Transl Res 2018;11(3):259–67.

55. Sato T, Aizawa Y, Yuasa S, et al. The effect of dapagliflozin treatment on epicardial adipose tissue volume. Cardiovasc Diabetol 2018;17(1):6.

56. Sha S, Polidori D, Heise T, et al. Effect of the sodium glucose co-transporter 2 inhibitor canagliflozin on plasma volume in patients with type 2 diabetes mellitus. Diabetes Obes Metab 2014;16(11):1087–95.

57. Croteau D, Qin F, Chambers JM, et al. Differential effects of sacubitril/valsartan on diastolic function in mice with obesity-related metabolic heart disease. JACC Basic Transl Sci 2020;5(9):916–27.

58. Aroor AR, Mummidi S, Lopez-Alvarenga JC, et al. Sacubitril/valsartan inhibits obesity-associated diastolic dysfunction through suppression of ventricular-vascular stiffness. Cardiovasc Diabetol 2021;20(1):80.

59. Douketis JD, Macie C, Thabane L, et al. Systematic review of long-term weight loss studies in obese adults: clinical significance and applicability to clinical practice. Int J Obes (Lond) 2005;29(10):1153–67.

60. Mikhalkova D, Holman SR, Jiang H, et al. Bariatric Surgery–induced cardiac and lipidomic changes in obesity-related heart failure with preserved ejection fraction. Obesity 2018;26(2):284–90.

61. Moussa O, Ardissino M, Heaton T, et al. Effect of bariatric surgery on long-term cardiovascular outcomes: a nationwide nested cohort study. Eur Heart J 2020;41(28):2660–7.

62. Shimada YJ, Tsugawa Y, Brown DFM, et al. Bariatric surgery and emergency department visits and hospitalizations for heart failure exacerbation: population-based, self-controlled series. J Am Coll Cardiol 2016;67(8):895–903.

63. Rush CJ, Berry C, Oldroyd KG, et al. Prevalence of coronary artery disease and coronary microvascular dysfunction in patients with heart failure with preserved ejection fraction. JAMA Cardiol 2021;6(10):1130–43.

64. Badar AA, Perez-Moreno AC, Hawkins NM, et al. Clinical characteristics and outcomes of patients with coronary artery disease and angina: analysis of the irbesartan in patients with heart failure and preserved systolic function trial. Circ Heart Fail 2015;8(4):717–24.

65. Rusinaru D, Houpe D, Szymanski C, et al. Coronary artery disease and 10-year outcome after hospital admission for heart failure with preserved and with reduced ejection fraction. Eur J Heart Fail 2014;16(9):967–76.

66. Oktay AA, Shah SJ. Diagnosis and management of heart failure with preserved ejection frac-tion: 10 key lessons. Curr Cardiol Rev 2015;11(1):42–52.

67. Yang JH, Obokata M, Reddy YNV, et al. Endothelium-dependent and independent coronary microvascular dysfunction in patients with heart failure with preserved ejection fraction. Eur J Heart Fail 2020;22(3):432–41.

68. Taqueti VR, Solomon SD, Shah AM, et al. Coronary microvascular dysfunction and future risk of heart failure with preserved ejection fraction. Eur Heart J 2018;39(10):840–9.

69. Ling HZ, Flint J, Damgaard M, et al. Calculated plasma volume status and prognosis in chronic heart failure. Eur J Heart Fail 2015;17(1):35–43.

70. Shah SJ, Lam CSP, Svedlund S, et al. Prevalence and correlates of coronary microvascular dysfunction in heart failure with preserved ejection fraction: PROMIS-HFpEF. Eur Heart J 2018;39(37):3439–50.

71. Taqueti VR, Di Carli MF. Coronary microvascular disease pathogenic mechanisms and therapeutic options: JACC state-of-the-art review. J Am Coll Cardiol 2018;72(21):2625–41.

72. Mohammed SF, Hussain S, Mirzoyev SA, et al. Coronary microvascular rarefaction and myocardial fibrosis in heart failure with preserved ejection fraction. Circulation 2015;131(6):550–9.

73. Massalha S, Walpot J, Dey D, et al. Epicardial adipose tissue. JACC Cardiovasc Imaging 2020;13(3):882–4.

74. Lopes RD, Alexander KP, Stevens SR, et al. Initial invasive versus conservative management of

stable ischemic heart disease in patients with a history of heart failure or left ventricular dysfunction. Circulation 2020;142(18):1725–35.

75. Lam CSP, Roger VL, Rodeheffer RJ, et al. Pulmonary hypertension in heart failure with preserved ejection fraction. a community-based study. J Am Coll Cardiol 2009;53(13):1119–26.

76. Tan YT, Wenzelburger F, Lee E, et al. The pathophysiology of heart failure with normal ejection fraction: exercise echocardiography reveals complex abnormalities of both systolic and diastolic ventricular function involving torsion, untwist, and longitudinal motion. J Am Coll Cardiol 2009;54(1):36–46.

77. Chamsi-Pasha MA, Zhan Y, Debs D, et al. CMR in the evaluation of diastolic dysfunction and phenotyping of HFpEF: current role and future perspectives. JACC Cardiovasc Imaging 2020;13(1 Pt 2): 283–96.

78. Borlaug BA, Olson TP, Lam CSP, et al. Global cardiovascular reserve dysfunction in heart failure with preserved ejection fraction. J Am Coll Cardiol 2010;56(11):845–54.

79. Dunlay SM, Roger VL, Weston SA, et al. Longitudinal changes in ejection fraction in heart failure patients with preserved and reduced ejection fraction. Circ Heart Fail 2012;5(6):720–6.

80. Shah AM, Claggett B, Sweitzer NK, et al. Prognostic importance of impaired systolic function in heart failure with preserved ejection fraction and the impact of spironolactone. Circulation 2015; 132(5):402–14.

81. Kosmala W, Przewlocka-Kosmala M, Rojek A, et al. Association of abnormal left ventricular functional reserve with outcome in heart failure with preserved ejection fraction. JACC Cardiovasc Imaging 2018;11(12):1737–46.

82. Solomon SD, Vaduganathan M, Claggett B L, et al. Sacubitril/valsartan across the spectrum of ejection fraction in heart failure. Circulation 2020;141(5): 352–61.

83. Solomon SD, Claggett B, Lewis EF, et al. Influence of ejection fraction on outcomes and efficacy of spironolactone in patients with heart failure with preserved ejection fraction. Eur Heart J 2016; 37(5):455–62.

84. Heidenreich PA, Bozkurt B, Aguilar D, et al. 2022 AHA/ACC/HFSA guideline for the management of heart failure: a report of the american college of cardiology/american heart association joint committee on clinical practice guidelines. Circulation 2022;145(18):e895–1032.

85. Park JJ, Choi H-M, Hwang I-C, et al. Myocardial strain for identification of β-blocker responders in heart failure with preserved ejection fraction. J Am Soc Echocardiogr 2019;32(11):1462–9.e8.

86. Reddy YNV, Obokata M, Egbe A, et al. Left atrial strain and compliance in the diagnostic evaluation of heart failure with preserved ejection fraction. Eur J Heart Fail 2019;21(7):891–900.

87. Obokata M, Negishi K, Kurosawa K, et al. Incremental diagnostic value of la strain with leg lifts in heart failure with preserved ejection fraction. JACC Cardiovasc Imaging 2013;6(7):749–58.

88. Shah SJ, Feldman T, Ricciardi MJ, et al. One-year safety and clinical outcomes of a transcatheter interatrial shunt device for the treatment of heart failure with preserved ejection fraction in the reduce elevated left atrial pressure in patients with heart failure (REDUCE LAP-HF I) trial: a ran. JAMA Cardiol 2018;3(10):968–77.

89. Feldman T, Mauri L, Kahwash R, et al. Transcatheter interatrial shunt device for the treatment of heart failure with preserved ejection fraction (REDUCE LAP-HF i [Reduce Elevated Left Atrial Pressure in Patients with Heart Failure]): a phase 2, randomized, sham-controlled trial. Circulation 2018;137(4):364–75.

90. Hanff TC, Kaye DM, Hayward CS, et al. Assessment of predictors of left atrial volume response to a transcatheter interatrial shunt device (from the REDUCE LAP-HF Trial). Am J Cardiol 2019; 124(12):1912–7.

91. Fukamachi K, Horvath DJ, Karimov JH, et al. Left atrial assist device to treat patients with heart failure with preserved ejection fraction: initial in vitro study. J Thorac Cardiovasc Surg 2021;162(1):120–6.

92. Solomon SD, Zile M, Pieske B, et al. The angiotensin receptor neprilysin inhibitor LCZ696 in heart failure with preserved ejection fraction: a phase 2 double-blind randomised controlled trial. Lancet 2012;380(9851):1387–95.

93. Aldaas OM, Lupercio F, Darden D, et al. Meta-analysis of the usefulness of catheter ablation of atrial fibrillation in patients with heart failure with preserved ejection fraction. Am J Cardiol 2021;142:66–73.

94. Rattka M, Kühberger A, Pott A, et al. Catheter ablation for atrial fibrillation in HFpEF patients-A propensity-score-matched analysis. J Cardiovasc Electrophysiol 2021;32(9):2357–67.

95. Packer DL, Piccini JP, Monahan KH, et al. Ablation versus drug therapy for atrial fibrillation in heart failure. Circulation 2021;143(14):1377–90.

96. Gorter TM, Hoendermis ES, van Veldhuisen DJ, et al. Right ventricular dysfunction in heart failure with preserved ejection fraction: a systematic review and meta-analysis. Eur J Heart Fail 2016; 18(12):1472–87.

97. Borlaug BA, Obokata M. Is it time to recognize a new phenotype? Heart failure with preserved ejection fraction with pulmonary vascular disease. Eur Heart J 2017;38(38):2874–8.

98. Fayyaz AU, Edwards WD, Maleszewski JJ, et al. Global pulmonary vascular remodeling in pulmonary hypertension associated with heart failure

and preserved or reduced ejection fraction. Circulation 2018;137(17):1796–810.

99. Hoeper MM, Meyer K, Rademacher J, et al. Diffusion capacity and mortality in patients with pulmonary hypertension due to heart failure with preserved ejection fraction. JACC Heart Fail 2016;4(6):441–9.

100. Olson TP, Johnson BD, Borlaug BA. Impaired pulmonary diffusion in heart failure with preserved ejection fraction. JACC Heart Fail 2016;4(6):490–8.

101. Gorter TM, van Veldhuisen DJ, Voors AA, et al. Right ventricular-vascular coupling in heart failure with preserved ejection fraction and pre- vs. post-capillary pulmonary hypertension. Eur Heart J Cardiovasc Imaging 2018;19(4):425–32.

102. Adamson PB, Abraham WT, Bourge RC, et al. Wireless pulmonary artery pressure monitoring guides management to reduce decompensation in heart failure with preserved ejection fraction. Circ Heart Fail 2014;7(6):935–44.

103. Obokata M, Reddy YNV, Shah SJ, et al. Effects of interatrial shunt on pulmonary vascular function in heart failure with preserved ejection fraction. J Am Coll Cardiol 2019;74(21):2539–50.

104. Guazzi M, Vicenzi M, Arena R, et al. Pulmonary hypertension in heart failure with preserved ejection fraction: a target of phosphodiesterase-5 inhibition in a 1-year study. Circulation 2011;124(2):164–74.

105. Redfield MM, Chen HH, Borlaug BA, et al. Effect of phosphodiesterase-5 inhibition on exercise capacity and clinical status in heart failure with preserved ejection fraction: a randomized clinical trial. JAMA 2013;309(12):1268–77.

106. Hoendermis ES, Liu LCY, Hummel YM, et al. Effects of sildenafil on invasive haemodynamics and exercise capacity in heart failure patients with preserved ejection fraction and pulmonary hypertension: a randomized controlled trial. Eur Heart J 2015;36(38):2565–73.

107. Borlaug BA, Koepp KE, Melenovsky V. Sodium nitrite improves exercise hemodynamics and ventricular performance in heart failure with preserved ejection fraction. J Am Coll Cardiol 2015;66(15):1672–82.

108. Redfield MM, Anstrom KJ, Levine JA, et al. Isosorbide mononitrate in heart failure with preserved ejection fraction. N Engl J Med 2015;373(24):2314–24.

109. Borlaug BA, Anstrom KJ, Lewis GD, et al. Effect of inorganic nitrite vs placebo on exercise capacity among patients with heart failure with preserved ejection fraction the INDIE-HFpEF randomized clinical trial. JAMA 2018;320(17):1764–73.

110. Armstrong PW, Lam CSP, Anstrom KJ, et al. Effect of vericiguat vs placebo on quality of life in patients with heart failure and preserved ejection fraction: the VITALITY-HFpEF randomized clinical trial. JAMA 2020;324(15):1512–21.

111. Melenovsky V, Hwang SJ, Lin G, et al. Right heart dysfunction in heart failure with preserved ejection fraction. Eur Heart J 2014;35(48):3452–62.

112. Ikoma T, Obokata M, Okada K, et al. Impact of right atrial remodeling in heart failure with preserved ejection fraction. J Card Fail 2021;27(5):577–84.

113. Nagata R, Harada T, Omote K, et al. Right atrial pressure represents cumulative cardiac burden in heart failure with preserved ejection fraction. ESC Heart Fail 2022;9(2):1454–62.

114. Asmarats L, Puri R, Latib A, et al. Transcatheter tricuspid valve interventions: landscape, challenges, and future directions. J Am Coll Cardiol 2018;71(25):2935–56.

115. Mesquita T, Zhang R, Cho JH, et al. Mechanisms of sinoatrial node dysfunction in heart failure with preserved ejection fraction. Circulation 2022;145(1):45–60.

116. Sarma S, Stoller D, Hendrix J, et al. Mechanisms of chronotropic incompetence in heart failure with preserved ejection fraction. Circ Heart Fail 2020;13(3):e006331.

117. Santos M, West E, Skali H, et al. Resting heart rate and chronotropic response to exercise: prognostic implications in heart failure across the left ventricular ejection fraction spectrum. J Card Fail 2018;24(11):753–62.

118. Kosmala W, Holland DJ, Rojek A, et al. Effect of If-channel inhibition on hemodynamic status and exercise tolerance in heart failure with preserved ejection fraction: a randomized trial. J Am Coll Cardiol 2013;62(15):1330–8.

119. Solomon SD, Rizkala AR, Lefkowitz MP, et al. Baseline characteristics of patients with heart failure and preserved ejection fraction in the PARAGON-HF trial. Circ Heart Fail 2018;11(7):e004962.

120. Zile MR, O'Meara E, Claggett B, et al. Effects of sacubitril/valsartan on biomarkers of extracellular matrix regulation in patients with HFrEF. J Am Coll Cardiol 2019;73(7):795–806.

121. Pal N, Sivaswamy N, Mahmod M, et al. Effect of selective heart rate slowing in heart failure with preserved ejection fraction. Circulation 2015;132(18):1719–25.

122. Komajda M, Isnard R, Cohen-Solal A, et al. Effect of ivabradine in patients with heart failure with preserved ejection fraction: the EDIFY randomized placebo-controlled trial. Eur J Heart Fail 2017;19(11):1495–503.

123. Nambiar L, Silverman D, VanBuren P, et al. Beta-Blocker cessation in stable outpatients with heart failure with a preserved ejection fraction. J Card Fail 2020;26(3):281–2.

124. Palau P, Seller J, Domínguez E, et al. Effect of β-blocker withdrawal on functional capacity in heart

failure and preserved ejection fraction. J Am Coll Cardiol 2021;78(21):2042–56.

125. Silverman DN, Rambod M, Lustgarten DL, et al. Heart rate–induced myocardial Ca 2+ Retention and Left ventricular volume loss in patients with heart failure with preserved ejection fraction. J Am Heart Assoc 2020;9(17):e017215.

126. Yeshwant SC, Zile MR, Lewis MR, et al. Safety and feasibility of a nocturnal heart rate elevation-exploration of a novel treatment concept. J Card Fail 2019;25(1):67–71.

127. Cohen JB, Schrauben SJ, Zhao L, et al. Clinical phenogroups in heart failure with preserved ejection fraction: detailed phenotypes, prognosis, and response to spironolactone. JACC Heart Fail 2020;8(3):172–84.

128. Shah SJ, Borlaug BA, Kitzman DW, et al. Research priorities for heart failure with preserved ejection fraction. Circulation 2020;141(12):1001–26.

129. Houstis NE, Eisman AS, Pappagianopoulos PP, et al. Exercise intolerance in heart failure with preserved ejection fraction. Circulation 2018;137(2): 148–61.

130. Jones E, Randall EB, Hummel SL, et al. Phenotyping heart failure using model-based analysis and physiology-informed machine learning. J Physiol 2021;599(22):4991–5013.

Approach to Echocardiography in Heart Failure with Preserved Ejection Fraction

C. Charles Jain, MD, Yogesh N.V. Reddy, MD, MSc*

KEYWORDS

- Doppler • Echocardiography • Heart failure • Strain

KEY POINTS

- Echocardiography is universally performed in the evaluation of suspected heart failure with preserved ejection fraction (HFpEF) and is helpful to delineate underlying phenotypic mechanisms and pathophysiology.
- In patients with overt volume overload or a prior heart failure hospitalization, the diagnosis of heart failure is already established clinically, and the primary goal of echocardiography is to exclude alternate causes of heart failure such as constrictive pericarditis, amyloidosis, valve disease or heart failure with reduced ejection fraction (EF).
- In contrast, among patients with exertional dyspnea and no volume overload, no single echo feature is pathognomonic for the diagnosis of HFpEF. In these patients, echo abnormalities should be considered along with clinical characteristics in a Bayesian manner to guide a shared decision-making approach with patients on the utility of gold standard exercise right heart catheterization.

INTRODUCTION

The echocardiogram is a universally performed test in the patient with suspected heart failure with preserved ejection fraction (HFpEF). The exclusion of alternate causes of HF–the most common being heart failure with reduced EF (HFrEF) – is the most crucial role of echocardiography. In patients with confirmed HFpEF, echocardiography provides important pathophysiological insight into atrial mechanics, right ventricular function, pericardial restraint, secondary atrial regurgitation, and pulmonary hypertension. In this review, we will provide an updated evidence-based framework for the optimal utilization of echocardiographic information in suspected HFpEF.

Approach to the Echocardiogram in a Patient with Suspected Heart Failure with Preserved Ejection Fraction

In clinical practice, an echocardiogram for HFpEF has typically performed in 2 distinct clinical settings (1) a patient with clear decompensated heart failure (elevated jugular venous pressure and gross volume overload) or (2) an otherwise clinically euvolemic patient with unexplained exertion dyspnea. For the first patient with obvious clinical heart failure, the diagnosis of HF is secure by history and physical examination. The role of echocardiography in this setting is to phenotype the HF, first by the ejection fraction (EF), and if the EF is preserved to rule out other HFpEF mimics

Cardiovascular Medicine, Mayo Clinic, 200 First St SW, Rochester, MN 55905, USA
* Corresponding author.
E-mail address: reddy.yogesh@mayo.edu
Twitter: @charliejainmd (C.C.J.); @yreddyhf (Y.N.V.R.)

Cardiol Clin 40 (2022) 431–442
https://doi.org/10.1016/j.ccl.2022.06.009

Table 1
HFpEF mimics

	Echo Clues
Dilated cardiomyopathy/HF with improved EF	Decreased EF. Subtle LV changes in HF with improved EF. Comparison with known prior echos.If prior echos not available, suspect a mild HFrEF phenotype with low-normal EF in presence of other risk factors such as coronary disease or prior myocardial infarction.
Valve disease	Standard valve disease criteria. Coexisting HFpEF may overestimate AS severity in paradoxical low gradient AS, and can overestimate mitral stenosis severity in mitral annular calcification
Amyloidosis	Reduced LV strain with apical sparing Markedly reduced tissue Doppler velocities Severe LA myopathy with atrial thrombi despite sinus rhythm
Hypertrophic cardiomyopathy	Asymmetric hypertrophy with dynamic outflow obstruction. May be challenging to differentiate from age and hypertension-related asymmetric hypertrophy in the elderly
High output heart failure	Elevated cardiac index > 3.5 L/min/m2
Precapillary PAH	Notching in RV outflow tract pulsed-wave Doppler Right heart remodeling with the abnormal coupling of RV function to afterload Cannot definitively differentiate from CpC PH without a right heart catheterization
Constrictive pericarditis	Ventricular interdependence visually and by Doppler. Subtler signs can be present in obese HFpEF, CpC PH HFpEF or permanent AF HFpEF

Abbreviations: HFpEF, heart failure with preserved ejection fraction; HFrEF, heart failure with reduced ejection fractoin; CpcPH, combined pre and post capillary pulmonary hypertension; PAH, pulmonary hypertension

(**Table 1**). Echo assessment of filling pressures is largely confirmatory of the clinical assessment in this setting, and right heart catheterization is typically not needed. Echo may also provide insight into underlying phenotypic mechanisms of an individual HFpEF patient's presentation as we will discuss later below.

For the second patient with unexplained exertional dyspnea, echocardiography may provide some suggestion of a structurally abnormal heart that may contribute to exertional pulmonary venous hypertension and occult HFpEF. However, the sensitivity of echocardiography (34%) [or even resting right heart catheterization (56%)] is poor for this euvolemic patient as filling pressures are often normal at rest and only increase abnormally during symptom onset with exertion.[1] The exertional increase in left atrial (LA) pressure is challenging to predict from resting studies alone, and the gold standard diagnostic test is an exercise right heart catheterization. Exercise Doppler echocardiography may improve accuracy based on a

single-center study but further multicenter validation of this approach is needed given the decreased specificity observed and substantial overlap in values between controls and HFpEF.[1] Given the emergence of treatment options for this cohort of very symptomatic patients,[2] more accurate diagnosis (or exclusion) of HFpEF may be desirable and should be factored in patient discussions about exercise right heart catheterization in a shared decision-making approach. This discussion is influenced by clinical factors and baseline echo abnormalities.[3] (**Fig. 1**).

Multiparametric Bayesian Approach to Echocardiographic Assessment of Heart Failure with Preserved Ejection Fraction

Unlike systolic HF, where the presence of a reduced EF by echo is pathognomonic of HF, there is no single echo measure that has sufficient sensitivity or specificity for the evaluation of HFpEF in isolation. Clinical trials and published

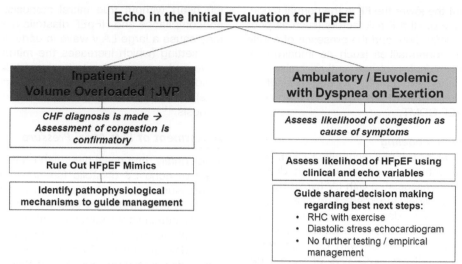

Fig. 1. Echo in the initial evaluation for HFpEF. The echocardiogram in the initial evaluation of heart failure with preserved ejection fraction (HFpEF) depends on the context of the patient's history and examination. Notably, in the outpatient/compensated setting (*right*), the echo is used in a multiparametric Bayesian approach to assess the likelihood of HFpEF and guide further decision-making.

HFpEF series have emphasized the multiple phenotypes of HFpEF (obese HFpEF, atrial fibrillation [AF] HFpEF, combined pre and postcapillary pulmonary hypertension [CpcPH] HFpEF among others)[4–6] which further contributes to echocardiographic heterogeneity. Therefore, the echo evaluation for HFpEF requires a Bayesian multiparametric approach with multiple echo and clinical parameters cumulatively providing an estimate of the probability that HFpEF is the diagnosis. Multiparametric scoring systems including the H$_2$FPEF and HFA-PEFF score use multiple echo parameters and clinical features to quantify this probability and can help guide decisions for further confirmatory invasive exercise testing.[3]

Clinical Parameters of Interest on Echocardiogram in Heart Failure with Preserved Ejection Fraction

Ejection fraction

Probably the most sought-after number from the echocardiogram report is the EF. As a fraction of stroke volume/end-diastolic volume, this does not necessarily reflect contractility, but is more accurately reflective of underlying chamber remodeling and the ventricular–vascular coupling relationship. Although it is clear that a patient with a reduced EF has cardiomyopathy, many patients with HFpEF may also have subtle abnormalities of left ventricular (LV) strain that may be masked by the small chamber size and wall thickening, and may therefore not be detected by the EF.[7] Furthermore, in clinical practice the biplane

Simpson method to directly measure end-diastolic and end-systolic volume to truly calculate SV/EDV for EF is not feasible in all patients, and many patients have either a "visual" estimate of EF by echocardiography or have volumes estimated by linear measurements in the parasternal view ignoring 3D geometry.[8] Even with central core lab measurements there is substantial variability in EF measurements by different modalities.[9] Therefore, excessive reliance on a single measurement of EF to phenotype patients should be avoided particularly in the borderline reduced EF range.

These practical limitations aside, recent studies have confirmed the important role of a reduction in EF as being a surrogate of a cardiomyopathic process that benefits from traditional guideline-directed medical therapy (GDMT). Many HFpEF trials have inadvertently included patients with milder forms of HFrEF (patients with EF 40–50%) and subsequent analyses of these trials have suggested the benefit of traditional GDMT up to an EF of 50–55% or so.[10] Furthermore, many patients with prior HFrEF often improve their EF to >50% but these patients have a persistent cardiomyopathic process termed HF with improved EF,[11] and are often incorrectly diagnosed with HFpEF if this prior history is unknown during their current echocardiogram. Therefore, although a reduced EF<50% remains a critical biomarker of the presence of an HFrEF cardiomyopathic remodeling process, there is a subset of patients with an EF >50% who may still have milder cardiomyopathy. How best to identify these patients remains unclear, but the lower the EF in the normal range, the presence of HFrEF risk factors (such as prior myocardial infarction) and the presence of subtle myocardial abnormalities (such as impaired LV strain and ventricular enlargement) may raise suspicion for this mild cardiomyopathy phenotype among a suspected HFpEF patient and prompt a trial of HFrEF GDMT.

Myocardial remodeling

In the early days of HFpEF recognition, HFpEF was considered primarily hypertensive heart disease and frequently associated with LV hypertrophy.[12] HFpEF is now widely regarded as an inflammatory disease with secondary myocardial remodeling driven by systemic factors.[13] Although there remains a subset of HFpEF with LV hypertrophy and vascular stiffness, <20–30% of current patients with HFpEF have ventricular hypertrophy (**Table 2**).[3,14] Clinical HFpEF phenotypes further confound geometry changes, where obesity may drive concentric remodeling and chamber enlargement independent of hypertension,[4] and permanent atrial fibrillation or CpC-PH HFpEF can cause chronic LV underfilling from pericardial restraint.[5,6] Therefore, ventricular remodeling patterns are heterogeneous and may even be frankly normal in HFpEF (**Fig. 2**).[14–16]

Assessment of chamber characteristics is also helpful in the exclusion of non-HFpEF causes of HF (see **Table 1**). Increased LV wall thickness particularly among older men should raise suspicion for transthyretin amyloidosis, especially with atrial abnormalities or the absence of substantial hypertension.[17] Some patients with age-related asymmetric septal hypertrophy and HFpEF may present with concern for LV outflow tract obstruction and may be challenging to differentiate from true hypertrophic cardiomyopathy. A high cardiac index by echocardiography (>3.5 L/min/m^2) may suggest an underlying high output heart failure state.[18] Exaggerated ventricular interdependence during breathing is seen in true constrictive pericarditis, but many patients with obese HFpEF, severe TR, permanent AF, and CpC-PH HFpEF may have subtler forms of echocardiographic ventricular interdependence that may mimic mild constriction.[4–6] Valvular calcification and remodeling is correlated with the underlying systemic HFpEF process and many patients with HFpEF may have otherwise incidental aortic valve sclerosis/mild stenosis that may be mistaken for severe AS as their HFpEF progress (pseudostenosis with paradoxical low gradient AS) (**Fig. 3**).[19,20] Calcification of the mitral valve is frequently a biomarker of the presence of underlying HFpEF physiology in the left heart without true mitral stenosis. The LA noncompliance and HFpEF diastolic dysfunction may cause a large LA v wave in early diastole in this setting (which increases the mitral valve E wave and associated mitral valve gradient) with rapid equalization of pressure (short deceleration time) (**Fig. 4**) resulting in "pseudo" mitral stenosis.[21]

Assessment of Left Atrial Pressure

Traditionally, emphasis has been on the assessment of echo LV diastolic function rather than LA pressure. LV diastolic function is assessed primarily by the mitral inflow velocity, but the ratio of early to late diastolic mitral flow (E/A ratio) poorly differentiates patients with heart failure from controls. Measuring tissue Doppler e' velocity allows better discrimination, but abnormalities in traditional diastolic function indices are not consistently present even in patients with proven HFpEF and so these measures are poorly sensitive (see **Table 2**). . The guidelines prioritize 4 parameters to diagnose diastolic dysfunction: (1) tissue Doppler e' velocity (medial <7 cm/s, lateral <10 cm/s), E/e' (average > 14), LA volume index >34 mL/m^2, and tricuspid regurgitant (TR) velocity >2.8 m/s.

The critical question of whether HFpEF is the cause of symptoms depends on the LA pressure (and not the LV end-diastolic pressure [EDP]) as it is the LA that is in direct communication with the pulmonary veins and can result in hydrostatic pulmonary edema.[22,23] In other words, the LVEDP may be high from diastolic dysfunction and LV noncompliance, but if atrial compliance is adequate with rest and exertion HFpEF may not manifest despite the presence of LV diastolic dysfunction. In a large community cohort from Olmsted county, <15% of patients with moderate–severe diastolic dysfunction had or developed incident HF in follow-up.[24] Therefore, diastolic abnormalities focused on the LV by echo correlate poorly with overt HFpEF. This with the frequent occurrence of elevated LA pressure only during exertion, and the dominant role of constrictive physiology in the LA pressure elevation in many phenotypes of HFpEF[4–6] explains the limited accuracy of traditional diastolic dysfunction grading for the diagnosis of HFpEF (**Fig. 5**).[3,14–16]

Doppler E/e'

Elevation in E/e' as a marker of the left heart filling pressures is relatively specific for the diagnosis of HFpEF when >13 (specificity 86%).[3] However, many patients with lower values still have HFpEF and therefore this is not a useful rule-out test

Table 2
Variability of echocardiographic assessment in HFpEF trials

	Charm-Preserved	I-Preserve	Relax	Topcat	Paragon
N	312	745	216	935	1097
LVEF	>40%	≥45%	>50%	≥45%	≥45%
Demographics					
Age (years)	75 (72, 79)	72 ± 7	69 (62, 77)	69.9 ± 9.7	73.7 ± 8.0
Female	56%	34%	48%	49%	53%
BMI (kg/m²)	29.6 ± 6.1	30 ± 5	32.9 (28.3, 39.1)	32.6 ± 7.5	29.9 ± 4.9
Atrial Fibrillation	29%	29%	51%	28%	32%
Left ventricle					
EDD (cm)	5.4 ± 0.7	4.8 ± 0.6	4.6 (4.3, 5.1)	4.8 (4.4, 5.2)	4.61 ± 0.65
ESD (cm)	3.6 ± 0.7	3.2 ± 0.7	-	3.4 (3.0, 4.7)	3.29 ± 0.68
EDVi (mL/m)	-	49 ± 14	-	47.2 (38.9, 58.2)	52.8 ± 16.8
ESVi (mL/m)	-	18 ± 9	-	18.6 (14.1, 24.0)	22.2 ± 10.6
Mass index (g/m²)	117 ± 42	-	78 (62, 94)	108 (90, 128)	87.3 ± 26.5
RWT	-	0.40 ± 0.08	-	0.47 (0.42, 0.53)	0.43 ± 0.12
Normal geometry	-	46%	54%	14%	46%
Concentric remodeling	-	25%	-	34%	33%
Concentric hypertrophy	-	29%	-	43%	12%
Eccentric hypertrophy	-	0%	-	9%	9%
EF (%)	50 ± 10	64 ± 9	60 (56, 65)	60.1 (55.6, 64.3)	58.6 ± 9.8
LAVI (mL/m²)	41.3 ± 14.7	66% LA enlargement	44 (36, 59)	27.9 (21.2, 35.1)	38.9 ± 15.5
Doppler					
TR velocity (m/sec)	-	-	-	2.7 (2.4, 3.0)	2.67 ± 0.46
RVSP (mm Hg)	-	37 ± 13	41 (33, 53)	29 + RAP	34 ± 10
Diastolic dysfunction (y/n)	67%	69%	-	66%	-
Grade 1	22%	29%	-	22%	-
Grade 2	37%	36%	-	34%	-
Grade 3	7%	4%	-	10%	-
Medial e' (cm/s)	-	7.2 ± 2.9	6 (5, 8)	5.6 (4.6, 7.3)	5.8 ± 1.8
Lateral e' (cm/s)	-	9.1 ± 3.4	-	7.6 (5.9, 9.8)	7.9 ± 2.5
Medial E/e'	-	-	16 (11, 24)	14.7 (10.5, 18.7)	16.8 ± 7.3
Lateral E/e'	-	10.0 ± 4.5	-	10.5 (7.9, 14.3)	12.6 ± 5.7

Abbreviations: BMI, body mass index; EDD, end-diastolic dimension; EDVi, end-diastolic volume index; EF, ejection fraction; ESD, end-systolic dimension; ESVi, end-systolic volume index; LAVI, left atrial volume index; LV, left ventricle; RAP, right atrial pressure; RV, right ventricle; RVSP, right ventricular systolic pressure; RWT, relative wall thickness; TR, tricuspid regurgitant.

with substantial overlap in values between HFpEF and controls (**Fig. 6**).[1] Therefore, as with other echo measures, the absolute value of E/e' is best viewed on a continual scale as an estimate of the probability of HFpEF (OR per unit increase in E/e' 1.22, CI 1.16–1.30, p < 0.0001) rather than a reliance on absolute cut-off values. The use of exercise E/e' appears to add diagnostic information at the cost of decreased specificity[1] but multicenter validation studies are lacking with other series reporting poorer diagnostic performance of E/e'.[25]

Prevalence of Normal LV Geometry

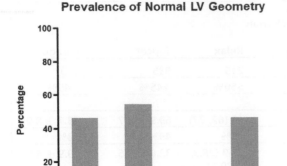

Fig. 2. Prevalence of normal LV geometry. This chart displays the reported prevalence of normal LV geometry as determined by the mass index and relative wall thickness in randomized controlled trials in patients with HFpEF with available data.

Right ventricular systolic pressure

The Doppler TR velocity provides the peak instantaneous gradient between the RV and right atrium (RA), and with the addition of estimated RA pressure to this gradient, pulmonary artery (PA) systolic pressure can be estimated. Mean PA pressure can then be estimated using the Chemla equation (0.61* PA systolic pressure + 2 mm Hg).[26] The PA pressure generally reflects downstream LA pressure in the absence of pulmonary vascular disease. Notching in the RV outflow tract pulsed-wave Doppler is suggestive of pulmonary vascular remodeling resulting in wave reflections decelerating PA flow during mid to late systole. This is the most reliable sign of elevated pulmonary vascular resistance by echocardiography,[27] and when present suggests either precapillary pulmonary arterial hypertension (as a mimic of HFpEF), or CpC-PH HFpEF and the possible need for right heart catheterization (**Fig. 7**).

The presence of a normal estimated PA systolic pressure at rest does not exclude HFpEF (sensitivity 46%) for a number of reasons.[3] Firstly, many patients have inadequate quality TR signals for measurement and this decreases feasibility[28] and diagnostic accuracy.[29] Secondly, even if PA systolic pressure is truly normal at rest, this does not exclude abnormalities during exertion. If high-quality TR signals can be obtained during exercise, there is reasonable accuracy for the RV-RA gradient, but underestimation of exercise RA pressure by echo will underestimate exercise pulmonary pressures (**Fig. 8**).[28] However, when there is any question of pulmonary vascular disease, this generally requires invasive catheterization for confirmation given the treatment implications regarding the use of pulmonary vasodilators.

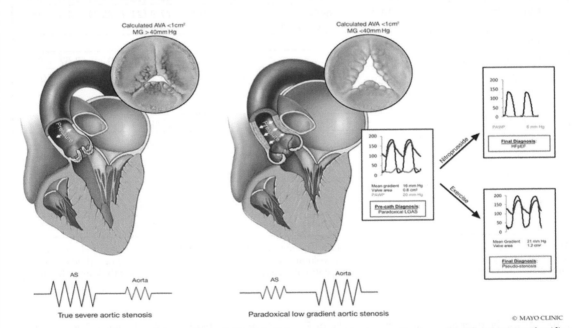

Fig. 3. Aortic valve disease in the setting of HFpEF. Left image shows severe aortic stenosis with a narrowed orifice opening, aortic valve area (AVA) < 1 cm2, mean gradient (MG) > 40 mmH, and valvular impedance. The heart on the right shows paradoxical normal flow low gradient aortic stenosis with AVA < 1 cm2 but MG < 40 mm Hg. Provocative maneuvers including nitroprusside to reduce afterload and exercise to increase preload reveal the true underlying HFpEF state rather than aortic valve disease as a driver of symptoms. (*From* Reddy YNV, Nishimura RA. Paradox of Low-Gradient Aortic Stenosis. Circulation. 2019 May 7;139(19):2195-2197.)

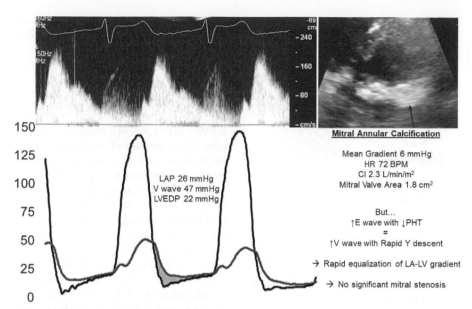

Fig. 4. Mitral annular calcification with reported mitral stenosis. Many patients with HFpEF develop mitral annular calcification (*top right, parasternal short axis view*) which can have an elevated diastolic transmitral gradient (top left) suggestive of stenosis. However, many of these patients do not have true mitral inflow obstruction, and instead the large LA V wave causes the gradient to be elevated in the absence of valvular impedance with the equalization of LA and LV pressures by middiastole.

Right atrial pressure

One of the most powerful physical exam findings to suggest left heart failure is an elevated jugular venous pressure or RA pressure. This reflects the general coupling of LA and RA pressure in most patients with HFpEF due to the physiology of pericardial restraint.[30,31] Thus, in those with elevated estimated RA pressure based on inferior vena cava, there is a high pretest probability of HFpEF.[3,32] However, a "normal" estimated RA pressure based on respiratory IVC collapse may be inaccurate in patients with prominent

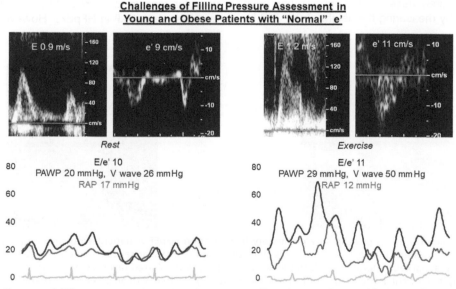

Fig. 5. Challenges of filling pressure assessment in young and/or obese patients with "normal" e′. Concurrent echocardiogram-catheterization of a 42-year-old- woman with a body mass index of 42 kg/m² assessment showing a normal estimate of LA pressure by E/e′ at rest and with exercise even though LA pressure was elevated at rest (*left*) and further so with exercise (*right*).

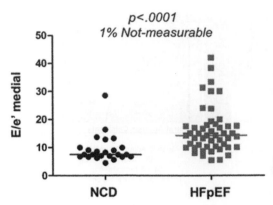

Fig. 6. Performance of resting E/e′ for diagnosis of HFpEF. This concurrent echocardiogram-catheterization study showed large overlap in resting E/e′ between HFpEF and controls limiting its role as an isolated diagnostic test for the evaluation of HFpEF. (*Reproduced with permission* Obokata M. Circulation 2017 Feb 28;135(9):825-838.)

intrathoracic pressure drops during inspiration such as obesity and lung disease where HFpEF may still be present. Transmural RA pressures should be measured at end-expiration (when intrathoracic pressure is zero), and therefore exaggerated intrathoracic pressure drops during inspiration can still collapse an IVC despite high end-expiratory transmural RA pressures (**Fig. 9**). Changes in venous compliance may also alter the area-pressure relationship for the IVC and associated RA pressures particularly in obesity leading to inaccuracies in RA pressure estimation by the IVC alone[33] A recent novel method to more accurately assess RA pressures has been proposed by measuring the height of the JVP by

ultrasound with high accuracy and this requires further study.[34] However, even if RA pressures truly are normal at rest, this does not exclude HFpEF during exertion as previously discussed.

Left atrial strain

LA enlargement with an LA volume index (LAVI) > 30 mL/m2 is a modestly sensitive and specific index for HFpEF evaluation, but merely reflects structural changes with LA enlargement being an imperfect surrogate of a decrease in LA compliance.[5,35] LAVI is particularly misleading in obese patients with HFpEF who have larger BSA that mathematically decreases LAVI even if absolute LA volumes may be abnormally increased.[36] The presence of atrial mitral regurgitation from annular enlargement also tends to reflect underlying HFpEF LA myopathic remodeling.[37]

Left atrial strain has shown promise for atrial function with LA reservoir strain best reflecting atrial operating compliance noninvasively by quantifying the distensibility of the LA.[35] LA reservoir strain at rest has shown predictive value for HFpEF during exercise.[35,38] In a single-center study that assessed LA strain during exercise by echo and MRI, there appeared to be the incremental value from exercise LA strain by MRI but not echo potentially due to greater image quality during exercise by MRI.[38] Assessment of changes in LA strain with volume load from leg elevation may also hold promise for diagnosis.[39] Abnormalities in LA strain also predict pulmonary vascular congestion during exercise,[22] worse pulmonary vascular reserve, abnormal RV-PA coupling and even new-onset AF in HFpEF.[5] However, optimal

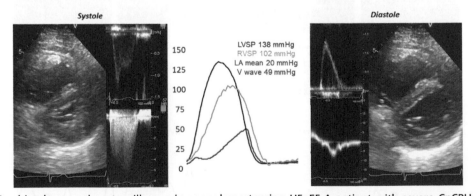

Fig. 7. Combined pre and postcapillary pulmonary hypertension HFpEF A patient with severe CpCPH HFpEF is shown. Left shows echo images during systole with D-shaped ventricular septum, notched RVOT pulsed-wave Doppler, and a markedly elevated TR continuous wave Doppler with slurred upstroke all suggestive of markedly elevated right ventricular afterload. Right shows images during diastole with an eccentric D-shaped left ventricle consistent with elevated biventricular filling pressures and pericardial restraint, elevated mitral E velocity consistent with a large E wave, and reduced tissue Doppler velocities suggestive myocardial disease. The catheterization tracings (*center*) confirm these echo findings with markedly elevated RVSP, elevated and equalized diastolic pressures, and a large LA V wave consistent with left heart diastolic dysfunction and noncompliance.

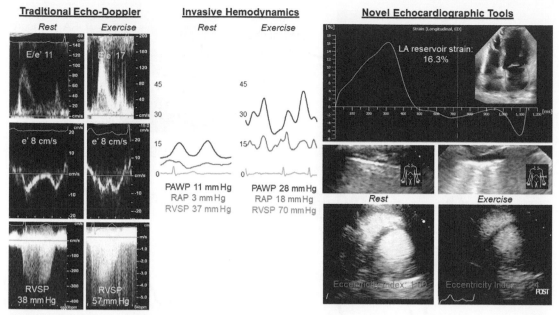

Fig. 8. Diastolic stress testing. Images from a patient undergoing simultaneous echo-catheterization testing (left, center) show normal filling pressures at rest, but elevated with exercise both noninvasively and invasively. Notably, the Doppler-estimated RVSP with exercise underestimated the true RVSP because it assumed an RA pressure of 5 mm Hg while invasively RA hypertension was seen. The right column shows the resting LA reservoir strain was markedly reduced consistent with impaired LA compliance. In addition, lung ultrasound was normal at rest but showed B-lines with exercise suggestive of pulmonary edema. There was also enhanced diastolic ventricular interaction with exercise in the setting of pericardial restraint as reflected by the increase in the eccentricity index.

cutpoints for diagnosis, standardization of strain packages for LA use and multicenter validation of its diagnostic accuracy are required before more widespread clinical use.

Lung ultrasound

Lung ultrasound B lines can evaluate for extravascular lung water, and dynamic B lines are associated with abnormal left heart filling pressures during exertion. The occurrence of B lines during exercise in HFpEF is associated not only with LA hypertension, but also with worse baseline right heart function and RA pressure which potentially impedes lung lymphatic drainage into the systemic veins worsening pulmonary edema.[22] However, as many as half of the patients with HFpEF do not develop B lines during exertion despite abnormal increases in exercise PCWP and dyspnea, and these findings suggest that the absence of B lines cannot exclude HFpEF during rest or exertion.[22]

Right Heart Function

Although usually considered a "left" heart disease, right heart remodeling is in fact highly prevalent in HFpEF, and in longitudinal follow-up the changes in right heart function and enlargement exceed those of left heart changes. This reflects not only the hemodynamic impact of LA hypertension and

associated pulsatile load on the right heart but also obesity, atrial fibrillation and systemic factors.[40] Simple visual assessment of RV dilation and dysfunction is, therefore, highly specific for the diagnosis of HFpEF in the absence of an alternate cause.[3] More quantitative assessment may also help for longitudinal follow-up using TAPSE, FAC or RV s' velocity although these imperfectly capture right heart functional reserve.

Some patients with HFpEF have CpC-PH which disproportionately affects right heart function and remodeling and echocardiography provides clues to its presence (abnormal RV function, right heart enlargement, pericardial restraint, and notching in the RV outflow tract Doppler) which may guide decisions about right heart catheterization.[6]

Pericardial restraint by echocardiography

The pericardium functions like an elastic rubber band around the heart, and with cardiomegaly, this can become stretched and restrain diastolic expansion of the ventricles. This will then exaggerate normal ventricular interdependence and result in a greater contribution of pericardial pressure to left heart filling pressures along with decreased LV end-diastolic volume (i.e., true preload).[30] This constriction-like physiology is common in HFpEF phenotypes with cardiomegalies

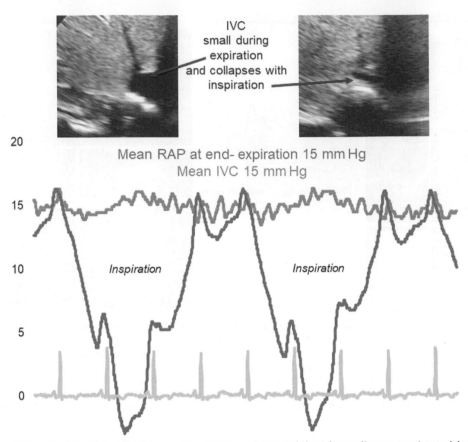

Fig. 9. Challenges in RA pressure assessment in obese patients. While echocardiogram estimated low/normal right atrial (RA) pressure in this patient with a body mass index of 45 kg/m², concurrent catheterization showed an elevated RA pressure at passive end-expiration with large respiratory swings due to prominent negative intra-thoracic pressure during inspiration. Concurrent measurement in the inferior vena cava demonstrated the true venous pressure independent of intrathoracic pressure swings. The intrathoracic IVC collapse at the RA junction in this patient despite high RA pressure was, therefore, reflective of the larger than normal intrathoracic pressure drop during inspiration which can overcome even a high transmural RA pressure (RA pressure–atmospheric pressure) and result in inspiratory collapse.

such as obese HFpEF,[4] CpC-PH HFpEF[6] and HFpEF with severe biatrial enlargement and AF.[5] This extrinsic compression from the compressive rubber band like pericardium around the heart preferentially decreases the septolateral dimension in the short axis view resulting in a D-shaped ventricular septum in diastole on the short axis. The eccentricity index (LV anteroposterior diameter divided by the septolateral diameter) correlates with the degree of pericardial restraint as it increases, and in many patients with HFpEF, this index may be elevated at rest and further with stress (see **Figs. 7** and **8**).

SUMMARY

The echocardiogram is universally performed in the evaluation of suspected HFpEF and provides the initial screen for alternate causes of heart failure. No single echo feature is pathognomonic for HFpEF

diagnosis and therefore echocardiographic abnormalities must be viewed in a probabilistic sense for the potential diagnosis of HFpEF. Dyspneic patients with HFpEF may not have obvious abnormalities at rest, and exercise testing is often required to confirm or refute the diagnosis. Once HFpEF has been confirmed, echocardiography is essential to provide structural and functional information to pathophysiologically phenotype patients.

CLINICS CARE POINTS

- There is significant heterogeneity of echo abnormalities in HFpEF.
- Echocardiography is critical to exclude alternative causes for heart failure symptoms in patients with preserved ejection fraction.

- E/e' should be viewed on a continual scale as modifying the probability of HFpEF. HFpEF is very common even with "normal" E/e' values.
- LA reservoir strain correlates with LA pressure at rest and exercise in suspected HFpEF.
- Echocardiographic measures frequently underestimate the diagnosis and severity of hemodynamic derangements in obese HFpEF.
- Pericardial restraint can be assessed by measuring the eccentricity index on the short axis and can help patients with phenotype HFpEF.

DISCLOSURE

The authors have nothing to disclose.

REFERENCES

1. Obokata M, Kane GC, Reddy YNV, et al. Role of diastolic stress testing in the evaluation for heart failure with preserved ejection fraction: a simultaneous invasive-echocardiographic study. Circulation 2017;135:825–38.
2. Nassif ME, Windsor SL, Borlaug BA, et al. The SGLT2 inhibitor dapagliflozin in heart failure with preserved ejection fraction: a multicenter randomized trial. Nat Med 2021. https://doi.org/10.1038/s41591-021-01536-x.
3. Reddy YNV, Carter RE, Obokata M, et al. A simple, evidence-based approach to help guide diagnosis of heart failure with preserved ejection fraction. Circulation 2018;138:861–70.
4. Obokata M, Reddy YNV, Pislaru SV, et al. Evidence supporting the existence of a distinct obese phenotype of heart failure with preserved ejection fraction. Circulation 2017;136:6–19.
5. Reddy YNV, Obokata M, Verbrugge FH, et al. Atrial dysfunction in patients with heart failure with preserved ejection fraction and atrial fibrillation. J Am Coll Cardiol 2020;76:1051–64.
6. Gorter TM, Obokata M, Reddy YNV, et al. Exercise unmasks distinct pathophysiologic features in heart failure with preserved ejection fraction and pulmonary vascular disease. Eur Heart J 2018;39:2825–35.
7. Stokke TM, Hasselberg NE, Smedsrud MK, et al. Geometry as a confounder when assessing ventricular systolic function: comparison between ejection fraction and strain. J Am Coll Cardiol 2017;70:942–54.
8. Wehner GJ, Jing L, Haggerty CM, et al. Routinely reported ejection fraction and mortality in clinical practice: where does the nadir of risk lie? Eur Heart J 2020;41:1249–57.
9. Pellikka PA, She L, Holly TA, et al. Variability in ejection fraction measured by echocardiography, gated single-photon emission computed tomography, and cardiac magnetic resonance in patients with coronary artery disease and left ventricular dysfunction. JAMA Netw Open 2018;1:e181456.
10. Kondo T, McMurray JJV. Re-emergence of heart failure with a normal ejection fraction? Eur Heart J 2022;43:427–9.
11. Basuray A, French B, Ky B, et al. Heart failure with recovered ejection fraction: clinical description, biomarkers, and outcomes. Circulation 2014;129:2380–7.
12. Topol EJ, Traill TA, Fortuin NJ. Hypertensive hypertrophic cardiomyopathy of the elderly. N Engl J Med 1985;312:277–83.
13. Schiattarella GG, Altamirano F, Tong D, et al. Nitrosative stress drives heart failure with preserved ejection fraction. Nature 2019;568:351–6.
14. Shah AM, Cikes M, Prasad N, et al. Echocardiographic features of patients with heart failure and preserved left ventricular ejection fraction. J Am Coll Cardiol 2019;74:2858–73.
15. Shah AM, Shah SJ, Anand IS, et al. Cardiac structure and function in heart failure with preserved ejection fraction: baseline findings from the echocardiographic study of the Treatment of Preserved Cardiac Function Heart Failure with an Aldosterone Antagonist trial. Circ Heart Fail 2014;7:104–15.
16. Zile MR, Gottdiener JS, Hetzel SJ, et al. Prevalence and significance of alterations in cardiac structure and function in patients with heart failure and a preserved ejection fraction. Circulation 2011;124:2491–501.
17. AbouEzzeddine OF, Davies DR, Scott CG, et al. Prevalence of transthyretin amyloid cardiomyopathy in heart failure with preserved ejection fraction. JAMA Cardiol 2021;6:1267–74.
18. Reddy YNV, Melenovsky V, Redfield MM, et al. High-output heart failure: a 15-year experience. J Am Coll Cardiol 2016;68:473–82.
19. Verbrugge FH, Reddy YNV, Eleid MF, et al. Mild aortic valve disease and the diastolic pressure-volume relationship in heart failure with preserved ejection fraction. Open Heart 2021;8:e001701.
20. Reddy YNV, Nishimura RA. Paradox of low-gradient aortic stenosis. Circulation 2019;139:2195–7.
21. Reddy YNV, Murgo JP, Nishimura RA. Complexity of defining severe 'stenosis' from mitral annular calcification. Circulation 2019;140:523–5.
22. Reddy YNV, Obokata M, Wiley B, et al. The haemodynamic basis of lung congestion during exercise in heart failure with preserved ejection fraction. Eur Heart J 2019;40:3721–30.
23. Reddy YNV, El-Sabbagh A, Nishimura RA. Comparing pulmonary arterial wedge pressure and

left ventricular end diastolic pressure for assessment of left-sided filling pressures. JAMA Cardiol 2018;3:453–4.

24. Kane GC, Karon BL, Mahoney DW, et al. Progression of left ventricular diastolic dysfunction and risk of heart failure. JAMA 2011;306:856–63.

25. Sharifov OF, Schiros CG, Aban I, et al. Diagnostic accuracy of tissue Doppler index E/e' for evaluating left ventricular filling pressure and diastolic dysfunction/heart failure with preserved ejection fraction: a systematic review and meta-analysis. J Am Heart Assoc 2016;5:e002530.

26. Chemla D, Castelain V, Humber M, et al. New formula for predicting mean pulmonary artery pressure using systolic pulmonary artery pressure. Chest 2004;126:1313–7.

27. Arkles JS, Opotowsky AR, Ojeda J, et al. Shape of the right ventricular Doppler envelope predicts hemodynamics and right heart function in pulmonary hypertension. Am J Respir Crit Care Med 2011; 183:268–76.

28. Obokata M, Kane GC, Sorimachi H, et al. Noninvasive evaluation of pulmonary artery pressure during exercise: the importance of right atrial hypertension. Eur Respir J 2020;55:1901617.

29. van Riel AC, Opotowsky AR, Santos M, et al. Accuracy of echocardiography to estimate pulmonary artery pressures with exercise: a simultaneous invasive-noninvasive comparison. Circ Cardiovasc Imaging 2017;10:e005711.

30. Borlaug BA, Reddy YNV. The role of the pericardium in heart failure: implications for pathophysiology and treatment. JACC Heart Fail 2019;7:574–85.

31. Horiuchi Y, Tanimoto S, Aoki J, et al. Mismatch between right- and left-sided filling pressures in heart failure patients with preserved ejection fraction. Int J Cardiol 2018;257:143–9.

32. Nagueh SF, Smiseth OA, Dokainish H, et al. Mean right atrial pressure for estimation of left ventricular filling pressure in patients with normal left ventricular ejection fraction: invasive and noninvasive validation. J Am Soc Echocardiogr 2018;31:799–806.

33. Sorimachi H, Burkhoff D, Verbrugge FH, et al. Obesity, venous capacitance, and venous compliance in heart failure with preserved ejection fraction. Eur J Heart Fail 2021. https://doi.org/10.1002/ejhf.2254.

34. Wang L, Harrison J, Dranow E, et al. Accuracy of ultrasound jugular venous pressure height in predicting central venous congestion. Ann Intern Med 2021. https://doi.org/10.7326/M21-2781.

35. Reddy YNV, Obokata M, Egbe A, et al. Left atrial strain and compliance in the diagnostic evaluation of heart failure with preserved ejection fraction. Eur J Heart Fail 2019;21:891–900.

36. Reddy YNV, Lewis GD, Shah SJ, et al. Characterization of the obese phenotype of heart failure with preserved ejection fraction: a RELAX trial ancillary study. Mayo Clin Proc 2019;94:1199–209.

37. Tamargo M, Obokata M, Reddy YNV, et al. Functional mitral regurgitation and left atrial myopathy in heart failure with preserved ejection fraction. Eur J Heart Fail 2020;22:489–98.

38. Backhaus SJ, Lange T, George EF, et al. Exercise-Stress Real-time Cardiac Magnetic Resonance Imaging for Non-Invasive Characterisation of Heart Failure with Preserved Ejection Fraction: The HFpEF Stress Trial. Circulation 2021;143(15):1484–98.

39. Obokata M, Negishi K, Kurosawa K, et al. Incremental diagnostic value of la strain with leg lifts in heart failure with preserved ejection fraction. JACC Cardiovasc Imaging 2013;6:749–58.

40. Obokata M, Reddy YNV, Melenovsky V, et al. Deterioration in right ventricular structure and function over time in patients with heart failure and preserved ejection fraction. Eur Heart J 2019;40:689–97.

The Role of Multimodality Imaging in the Evaluation of Heart Failure with Preserved Ejection Fraction

Mahesh K. Vidula, MD[a],*, Paco E. Bravo, MD[a,b], Julio A. Chirinos, MD, PhD[a,c]

KEYWORDS

- Heart failure with preserved ejection fraction • Multimodality imaging • Echocardiography
- Cardiac magnetic resonance imaging • Nuclear cardiology • Phenogroups

KEY POINTS

- Multimodality imaging helps establish the diagnosis of heart failure with preserved ejection fraction (HFpEF) and provides a noninvasive assessment of elevated left ventricular filling pressures.
- Multimodality imaging can identify specific etiologies of HFpEF that warrant targeted therapies.
- Multimodality imaging has the potential to enhance our mechanistic phenotypic characterization of patients with HFpEF, which will aid in the development of targeted therapies for this heterogeneous population.

Heart failure with preserved ejection fraction (HFpEF) is highly prevalent, affecting approximately half of all patients with heart failure.[1] It is a significantly heterogeneous condition with a complex pathophysiology and a variety of proposed mechanisms, including abnormal left ventricular (LV) diastolic function, cardiometabolic derangements, myocardial ischemia, large artery stiffening with adverse pulsatile hemodynamics, abnormal ventricular–arterial interactions, systemic and local inflammation, pulmonary vascular abnormalities, peripheral microvascular abnormalities, abnormalities in the cardiorenal axis, and skeletal muscle abnormalities.[2] Several risk factors for HFpEF have been identified, including older age, female sex, obesity, diabetes, hypertension, coronary artery disease (CAD), and atrial fibrillation.[3] The heterogeneity in mechanisms and phenotypes of HFpEF likely underlies the failure of most therapies evaluated in randomized controlled trials (RCTs).

The diagnosis of HFpEF can be notoriously challenging in clinical practice, given the many overlapping etiologies of dyspnea or reduced exercise tolerance in patients at risk for HFpEF. Therefore, the diagnosis of HFpEF relies on clinical signs and symptoms consistent with heart failure, with an ejection fraction (EF) greater than or equal to 50%, and objective evidence of elevated LV filling pressures at rest or with exercise.[4] Multimodality imaging has an important role in establishing the diagnosis of HFpEF and elevated LV filling pressures, identifying specific etiologies of HFpEF (such as cardiac amyloidosis) that can benefit from approved therapies, and discerning distinct phenogroups of patients, or discrete mechanistic abnormalities (such as tissue fibrosis) that may benefit from specific treatments, thus enhancing the design of RCTs for novel therapeutics (**Fig. 1**).[5]

INITIAL EVALUATION AND ESTABLISHING THE DIAGNOSIS OF HFpEF

Echocardiography is the primary imaging modality for the initial evaluation of patients with suspected heart failure[6] and for establishing the diagnosis of

[a] Division of Cardiovascular Medicine, Department of Medicine, Hospital of the University of Pennsylvania, 3400 Civic Center Boulevard, 11-125 South Pavilion, Philadelphia, PA, 19104, USA; [b] Division of Nuclear Medicine, Department of Radiology, Hospital of the University of Pennsylvania, 3400 Civic Center Boulevard, 11-154 South Pavilion, Philadelphia, PA 19104, USA; [c] University of Pennsylvania Perelman School of Medicine, 3400 Civic Center Boulevard, 11-154 South Pavilion, Philadelphia, PA 19104, USA
* Corresponding author.
E-mail address: Mahesh.Vidula@pennmedicine.upenn.edu

Cardiol Clin 40 (2022) 443–457
https://doi.org/10.1016/j.ccl.2022.06.002
0733-8651/22/© 2022 Elsevier Inc. All rights reserved.

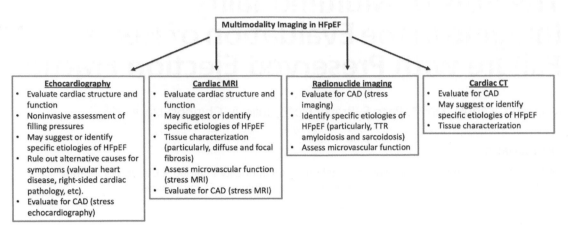

Fig. 1. The role of echocardiography, cardiac MRI, radionuclide imaging, and cardiac CT in the multimodality imaging of patients with HFpEF. CAD, coronary artery disease.

HFpEF. Echocardiographic parameters are incorporated into diagnostic algorithms and risk scores to enhance the diagnosis of HFpEF.[7,8] The H$_2$FPEF score incorporates clinical and echocardiographic variables (body mass index>30 kg/m^2, hypertension, atrial fibrillation, pulmonary hypertension defined as PASP>35 mm Hg, age>60 years, and E/e'>9) to estimate the odds of HFpEF, and performs well in patients with EF $\geq$ 50% (**Fig. 2**A).[8,9] The HFA-PEFF score consists of functional and morphological criteria obtained by echocardiography including septal and lateral tissue velocities, E/e', tricuspid regurgitation (TR) velocity, longitudinal strain, left atrial volume, LV mass, and wall thickness (see **Fig. 2**B).

Echocardiography fulfills three main roles in the assessment of patients with suspected or established HFpEF. First, it has a key role in evaluating cardiac structure and function in patients with

HFpEF. In addition to establishing the presence of a preserved LV EF (i.e., $\geq$50%), echocardiography can assess LV geometry, pulmonary artery systolic pressure, right ventricular structure and function, left atrial structure and function, valvular structure and function, as well as pericardial disease.[10–16] Second, echocardiography has a crucial role in the noninvasive estimation of left-sided filling pressures and is the primary method of establishing the presence of elevated filling pressures at rest or with exercise in patients with suspected HFpEF in most centers.[17–27] Assessment of diastolic function (**Table 1**) and estimation of LV filling pressures by echocardiography require the integration of multiple echocardiographic parameters, which are described in detail in the 2016 American Society of Echocardiography (ASE)/European Association of Cardiovascular Imaging (EACVI) guidelines.[17] Lastly, as discussed in

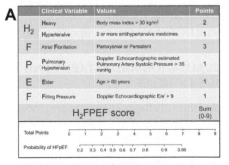
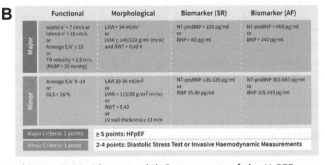

Fig. 2. Echocardiographic parameters incorporated into HFpEF risk scores. (*A*) Components of the H$_2$PEF score. and (*B*) Components of the HFA-PEFF score. (*From* [A] Reddy YNV, Carter RE, Obokata M, Redfield MM, Borlaug BA. A Simple, Evidence-Based Approach to Help Guide Diagnosis of Heart Failure With Preserved Ejection Fraction. Circulation. 2018 Aug 28;138(9):861-870.) and (*B*) Components of the HFA-PEFF score; and [B] Pieske B, Tschöpe C, de Boer RA, Fraser AG, Anker SD, Donal E, Edelmann F, Fu M, Guazzi M, Lam CSP, Lancellotti P, Melenovsky V, Morris DA, Nagel E, Pieske-Kraigher E, Ponikowski P, Solomon SD, Vasan RS, Rutten FH, Voors AA, Ruschitzka F, Paulus WJ, Seferovic P, Filippatos G. How to diagnose heart failure with preserved ejection fraction: the HFA-PEFF diagnostic algorithm: a consensus recommendation from the Heart Failure Association (HFA) of the European Society of Cardiology (ESC). Eur Heart J. 2019 Oct 21;40(40):3297-3317.)

Table 1
Key features of the different grades of diastolic dysfunction

Diastolic Function	Typical Features
Normal	• E/A $\geq$ 0.8 • Average E/é < 10 • Normal left atrial volume index • Peak TR velocity < 2.8 m/s • Normal LV relaxation • Normal left atrial pressure
Grade I (Impaired Relaxation)	• E/A $\leq$ 0.8 • Average E/é < 10 • Normal/increased left atrial volume index • Peak TR velocity < 2.8 m/s • Abnormal LV relaxation • Normal left atrial pressure
Grade II (Pseudonormal)	• 0.8 < E/A < 2 • Average E/é 10–14 • Increased left atrial volume index • Peak TR velocity > 2.8 m/s • Abnormal LV relaxation • Elevated left atrial pressure
Grade III (Restrictive)	• E/A > 2 • Average E/é > 14 • Increased left atrial volume index • Peak TR velocity > 2.8 m/s • Abnormal LV relaxation • Elevated left atrial pressure
Supranormal (Athletes)	• Typically seen in the athlete's heart • E/A > 2 • Increased é • Low E/é

the remaining sections of this article, echocardiography has the ability to identify specific etiologies and phenotypes of HFpEF that may benefit from targeted therapies.

For more information on the use of echocardiography in HFpEF, please see Chapter 11.

IDENTIFICATION OF SPECIFIC PHENOTYPES OF HFpEF

Once the diagnosis of HFpEF has been established, multimodality imaging can potentially identify specific etiologies and phenotypes of HFpEF that may benefit from specific therapies. While echocardiography is an initial tool to assess cardiac structure and function, echocardiography, cardiac magnetic resonance (CMR), and radionuclide imaging also have important roles in the evaluation of patients with suspected HFpEF.

Coronary Artery Disease

CAD is a common comorbidity in patients with HFpEF. One study identified angiographically proven epicardial CAD in 68% of HFpEF patients,[28] and another study found evidence of epicardial or microvascular disease in 91% of patients hospitalized with HFpEF.[29] Both epicardial and microvascular diseases can contribute to the pathophysiology of HFpEF, with ischemia leading to supply–demand mismatch, inflammation, fibrosis, and myocardial dysfunction.[30] In the study by Hwang and colleagues,[28] patients with angiographically proven CAD (defined as >50% in $\geq$1 epicardial artery), had similar HF and anginal symptoms as patients without CAD, but patients with CAD were at higher risk of worsening EF and increased mortality. Furthermore, patients who underwent complete revascularization (defined as either percutaneous coronary intervention or coronary bypass grafting of all stenoses >50%) experienced improved mortality and less reduction in EF than patients who were incompletely revascularized.[28] Therefore, it is important to identify both epicardial and microvascular diseases and evaluate the need for antiischemic therapies (including revascularization) as appropriate. Furthermore, since dyspnea can be an anginal equivalent, it is important to differentiate patients with exertional dyspnea resulting purely or predominantly from CAD, as symptom relief can be potentially achieved with coronary revascularization.

Several modalities are commonly used in clinical practice for the noninvasive assessment of hemodynamically significant epicardial CAD, including exercise or pharmacologic stress echocardiography, exercise or pharmacologic stress single-photon emission computed tomography (SPECT), pharmacologic stress PET, pharmacologic stress CMR, and coronary computed tomographic angiography. Coronary microvascular dysfunction (CMD) is noninvasively evaluated by assessing for impaired coronary flow reserve (CFR), which is determined by calculating the ratio of myocardial blood flow (MBF) at peak stress to MBF at rest. Currently, radionuclide imaging techniques, contrast echocardiography, and CMR can be used to calculate CFR, but the modality most commonly used in clinical practice is pharmacologic stress PET due to the extensive evidence and experience with this modality.[31] Pharmacologic stress PET may be the preferred test for the evaluation of patients with HFpEF, given its high accuracy in diagnosing both flow-limiting epicardial lesions and microvascular disease.[32] PET-derived CFR can be calculated using a variety of radionuclide tracers, most commonly Rubidium-82, O-15 water, and N-13 ammonia.[31] CMD is defined as an impaired CFR (<2) in the absence of epicardial flow-limiting CAD, and a prior study has shown that impaired CFR correlates with diastolic dysfunction and adverse cardiovascular outcomes in patients with HFpEF.[33] However, it is unknown whether this is a causal relationship. Examples of an HFpEF patient with obstructive CAD and a patient with microvascular dysfunction are shown in **Fig. 3**.

It is important to note that aortic stiffening, which is discussed in detail in the section titled, "aorta," can result in a reduction in coronary perfusion. As the aorta becomes less compliant and its pulse wave velocity (PWV) increases, wave reflections arrive earlier in the proximal aorta, augmenting systolic rather than diastolic pressure, which results in a steep diastolic pressure decay, thereby reducing the diastolic perfusion pressure that drives microvascular flow in diastole.[34] Therefore, the phenotypic presentation and potentially, the clinical consequences of epicardial or microvascular CAD can be modified by aortic stiffening, an issue that should be addressed in future studies.

Hypertrophic Cardiomyopathy

Hypertrophic cardiomyopathy (HCM) is an important cause of LV hypertrophy and is important to recognize in patients with suspected HFpEF to ensure appropriate diagnosis, risk stratification, treatment, and screening of family members. On imaging, HCM is defined as wall thickness greater than or equal to 15 mm in any segment, which cannot be explained by abnormal loading conditions (such as arterial hypertension or aortic valve stenosis). In patients with a family history of HCM or with a positive genotype, an unexplained wall thickness of greater than 13 mm can be consistent with the diagnosis.[35] Echocardiography and CMR are the primary imaging modalities utilized for the diagnosis of HCM. Supportive morphologic features of HCM include elongated mitral valve leaflets, abnormal papillary muscle insertion and placement, and systolic anterior motion of the mitral valve, contributing to LV outflow tract obstruction. However, these findings are nonspecific and may be present in non-HCM conditions

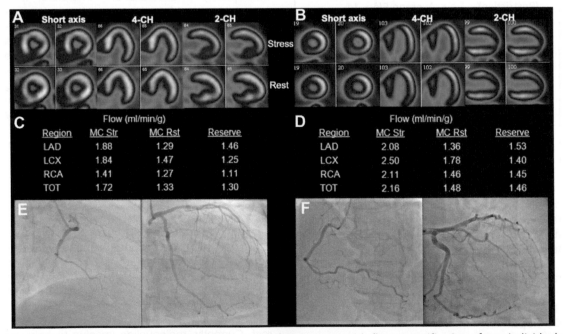

Fig. 3. Selected stress and rest Rubidium-82 myocardial PET images with flow quantification of two individuals with HFpEF complaining of worsening dyspnea. In both the cases, myocardial perfusion (*A, B*) and CFR (*C, D*) were abnormal. The first individual showed single vessel angiographic disease in the right coronary artery (*E*), which was amenable to revascularization, whereas the second individual showed angiographically normal coronary arteries (*F*) but with markedly reduced CFR, consistent with severe microvascular dysfunction.

as well.[36] Patients with suspected HCM on echo-cardiography typically undergo subsequent imaging with CMR, which offers a greater anatomic definition and a more complete evaluation of the entire heart. Late gadolinium enhancement (LGE) sequences on CMR identify regions of replacement fibrosis and scar in the myocardium, which can help inform risk stratification for sudden cardiac death.[37]

Infiltrative Cardiomyopathies

Patients diagnosed with HFpEF must be evaluated for the presence of infiltrative cardiomyopathies since specific medical treatments can be initiated to modify the disease course and outcomes. In a framework that has been previously described,[38,39] infiltrative cardiomyopathies have been divided into two categories: (1) infiltrative cardiomyopathies characterized by increased wall thickness and (2) infiltrative cardiomyopathies with normal wall thickness. In the following section, we briefly discuss the infiltrative cardiomyopathies that are important to recognize in patients undergoing evaluation for HFpEF.

Increased wall thickness

Amyloidosis Cardiac amyloidosis results from the deposition of amyloid fibrils in the myocardium, and the two main types are light-chain amyloidosis (AL) and transthyretin amyloidosis (ATTR). Accurate diagnosis of cardiac amyloidosis, and differentiation of AL and ATTR amyloidosis, is critical to ensure the initiation of appropriate medical therapies. Multimodality imaging plays a central role in the evaluation of suspected amyloidosis. In general, echocardiography and CMR are utilized to support a diagnosis of cardiac amyloidosis, whereas radionuclide imaging with bone scintigraphy is used to differentiate between AL and ATTR amyloidosis.[38]

On echocardiography, patients with cardiac amyloidosis can exhibit increased biventricular wall thickness and mass, thickened valves and interatrial septum, biatrial enlargement and thickening, stasis/thrombi in the left atrium or appendage, reduced left atrial function, and pericardial effusions.[40,41] An apical sparing pattern on longitudinal strain mapping, known as the "cherry-on-top" pattern, has been reported to have high sensitivity and specificity for diagnosing amyloidosis in patients with increased wall thickness.[42] On CMR, infiltration of the amyloid fibrils in the myocardium results in expansion of the extracellular space, leading to abnormal gadolinium kinetics, which can have effects on the inversion time and contrast in inversion recovery scout sequences,[43] which are typically performed prior to

phase-sensitive inversion recovery imaging to detect LGE. However, LGE patterns vary with increasing severity of disease, beginning with no visible LGE in the LV early in the disease course, progressing to diffuse, circumferential subendocardial, and transmural LGE, with potential involvement of the atria and RV, in advanced stages (**Fig. 4**). The native T1 relaxation time, which measures the recovery time of the longitudinal magnetization of myocardial tissue, is prolonged in patients with amyloidosis (see **Fig. 4**).[44] Myocardial extracellular volume (ECV) can be quantified using pre- and post-gadolinium-based contrast T1 relaxation times of the myocardium and blood pool. An elevation in ECV is also commonly seen in patients with cardiac amyloidosis.[45]

If there is suspicion of cardiac amyloidosis by clinical history, echocardiography, and/or CMR, current guidelines recommend beginning with screening for the presence of a monoclonal immunoglobulin light chain with serum and urine immunofixation electrophoresis and serum kappa/lambda free light chain ratio.[46] If a monoclonal protein is detected, a biopsy is recommended to identify AL amyloidosis.[46] If a monoclonal protein is not detected, bone scintigraphy is performed to identify ATTR amyloidosis.[41,46] The most common bone tracers utilized are [99m]Technetium (Tc)-pyrophosphate (PYP) and

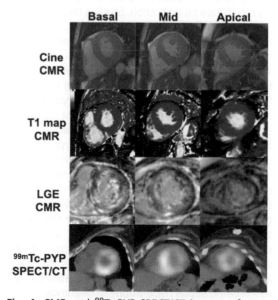

Fig. 4. CMR and ^{99}Tc-PYP SPECT/CT images of a patient with ATTR amyloidosis. *Top row,* cine CMR demonstrating increased wall thickness, (*second row*) T1 maps demonstrating elevated T1 times in the myocardium, (*third row*) LGE sequences revealing diffuse LGE throughout the myocardium, and (*bottom row*) ^{99}Tc-PYP SPECT/CT images demonstrating diffuse PYP uptake in the myocardium, consistent with ATTR amyloidosis.

^{99m}Tc-3,3-diphosphono-1,2-propanodiacarboxylic acid, which bind to microcalcifications associated with TTR fibrils, and these bone tracers are used in combination with planar or SPECT imaging.[41] In the absence of a detectable monoclonal protein, significant uptake of the bone radiotracer in the heart as compared to the ribs has a specificity and positive predictive value approaching 100% for the diagnosis of ATTR, thus eliminating the need for myocardial biopsy (see **Fig. 4**).[41] However, in the presence of a monoclonal protein, the diagnostic accuracy is reduced, and therefore serum/urine testing for monoclonal proteins should always be performed prior to proceeding with bone scintigraphy. Once a diagnosis of ATTR amyloidosis is confirmed, genotyping must be performed to identify mutant or wild-type forms of ATTR.

Anderson–Fabry disease Anderson–Fabry disease (AFD) is an X-linked lysosomal storage disorder caused by mutations of the GLA gene that encodes alpha-galactosidase A. It is characterized by glycosphingolipid accumulation.[47] On echocardiography, patients may have increased biventricular wall thickness, left atrial dilation and dysfunction, and abnormal longitudinal strain in the basal inferolateral wall, a common site of myocardial fibrosis.[48] CMR can reveal mid-myocardial LGE in the basal inferolateral wall and reduced native T1 relaxation time due to diffuse fat infiltration. Studies have also proposed that there may be an inflammatory component in AFD since some patients were found to have elevated T2 values and increased signal on T2 short inversion time inversion recovery, with uptake on PET with fludeoxyglucose F 18 (^{18}F FDG-PET).[49–52] In contrast to HFpEF, the symptom onset of Fabry's disease typically occurs in late childhood or early adulthood and includes extracardiac manifestations (such as neuropathic pain, hypohidrosis, and gastrointestinal symptoms).[53] Diagnosis, however, can be delayed for decades, and patients may present in middle age with advanced disease, characterized by renal involvement (proteinuria progressing to renal failure), cardiovascular manifestations (including heart failure and ventricular arrhythmias), and stroke.[54] In late-stage patients with AFD, localized relative thinning of the basal inferolateral wall is seen, which can result in an asymmetric septal hypertrophy appearance.

Interestingly, a cardiac variant of AFD with late-onset isolated cardiac manifestation has been recognized.[55] In this form, cardiac manifestations occur after middle age without any other signs of AFD. Nakao and colleagues[55] reported a 3% prevalence of this atypical variant of AFD in male patients with LVH (septal or posterior wall thickness ≥13 mm) referred to the cardiology section of an academic medical center for evaluation of cardiac abnormalities. The age of patients with this form of AFD ranged from 55 years to 72 years and 28% exhibited dyspnea. The prevalence of this form of AFB in unselected patients with LVH remains unclear. AFB should be considered in the differential diagnosis of HFpEF given the availability of disease-specific enzyme replacement therapy.

Normal wall thickness

Sarcoidosis Sarcoidosis, a multisystem, granulomatous, inflammatory disease, results in granulomatous infiltration of the heart in up to 25%–58% of cases and is an important disease process to identify in patients diagnosed with HfpEF.[56] Patients may present with ventricular arrhythmias, conduction block, sudden cardiac death, or heart failure. Early stages of cardiac sarcoidosis (CS) are characterized by active inflammation requiring immunosuppression, and late stages are characterized by fibrosis. Multimodality cardiac imaging with echocardiography, CMR, and nuclear imaging aid in the diagnosis of CS, and nuclear imaging is essential for monitoring disease activity.

Echocardiography is the initial modality recommended for the evaluation of CS, but findings can be notoriously nonspecific.[57] Findings suspicious of CS include regional wall motion abnormalities in noncoronary distributions, basal septal thinning and akinesis, and inferolateral wall aneurysms.[57] CMR findings can increase the diagnostic accuracy of CS, but unfortunately, there are no pathognomonic tissue characteristics that can definitively diagnose CS. Areas of inflammation can be detected by T1 and T2 mapping, and LGE patterns can be multifocal and involve any portion of the myocardium (**Fig. 5**).

^{18}F FDG-PET is utilized to monitor inflammation and assess disease activity.[57] Patients must follow a high-fat, low-carbohydrate diet to suppress normal myocardial glucose uptake prior to their study, enabling the FDG taken up by the inflamed regions to be visualized on PET (see **Fig. 5**). Perfusion imaging can be performed as well to identify regions of the scar. While multimodality imaging is helpful in increasing the probability of a diagnosis of CS, the gold standard of diagnosis is a cardiac biopsy, which is, however, limited by the patchy nature of the granulomatous infiltration. Therefore, a thoughtful approach to the diagnosis of CS is mandatory to ensure accurate diagnosis and appropriate initiation/escalation of immunosuppressive therapy.

Iron overload cardiomyopathy Patients who require or have required frequent blood transfusions, or have genetic hemochromatosis, are at

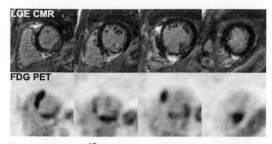

Fig. 5. CMR and ^{18}F FDG-PET images of a patient with CS. *Top row,* CMR LGE images demonstrating multifocal LGE. *Bottom row,* FDG-PET images revealing FDG uptake corresponding to the same regions of LGE.

risk for iron overload cardiomyopathy, which can result in HF. On CMR, T2* mapping values correlate with the degree of myocardial iron deposition.[58] Myocardial T2* mapping value of <10 ms indicates a high risk of heart failure and T2* mapping value of <20 ms is associated with an increased risk of arrhythmias, and therefore T2* mapping is used to guide the initiation of iron chelation therapy in this group of patients.[59] Reduction in native T1 relaxation times can also be seen with myocardial iron deposition.[60]

Diffuse Myocardial Fibrosis

Many of the risk factors and pathways involved in the pathophysiology of HFpEF, including diabetes and hypertension, are hypothesized to culminate in the activation of fibrotic processes and expansion of the myocardial extracellular matrix.[61] The degree of diffuse interstitial fibrosis can be assessed by T1 mapping on CMR since fibrosis prolongs myocardial T1 relaxation times. Myocardial ECV (calculated from pre- and postcontrast T1 maps) will also be elevated in the presence of diffuse interstitial fibrosis, and studies have shown that both T1 mapping and ECV correlate with myocardial fibrosis on biopsy and with diastolic dysfunction.[62-64] Furthermore, fibrosis detected by CMR is associated with worse outcomes in HFpEF patients.[65] Care must be taken when interpreting T1 maps on CMR since elevated T1 values can be seen in other disease states, such as edema, inflammation, and infiltration. While CMR is the most commonly used noninvasive modality for the assessment of diffuse myocardial fibrosis, cardiac computed tomography (CT) can also be used to calculate ECV.[66]

It is important to note that while average ECV values are significantly higher in HFpEF patients than in controls, only a minority (~ one-third) of patients with HFpEF exhibit abnormal levels of ECV. Su and colleagues[64] found that patients with HFpEF

had a median ECV of 28.9% (interquartile range (IQR): 27.8% to 31.3%) and healthy controls had a median ECV of 27.9% (IQR: 26.2% to 29.4%; $P = .006$). Furthermore, a biopsy study found that moderate-severe fibrosis is present in 27% of HFpEF patients, and mild or patchy fibrosis is present in 66% of HFpEF patients.[67] These results indicate that significant fibrosis appears to only be present in a subset of HFpEF patients, and therefore, the accurate identification of this subset may have an impact on potential eligibility for antifibrotic therapies. However, it is currently unclear whether antifibrotic therapies are effective in reducing the risk of adverse outcomes for HFpEF patients with evidence of interstitial fibrosis. Pirfenidone, an antifibrotic agent, was recently studied in patients with heart failure, $EF \geq 45\%$ and myocardial $ECV \geq 27\%$.[68] After 52 weeks, there was a significant reduction in ECV in the patients randomized to pirfenidone (between-group difference −1.21%; 95% confidence interval −2.12 to −0.31, $P = .009$).[68] Further studies are required to determine whether this reduction in ECV leads to improvement in clinical outcomes.

IMAGING OF EXTRACARDIAC ORGANS IN HFpEF

Several extracardiac organs have been implicated in the pathogenesis of HFpEF. In this final section, we briefly review imaging of the aorta, body composition, skeletal muscle, liver, and kidneys in patients with HFpEF.

Aorta

Prior studies have demonstrated that large artery stiffness is associated with increased afterload, diastolic dysfunction, heart failure symptoms, and worse outcomes.[69-71]

Measuring PWV is the most common method of quantifying aortic stiffness. PWV is computed by dividing the distance between two sites of the aorta by the time it takes for the pulse to travel between those sites. With MRI, anatomic imaging of the aorta can be performed to obtain the aortic length, and phase-contrast images can be obtained to measure the transit time. This is typically done via the plane phase-contrast acquisition of the thoracic aorta in which the ascending and descending aorta are simultaneously imaged (**Fig. 6**A). However, effectiveness of this method may be limited in the presence of stiff aortas *with* very short transit times between these two locations. Carotid-femoral PWV can also be measured using applanation tonometry or Doppler ultrasound.[34,72,73] Echocardiography can also be used to assess aortic stiffness, and specifically measure aortic PWV.[34] Pulse wave Doppler

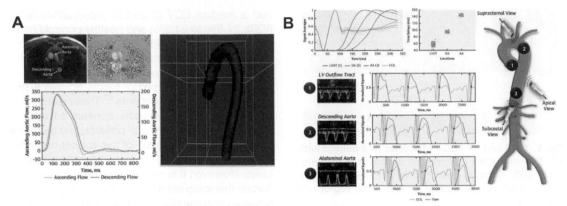

Fig. 6. (*A*) PWV measurements by MRI. Two planes perpendicular to the thoracic aorta are placed at a fixed distance of 15 cm. The total distance between region of interest (ROI)$_1$ and ROI$_3$ is the sum of dist$_1$ and dist$_2$ (*left*). Velocity–time curves are generated at the two ROIs (right), and time-delay calculation is performed. (*B*) Assessment of PWV by echocardiography. Pulse wave Doppler interrogation of the LV outflow tract, descending aorta, and abdominal aorta can be obtained (panels 1–3). These waveforms are signal-averaged, and transit time can be calculated (*top panels*). (*From* Chirinos JA, Segers P, Hughes T, Townsend R. Large-Artery Stiffness in Health and Disease: JACC State-of-the-Art Review. J Am Coll Cardiol. 2019 Sep 3;74(9):1237-1263.

interrogations of blood flow can be obtained at the LV outflow tract, proximal descending aorta, and proximal abdominal aorta, and the time it takes for the pulse wave to travel between these three sites can be measured using the electrocardiogram as a fiducial point (see **Fig. 6**B), thus providing a means to measure thoracic aortic wall stiffness.[34,74] Cardiac-to-ankle PWV can also be measured using a combination of phonocardiography, brachial and ankle cuff waveforms.[75–77] The reader is referred to recent publications for comprehensive reviews on methods to measure aortic stiffness.[34,73,78]

Although aortic stiffness is a relevant phenotype in HFpEF, a more direct assessment of cardiac load can be obtained via analyses of central pressure-flow relations. This has been the topic of previous reviews[79–84] and only a brief summary is presented here. The carotid pressure waveform derived from carotid arterial tonometry recordings can be considered to be a close surrogate of the aortic pressure waveform. Pulse wave Doppler interrogation through the LV outflow tract provides a noninvasive measurement of LV outflow, which equals aortic inflow. These waveforms undergo signal averaging, and the processed central pressure versus time and central flow versus time waveforms are aligned to provide a more direct assessment of arterial load through various quantitative and modeling techniques, including input impedance analysis (which assesses pulsatile arterial load in the frequency domain), wave separation analysis (which quantifies wave reflection), Windkessel modeling (which is used predominantly to quantify total arterial compliance), and wave intensity/wave power analysis (which is

used to assess discrete wavefronts arising ventricular–arterial interactions at various times in the cardiac cycle).[79–84]

Body composition

Obesity has been hypothesized to increase inflammation, worsen insulin resistance and hypertension, contribute to abnormal hemodynamics, and lead to ventricular stiffening.[85–87] A study by Selvaraj and colleagues[85] found that patients with HFpEF had increased pericardial, subcutaneous, and visceral fat. In another study, patients with epicardial fat were found to have higher filling pressures, increased pericardial restraint, and worse exercise capacity than patients without epicardial fat.[88] Fat thickness (subcutaneous, visceral, and paracardiac) measurements can be performed on MRI or CT, and echocardiography has also been used to measure the epicardial fat thickness.[85,88] Dual-energy X-ray absorptiometry can also be used to noninvasively measure muscle mass.[89]

Skeletal muscle

Skeletal muscle abnormalities have been demonstrated in patients with HFpEF, which may contribute to the exercise intolerance seen in this patient population. Haykowsky and colleagues[90] used MRI to demonstrate increased intermuscular fat infiltration in the thighs of participants with HFpEF, which was associated with reduced oxygen consumption at peak exercise. Needle biopsies have revealed that patients with HFpEF exhibit reduced type I oxidative muscle fibers and reduced capillary-to-fiber ratios in skeletal muscle compared to healthy controls, which correlated with the reduction in exercise capacity.[91] Creatine (Cr) chemical exchange-saturation transfer (CrCEST) is a novel MRI technique, which utilizes the magnetic saturation of Cr to measure Cr concentrations in tissues, and this method has been used to noninvasively assess oxidative phosphorylation capacity in skeletal muscle mitochondria.[92,93] Using this imaging technique, patients with HFpEF were found to have abnormal skeletal muscle oxidative phosphorylation capacity, which may contribute to impaired exercise tolerance (**Fig. 7**).[94] Furthermore, smaller axial muscle size, as measured by MRI, has been shown to be associated with death in patients with heart failure, suggesting that targeting sarcopenia in this patient population may improve outcomes.[95] Interestingly, in the study by Selvaraj and colleagues[85] mentioned earlier, lower axial skeletal muscle size, but not fat, was significantly and independently associated with mortality and more closely associated with N-terminal pro-brain natriuretic peptide levels than fat distribution or body mass index. The biological interrelationships between skeletal muscle and the natriuretic peptide system require further study.

Liver

Liver disease, particularly nonalcoholic fatty liver disease, is associated with cardiac remodeling and adverse hemodynamic consequences and may contribute to certain phenotypes of HFpEF.[96] In addition to its key metabolic function, under normal conditions, the liver has a key role as a venous reservoir, increasing venous compliance to sequester blood volume when faced with increased central venous pressures.[97] However, in patients with advanced liver disease and fibrosis, hepatic sinusoidal resistance may increase, resulting in an increase in the hepatic venous pressure gradient, reduction in compliance, and a reduction in hepatic blood flow during exercise. This may result in reduction in abnormal preload delivered to the right ventricle during exercise, contributing to impairment in exercise capacity.[96,98] Furthermore, systemic inflammation and abnormalities in hepatic metabolism are common in patients with liver disease, which may contribute to diastolic dysfunction and endothelial dysfunction.[96] Evaluation of liver disease in patients with HFpEF using multimodality imaging can identify specific phenogroups, which may ultimately guide therapies targeted toward these specific pathophysiologic pathways. Elastography is a powerful tool to evaluate liver tissue stiffness and assess for the presence of fibrosis, and studies have shown that liver stiffness is associated with progression of liver fibrosis and outcomes.[99] Shear wave elastography is a commonly used technique, where the propagation of shear waves through the liver is measured using ultrasound or MRI, and the shear wave velocity is used to calculate the stiffness of the liver tissue.[100,101] MRI elastography and some ultrasound devices utilize external mechanical stimulation to generate shear waves, whereas other ultrasound techniques utilize shear waves induced by ultrasound. An example of shear wave ultrasound elastography from our research group is shown in **Fig. 8**.

Kidneys

Renal dysfunction is common in patients with HFpEF, with several proposed mechanistic links between renal disease and the development of

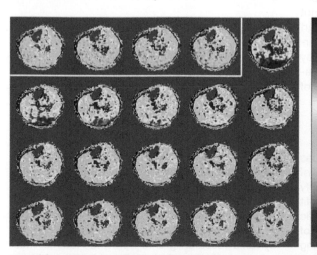

Fig. 7. CrCEST maps of skeletal muscle Cr concentration in a healthy male after plantar flexion exercises. The white box shows CrCEST maps prior to exercise. Following exercise, there is increase in free Cr, in an effort to generate adenosine triphosphate, indicated by the increase in red. Free Cr decreases during recovery. (*From* Zamani P, Proto EA, Wilson N, Fazelinia H, Ding H, Spruce LA, Davila A Jr, Hanff TC, Mazurek JA, Prenner SB, Desjardins B, Margulies KB, Kelly DP, Arany Z, Doulias PT, Elrod JW, Allen ME, McCormack SE, Schur GM, D'Aquilla K, Kumar D, Thakuri D, Prabhakaran K, Langham MC, Poole DC, Seeholzer SH, Reddy R, Ischiropoulos H, Chirinos JA. Multimodality assessment of heart failure with preserved ejection fraction skeletal muscle reveals differences in the machinery of energy fuel metabolism. ESC Heart Fail. 2021 Aug;8(4):2698-2712.)

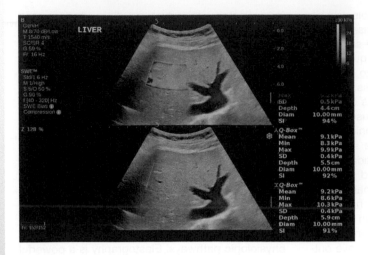

Fig. 8. An example of shear wave liver elastography from our research group. Measurements are obtained 1.5 cm–2.0 cm from the liver capsule. The mean liver stiffness of 9.1 kPa–9.2 kPa in this patient is suggestive of advanced chronic liver disease.[100].

HFpEF, including inflammation, alterations to mineral metabolism, neurohormonal activation, arterial stiffening, and microvascular disease.[102] Intrarenal Doppler ultrasonography is a noninvasive method to evaluate intrarenal hemodynamics and was initially studied in patients with intrinsic renal diseases and obstructive uropathy.[103,104] Recent studies have found that intrarenal venous flow patterns were associated with right atrial pressure in patients with heart failure.[103,105] Discontinuous (biphasic or monophasic) flow patterns were associated with elevated right atrial pressures when compared with continuous flow patterns, and discontinuous patterns were associated with worse outcomes. The renal resistive index has also been shown to be higher in patients with HFpEF and is associated with worse outcomes.[106] T1 mapping of the kidneys and kidney shear wave elastography are promising techniques to evaluate for renal fibrosis but have not yet been extensively studied in patients with heart failure.[107] Further research is required to determine how multimodality imaging of the kidney may identify specific phenogroups of HFpEF patients, and potentially guide the development of novel therapies.

SUMMARY

Multimodality imaging of patients with HFpEF has multiple goals: (1) establish the diagnosis of HFpEF and assess filling pressures, (2) identify specific etiologies of HFpEF that may benefit from targeted therapies, and (3) identify specific phenogroups that can guide the development of future therapies. Future advancements in imaging will likely further our understanding of the pathophysiology of HFpEF and enable the development of personalized therapies to improve outcomes in this heterogeneous population.

CLINICS CARE POINTS

- The diagnosis of HFpEF relies on clinical signs and symptoms consistent with heart failure, with an ejection fraction (EF) greater than or equal to 50%, and objective evidence of elevated LV filling pressures at rest or with exercise.

- Echocardiography, cardiac magnetic resonance, and radionuclide imaging should be used to identify specific etiologies of HFpEF, which may benefit from targeted therapies.

CONFLICT OF INTEREST/DISCLOSURES

M.K. Vidula: None. P.E. Bravo: None. J.A. Chirinos is supported by the National Institutes of Health (NIH) grants R01-HL 121510, U01-TR003734, 3U01TR003734 - 01W1, U01-HL160277, R33-HL-146390, R01-HL153646, K24-AG070459, R01-AG058969, R01-HL104106, P01-HL094307, R03-HL146874, R56-HL136730, R01 HL155599, R01 HL157264, R01HL155, and 1R01HL153646-01. He has recently consulted for Bayer, Sanifit, Fukuda-Denshi, Bristol-Myers Squibb, JNJ, Edwards Life Sciences, Merck, NGM Biopharmaceuticals, and the Galway-Mayo Institute of Technology. He received the University of Pennsylvania research grants from the National Institutes of Health, Fukuda-Denshi, Bristol-Myers Squibb, Microsoft, and Abbott. He is named as the inventor in a University of Pennsylvania patent for the use of inorganic nitrates/nitrites for the treatment of heart failure and preserved ejection fraction and for the use of biomarkers in heart failure with preserved ejection fraction. He has received payments for editorial roles from the American Heart Association, the American College of Cardiology, and Wiley. He has received research device loans from Atcor Medical, Fukuda-Denshi, Uscom, NDD Medical Technologies, Microsoft, and MicroVision Medical.

REFERENCES

1. Dunlay SM, Roger VL, Redfield MM. Epidemiology of heart failure with preserved ejection fraction. Nat Rev Cardiol 2017;14:591–602.

2. Obokata M, Reddy YNV, Borlaug BA. Diastolic dysfunction and heart failure with preserved ejection fraction: understanding mechanisms by using noninvasive methods. JACC Cardiovasc Imaging 2020;13:245–57.

3. Chirinos JA, Orlenko A, Zhao L, et al. Multiple plasma biomarkers for risk stratification in patients with heart failure and preserved ejection fraction. J Am Coll Cardiol 2020;75:1281–95.

4. Pfeffer MA, Shah AM, Borlaug BA. Heart failure with preserved ejection fraction in perspective. Circ Res 2019;124:1598–617.

5. Smiseth OA, Morris DA, Cardim N, et al. Multimodality imaging in patients with heart failure and preserved ejection fraction: an expert consensus document of the European Association of Cardiovascular Imaging. Eur Heart J Cardiovasc Imaging 2022;23:e34–61.

6. Yancy CW, Jessup M, Bozkurt B, et al. 2013 ACCF/AHA guideline for the management of heart failure: a report of the American College of Cardiology Foundation/American Heart Association Task Force on practice guidelines. Circulation 2013;128. e240–327.

7. Pieske B, Tschöpe C, de Boer RA, et al. How to diagnose heart failure with preserved ejection fraction: the HFA-PEFF diagnostic algorithm: a consensus recommendation from the Heart Failure Association (HFA) of the European Society of Cardiology (ESC). Eur Heart J 2019;40: 3297–317.

8. Reddy YNV, Carter RE, Obokata M, et al. A Simple, evidence-based approach to help guide diagnosis of heart failure with preserved ejection fraction. Circulation 2018;138:861–70.

9. Sepehrvand N, Alemayehu W, Dyck GJB, et al. External validation of the H(2)F-PEF model in diagnosing patients with heart failure and preserved ejection fraction. Circulation 2019;139:2377–9.

10. Lang RM, Badano LP, Mor-Avi V, et al. Recommendations for cardiac chamber quantification by echocardiography in adults: an update from the American Society of Echocardiography and the European Association of Cardiovascular Imaging. J Am Soc Echocardiogr 2015;28:1–39.e14.

11. Zile MR, Gottdiener JS, Hetzel SJ, et al. Prevalence and significance of alterations in cardiac structure and function in patients with heart failure and a preserved ejection fraction. Circulation 2011;124: 2491–501.

12. Lam CS, Roger VL, Rodeheffer RJ, et al. Cardiac structure and ventricular-vascular function in persons with heart failure and preserved ejection fraction from Olmsted County, Minnesota. Circulation 2007;115:1982–90.

13. Morris DA, Ma XX, Belyavskiy E, et al. Left ventricular longitudinal systolic function analysed by 2D speckle-tracking echocardiography in heart failure with preserved ejection fraction: a meta-analysis. Open Heart 2017;4:e000630.

14. Wang J, Khoury DS, Yue Y, et al. Preserved left ventricular twist and circumferential deformation, but depressed longitudinal and radial deformation in patients with diastolic heart failure. Eur Heart J 2008;29:1283–9.

15. Lumens J, Delhaas T, Arts T, et al. Impaired subendocardial contractile myofiber function in asymptomatic aged humans, as detected using MRI. Am J Physiol Heart Circ Physiol 2006;291: H1573–9.

16. Martinez DA, Guhl DJ, Stanley WC, et al. Extracellular matrix maturation in the left ventricle of normal and diabetic swine. Diabetes Res Clin Pract 2003; 59:1–9.

17. Nagueh SF, Smiseth OA, Appleton CP, et al. Recommendations for the evaluation of left ventricular diastolic function by echocardiography: an update from the american society of echocardiography and the european association of cardiovascular imaging. J Am Soc Echocardiogr 2016;29:277–314.

18. Hoit BD. Left atrial size and function: role in prognosis. J Am Coll Cardiol 2014;63:493–505.

19. Inoue K, Khan FH, Remme EW, et al. Determinants of left atrial reservoir and pump strain and use of atrial strain for evaluation of left ventricular filling pressure. Eur Heart J Cardiovasc Imaging 2021; 23:61–70.

20. Morris DA, Belyavskiy E, Aravind-Kumar R, et al. Potential usefulness and clinical relevance of adding left atrial strain to left atrial volume index in the detection of left ventricular diastolic dysfunction. JACC Cardiovasc Imaging 2018;11:1405–15.

21. Lam CS, Roger VL, Rodeheffer RJ, et al. Pulmonary hypertension in heart failure with preserved ejection fraction: a community-based study. J Am Coll Cardiol 2009;53:1119–26.

22. Andersen OS, Smiseth OA, Dokainish H, et al. Estimating left ventricular filling pressure by echocardiography. J Am Coll Cardiol 2017;69:1937–48.

23. Lancellotti P, Galderisi M, Edvardsen T, et al. Echo-Doppler estimation of left ventricular filling pressure: results of the multicentre EACVI Euro-Filling study. Eur Heart J Cardiovasc Imaging 2017;18:961–8.

24. Williams B, Mancia G, Spiering W, et al. 2018 ESC/ESH Guidelines for the management of arterial hypertension. Eur Heart J 2018;39:3021–104.

25. Olsen FJ, Møgelvang R, Modin D, et al. Association between isometric and allometric height-indexed left atrial size and atrial fibrillation. J Am Soc Echocardiogr 2022;35:141–50.e4.

26. Nagueh SF, Chang SM, Nabi F, et al. Cardiac imaging in patients with heart failure and preserved ejection fraction. Circ Cardiovasc Imaging 2017;10(9):e006547.

27. Obokata M, Kane GC, Reddy YN, et al. Role of diastolic stress testing in the evaluation for heart failure with preserved ejection fraction: a simultaneous invasive-echocardiographic study. Circulation 2017;135:825–38.

28. Hwang SJ, Melenovsky V, Borlaug BA. Implications of coronary artery disease in heart failure with preserved ejection fraction. J Am Coll Cardiol 2014;63:2817–27.

29. Rush CJ, Berry C, Oldroyd KG, et al. Prevalence of coronary artery disease and coronary microvascular dysfunction in patients with heart failure with preserved ejection fraction. JAMA Cardiol 2021;6:1130–43.

30. Obokata M, Reddy YNV, Melenovsky V, et al. Myocardial injury and cardiac reserve in patients with heart failure and preserved ejection fraction. J Am Coll Cardiol 2018;72:29–40.

31. Bravo PE, Di Carli MF, Dorbala S. Role of PET to evaluate coronary microvascular dysfunction in non-ischemic cardiomyopathies. Heart Fail Rev 2017;22:455–64.

32. Jaarsma C, Leiner T, Bekkers SC, et al. Diagnostic performance of noninvasive myocardial perfusion imaging using single-photon emission computed tomography, cardiac magnetic resonance, and positron emission tomography imaging for the detection of obstructive coronary artery disease: a meta-analysis. J Am Coll Cardiol 2012;59:1719–28.

33. Taqueti VR, Solomon SD, Shah AM, et al. Coronary microvascular dysfunction and future risk of heart failure with preserved ejection fraction. Eur Heart J 2018;39:840–9.

34. Chirinos JA, Segers P, Hughes T, et al. Large-artery stiffness in Health and disease: JACC state-of-the-art review. J Am Coll Cardiol 2019;74:1237–63.

35. Maron BJ, Desai MY, Nishimura RA, et al. Diagnosis and evaluation of hypertrophic cardiomyopathy: JACC state-of-the-art review. J Am Coll Cardiol 2022;79:372–89.

36. Rowin EJ, Maron BJ, Maron MS. The hypertrophic cardiomyopathy phenotype viewed through the prism of multimodality imaging: clinical and etiologic implications. JACC Cardiovasc Imaging 2020;13:2002–16.

37. Chan RH, Maron BJ, Olivotto I, et al. Prognostic value of quantitative contrast-enhanced cardiovascular magnetic resonance for the evaluation of sudden death risk in patients with hypertrophic cardiomyopathy. Circulation 2014;130:484–95.

38. Vidula MK, Bravo PE. Multimodality imaging for the diagnosis of infiltrative cardiomyopathies. Heart 2022;108:98–104.

39. Seward JB, Casaclang-Verzosa G. Infiltrative cardiovascular diseases: cardiomyopathies that look alike. J Am Coll Cardiol 2010;55:1769–79.

40. Nochioka K, Quarta CC, Claggett B, et al. Left atrial structure and function in cardiac amyloidosis. Eur Heart J Cardiovasc Imaging 2017;18:1128–37.

41. Dorbala S, Ando Y, Bokhari S, et al. ASNC/AHA/ASE/EANM/HFSA/ISA/SCMR/SNMMI expert consensus recommendations for multimodality imaging in cardiac amyloidosis: Part 1 of 2-evidence base and standardized methods of imaging. J Nucl Cardiol 2019;26:2065–123.

42. Phelan D, Collier P, Thavendiranathan P, et al. Relative apical sparing of longitudinal strain using two-dimensional speckle-tracking echocardiography is both sensitive and specific for the diagnosis of cardiac amyloidosis. Heart 2012;98:1442–8.

43. Fontana M, Chung R, Hawkins PN, et al. Cardiovascular magnetic resonance for amyloidosis. Heart Fail Rev 2015;20:133–44.

44. Baggiano A, Boldrini M, Martinez-Naharro A, et al. Noncontrast magnetic resonance for the diagnosis of cardiac amyloidosis. JACC Cardiovasc Imaging 2020;13:69–80.

45. Fontana M, Banypersad SM, Treibel TA, et al. Differential myocyte responses in patients with cardiac transthyretin amyloidosis and light-chain amyloidosis: a cardiac mr imaging study. Radiology 2015;277:388–97.

46. Kittleson MM, Maurer MS, Ambardekar AV, et al. Cardiac amyloidosis: evolving diagnosis and management: a scientific statement from the american heart association. Circulation 2020;142:e7–22.

47. Perry R, Shah R, Saiedi M, et al. The role of cardiac imaging in the diagnosis and management of anderson-fabry disease. JACC Cardiovasc Imaging 2019;12:1230–42.

48. Linhart A, Kampmann C, Zamorano JL, et al. Cardiac manifestations of Anderson-Fabry disease: results from the international Fabry outcome survey. Eur Heart J 2007;28:1228–35.

49. Kozor R, Grieve SM, Tchan MC, et al. Cardiac involvement in genotype-positive Fabry disease patients assessed by cardiovascular MR. Heart 2016;102:298–302.

50. Thompson RB, Chow K, Khan A, et al. T_1 mapping with cardiovascular MRI is highly sensitive for Fabry disease independent of hypertrophy and sex. Circ Cardiovasc Imaging 2013;6:637–45.

51. Augusto JB, Nordin S, Vijapurapu R, et al. Myocardial edema, myocyte injury, and disease severity in fabry disease. Circ Cardiovasc Imaging 2020;13: e010171.

52. Nappi C, Altiero M, Imbriaco M, et al. First experience of simultaneous PET/MRI for the early detection of cardiac involvement in patients with Anderson-Fabry disease. Eur J Nucl Med Mol Imaging 2015;42:1025–31.

53. Waldek S, Patel MR, Banikazemi M, et al. Life expectancy and cause of death in males and females with Fabry disease: findings from the Fabry Registry. Genet Med 2009;11:790–6.

54. Kubo T. Fabry disease and its cardiac involvement. J Gen Fam Med 2017;18:225–9.

55. Nakao S, Takenaka T, Maeda M, et al. An atypical variant of Fabry's disease in men with left ventricular hypertrophy. N Engl J Med 1995;333:288–93.

56. Trivieri MG, Spagnolo P, Birnie D, et al. Challenges in cardiac and pulmonary sarcoidosis: JACC state-of-the-art review. J Am Coll Cardiol 2020;76: 1878–901.

57. Slart R, Glaudemans A, Lancellotti P, et al. A joint procedural position statement on imaging in cardiac sarcoidosis: from the cardiovascular and inflammation & infection committees of the European association of nuclear medicine, the European association of cardiovascular imaging, and the American society of nuclear cardiology. J Nucl Cardiol 2018;25:298–319.

58. Anderson LJ, Holden S, Davis B, et al. Cardiovascular T2-star (T2*) magnetic resonance for the early diagnosis of myocardial iron overload. Eur Heart J 2001;22:2171–9.

59. Kirk P, Roughton M, Porter JB, et al. Cardiac T2* magnetic resonance for prediction of cardiac complications in thalassemia major. Circulation 2009; 120:1961–8.

60. Torlasco C, Cassinerio E, Roghi A, et al. Role of T1 mapping as a complementary tool to T2* for non-invasive cardiac iron overload assessment. PLoS One 2018;13:e0192890.

61. Sweeney M, Corden B, Cook SA. Targeting cardiac fibrosis in heart failure with preserved ejection fraction: mirage or miracle? EMBO Mol Med 2020;12: e10865.

62. Mascherbauer J, Marzluf BA, Tufaro C, et al. Cardiac magnetic resonance postcontrast T1 time is associated with outcome in patients with heart failure and preserved ejection fraction. Circ Cardiovasc Imaging 2013;6:1056–65.

63. Duca F, Kammerlander AA, Zotter-Tufaro C, et al. Interstitial fibrosis, functional status, and outcomes in heart failure with preserved ejection fraction: insights from a prospective cardiac magnetic resonance imaging study. Circ Cardiovasc Imaging 2016;9(12):e005277.

64. Su MY, Lin LY, Tseng YH, et al. CMR-verified diffuse myocardial fibrosis is associated with diastolic dysfunction in HFpEF. JACC Cardiovasc Imaging 2014;7:991–7.

65. Assadi H, Jones R, Swift AJ, et al. Cardiac MRI for the prognostication of heart failure with preserved ejection fraction: a systematic review and meta-analysis. Magn Reson Imaging 2021;76:116–22.

66. Nacif MS, Liu Y, Yao J, et al. 3D left ventricular extracellular volume fraction by low-radiation dose cardiac CT: assessment of interstitial myocardial fibrosis. J Cardiovasc Comput Tomogr 2013;7:51–7.

67. Hahn VS, Yanek LR, Vaishnav J, et al. Endomyocardial biopsy characterization of heart failure with preserved ejection fraction and prevalence of cardiac amyloidosis. JACC Heart Fail 2020;8:712–24.

68. Lewis GA, Dodd S, Clayton D, et al. Pirfenidone in heart failure with preserved ejection fraction: a randomized phase 2 trial. Nat Med 2021;27:1477–82.

69. Chirinos JA, Kips JG, Jacobs DR Jr, et al. Arterial wave reflections and incident cardiovascular events and heart failure: MESA (Multiethnic Study of Atherosclerosis). J Am Coll Cardiol 2012;60: 2170–7.

70. Karagodin I, Aba-Omer O, Sparapani R, et al. Aortic stiffening precedes onset of heart failure with preserved ejection fraction in patients with asymptomatic diastolic dysfunction. BMC Cardiovasc Disord 2017;17:62.

71. Chi C, Liu Y, Xu Y, et al. Association between arterial stiffness and heart failure with preserved ejection fraction. Front Cardiovasc Med 2021;8: 707162.

72. Chirinos JA, Segers P. Noninvasive evaluation of left ventricular afterload: part 1: pressure and flow measurements and basic principles of wave conduction and reflection. Hypertension 2010;56: 555–62.

73. Segers P, Rietzschel ER, Chirinos JA. How to measure arterial stiffness in humans. Arterioscler Thromb Vasc Biol 2020;40:1034–43.

74. Chirinos JA. Echocardiographic assessment of large artery stiffness. J Am Soc Echocardiogr 2016;29:1117–21.

75. Matsushita K, Ding N, Kim ED, et al. Cardio-ankle vascular index and cardiovascular disease: systematic review and meta-analysis of prospective and cross-sectional studies. J Clin Hypertens (Greenwich) 2019;21:16–24.

76. Budoff MJ, Alpert B, Chirinos JA, et al. Clinical applications measuring arterial stiffness: an expert consensus for the application of cardio-ankle vascular index (CAVI). Am J Hypertens 2022;35(5):441–53.

77. Spronck B, Obeid MJ, Paravathaneni M, et al. Predictive ability of pressure-corrected arterial stiffness indices: comparison of pulse wave velocity, cardio-ankle vascular index (CAVI), and CAVI0. Am J Hypertens 2022;35:272–80.

78. Segers P, Chirinos JA. Arterial wall stiffness: basic principles and methods of measurement in vivo. London, UK: Elsevier/Academic Press; 2022.

79. Weber T, Chirinos JA. Pulsatile arterial haemodynamics in heart failure. Eur Heart J 2018;39: 3847–54.

80. Ikonomidis I, Aboyans V, Blacher J, et al. The role of ventricular-arterial coupling in cardiac disease and heart failure: assessment, clinical implications and therapeutic interventions. A consensus document of the European Society of Cardiology Working Group on Aorta & Peripheral Vascular Diseases, European Association of Cardiovascular Imaging, and Heart Failure Association. Eur J Heart Fail 2019;21:402–24.

81. Chirinos JA, Sweitzer N. Ventricular-arterial coupling in chronic heart failure. Card Fail Rev 2017;3:12–8.

82. Chirinos JA. Ventricular-arterial coupling: invasive and non-invasive assessment. Artery Res 2013;7.

83. Segers P, Chirinos JA. Essential principles of pulsatile pressure-flow relations in the arterial tree. In: Chirinos JA, editor. Textbook of arterial stiffness and pulsatile hemodynamics in Health and disease. London, UK: Academic Press/Elsevier; 2022. p. 49–65.

84. Mitchell GF. Assessment of ventricular arterial interactions via arterial pressure-flow relations in humans. London. UK: Academic Press/Elsevier.

85. Selvaraj S, Kim J, Ansari BA, et al. Body composition, natriuretic peptides, and adverse outcomes in heart failure with preserved and reduced ejection fraction. JACC Cardiovasc Imaging 2021;14:203–15.

86. Kitzman DW, Shah SJ. The HFpEF obesity phenotype: the elephant in the room. J Am Coll Cardiol 2016;68:200–3.

87. Obokata M, Reddy YNV, Pislaru SV, et al. Evidence supporting the existence of a distinct obese phenotype of heart failure with preserved ejection fraction. Circulation 2017;136:6–19.

88. Koepp KE, Obokata M, Reddy YNV, et al. Hemodynamic and functional impact of epicardial adipose tissue in heart failure with preserved ejection fraction. JACC Heart Fail 2020;8:657–66.

89. Cruz-Jentoft AJ, Bahat G, Bauer J, et al. Sarcopenia: revised European consensus on definition and diagnosis. Age Ageing 2019;48:16–31.

90. Haykowsky MJ, Kouba EJ, Brubaker PH, et al. Skeletal muscle composition and its relation to exercise intolerance in older patients with heart failure and preserved ejection fraction. Am J Cardiol 2014;113:1211–6.

91. Kitzman DW, Nicklas B, Kraus WE, et al. Skeletal muscle abnormalities and exercise intolerance in older patients with heart failure and preserved ejection fraction. Am J Physiol Heart Circ Physiol 2014;306:H1364–70.

92. Kogan F, Hariharan H, Reddy R. Chemical exchange saturation transfer (CEST) imaging: description of technique and potential clinical applications. Curr Radiol Rep 2013;1:102–14.

93. Kumar AA, Kelly DP, Chirinos JA. Mitochondrial dysfunction in heart failure with preserved ejection fraction. Circulation 2019;139:1435–50.

94. Zamani P, Proto EA, Wilson N, et al. Multimodality assessment of heart failure with preserved ejection fraction skeletal muscle reveals differences in the machinery of energy fuel metabolism. ESC Heart Fail 2021;8:2698–712.

95. Kumar A, Ansari BA, Kim J, et al. Axial muscle size as a strong predictor of death in subjects with and without heart failure. J Am Heart Assoc 2019;8: e010554.

96. Salah HM, Pandey A, Soloveva A, et al. Relationship of nonalcoholic fatty liver disease and heart failure with preserved ejection fraction. JACC Basic Transl Sci 2021;6:918–32.

97. Lautt WW, Greenway CV. Hepatic venous compliance and role of liver as a blood reservoir. Am J Physiol 1976;231:292–5.

98. Fudim M, Sobotka PA, Dunlap ME. Extracardiac abnormalities of preload reserve: mechanisms underlying exercise limitation in heart failure with preserved ejection fraction, autonomic dysfunction, and liver disease. Circ Heart Fail 2021;14: e007308.

99. Gherlan GS. Liver ultrasound elastography: more than staging the disease. World J Hepatol 2015; 7:1595–600.

100. Barr RG, Wilson SR, Rubens D, et al. Update to the society of radiologists in ultrasound liver elastography consensus statement. Radiology 2020;296: 263–74.

101. Guglielmo FF, Venkatesh SK, Mitchell DG. Liver MR elastography technique and image interpretation: pearls and pitfalls. Radiographics 2019;39: 1983–2002.

102. van de Wouw J, Broekhuizen M, Sorop O, et al. Chronic kidney disease as a risk factor for heart failure with preserved ejection fraction: a focus on microcirculatory factors and therapeutic targets. Front Physiol 2019;10:1108.

103. Iida N, Seo Y, Sai S, et al. Clinical implications of intrarenal hemodynamic evaluation by Doppler ultrasonography in heart failure. JACC Heart Fail 2016; 4:674–82.

104. de la Espriella-Juan R, Núñez E, Miñana G, et al. Intrarenal venous flow in cardiorenal syndrome: a shining light into the darkness. ESC Heart Fail 2018;5:1173–5.

105. Puzzovivo A, Monitillo F, Guida P, et al. Renal venous pattern: a new parameter for predicting prognosis in heart failure outpatients. J Cardiovasc Dev Dis 2018;5.

106. Ennezat PV, Maréchaux S, Six-Carpentier M, et al. Renal resistance index and its prognostic significance in patients with heart failure with preserved ejection fraction. Nephrol Dial Transpl 2011;26:3908–13.

107. Wu J, Shi Z, Zhang Y, et al. Native T1 mapping in assessing kidney fibrosis for patients with chronic glomerulonephritis. Front Med (Lausanne) 2021;8: 772326.

Hemodynamic Assessment in Heart Failure with Preserved Ejection Fraction

Kazunori Omote, MD, PhD[a], Steven Hsu, MD[b], Barry A. Borlaug, MD[a],*

KEYWORDS

- Cardiac output • Echocardiography • Heart failure • HFpEF

KEY POINTS

- Heart failure (HF) with preserved ejection fraction (HFpEF) is characterized by a reduced capacity of the heart to pump blood adequately without pathologic increases in filling pressure.
- The diagnosis of HFpEF is often challenging and requires the demonstration of objective evidence of congestion or impairment in cardiac output using assessment of clinical history, physical examination, blood tests, echocardiography, or invasive exercise testing when less invasive results are equivocal.
- The pretest probability of HFpEF scoring systems based on clinical data (the H_2FPEF score and the HFA-PEFF score) are useful to help inform decision making to refer for invasive exercise testing in patients with unexplained dyspnea.
- In addition to its role as the gold standard for diagnosis, invasive cardiopulmonary exercise testing can provide valuable information to guide clinical phenotyping, particularly when paired with echocardiography and blood sampling.

INTRODUCTION

Heart failure (HF) with preserved ejection fraction (HFpEF) can be defined hemodynamically as a reduced capacity of the heart to pump blood to the body at a rate commensurate with its needs at normal diastolic filling pressures.[1–4] HFpEF manifests by elevations in left ventricular (LV) filling pressure during exercise, often associated with blunted cardiac output (CO) reserve,[5,6] impaired peripheral oxygen extraction,[7,8] and impaired pulmonary vasodilator reserve.[9] This definition requires invasive measurements, but in many patients the diagnosis can be made using noninvasive indices including natriuretic peptide testing[10] and echocardiography.[11] Many patients with HFpEF have hemodynamic abnormalities only during exercise and would be considered to be normal based on resting data alone.[12] Invasive exercise testing provides the most robust and direct method to evaluate the causes for symptoms of HF and serves as the gold standard to confirm or refute the presence of HFpEF.[2,8,11,12] This review focuses on the emerging utility and interpretation of the hemodynamic assessment for patients with HFpEF in modern clinical practice.

Diagnostic Uncertainty in Heart Failure with Preserved Ejection Fraction

In contrast to HF with reduced ejection fraction (HFrEF), the diagnosis of HFpEF is much more challenging because ejection fraction is preserved and many of the additional echo-Doppler findings overlap with findings observed in patients with noncardiac dyspnea (NCD). Clinical history, physical examination, blood tests, and imaging tools are useful to diagnose HFpEF, but in many cases, these measures are poorly sensitive,[10,13] at least in

[a] Department of Cardiovascular Medicine, Mayo Clinic and Foundation, 200 First Street Southwest, Rochester, MN 55905, USA; [b] Division of Cardiology, Department of Medicine, Johns Hopkins University, 700 Rutland Avenue, Baltimore, MD 21205, USA
* Corresponding author.
E-mail address: borlaug.barry@mayo.edu

Cardiol Clin 40 (2022) 459–472
https://doi.org/10.1016/j.ccl.2022.06.010
0733-8651/22/© 2022 Elsevier Inc. All rights reserved.

part because hemodynamics may be normal at rest. Plasma natriuretic peptide levels increase in response to elevation in cardiac wall stress, which is related to chamber dimension and distending pressure. However, compared with patients with HFrEF, patients with HFpEF have lower wall stress owing to smaller cavity size and thicker ventricular walls.[14] Moreover, many patients with HFpEF have normal distending cardiac pressures at rest and increased distending pressures only during exercise. Therefore, resting plasma natriuretic peptide levels are substantially lower in patients with HFpEF, and in fact often fall within the normal range used by clinical diagnostic laboratories.[10,15] Noninvasive tests such as echocardiography are specific when frankly abnormal (eg, clearly elevated markers of congestion) but have low sensitivity to identify elevated filling pressures.[11,16]

Given the challenges of diagnosing patients with HFpEF in the resting state, more sensitive diagnostic approaches have been developed. Stressing the patient with occult HFpEF uncovers abnormalities with exertion that may be unapparent at rest. Even the patient with HFpEF with clinical euvolemia, normal natriuretic peptide levels, normal echocardiography, and normal resting filling pressures at rest will display greater hemodynamic abnormalities during exercise when compared with those with NCD (**Fig. 1**). Given its definitive and comprehensive nature, invasive exercise test has emerged as the gold-standard method to evaluate patients with unexplained dyspnea and preserved ejection fraction.[3,11,12]

A Bayesian Approach to Invasive Exercise Testing

In the patient with unexplained dyspnea, assessment of the pretest probability of HFpEF is first performed by noninvasive tests (clinical, echocardiography, and natriuretic peptides). Recently, 2 novel scoring systems (the H_2FPEF score[13] and the HFA-PEFF score[3]) have been developed as approaches for the diagnostic workup of HFpEF. With either system, patients deemed at high and low probability are generally diagnosed as having or not having HFpEF, respectively, without further testing. In patients with intermediate pretest likelihood for HFpEF based on these scoring tools, current guidelines recommend exercise stress testing,[3] which can be performed using cardiac catheterization or stress echocardiography. If exercise echocardiography is of inadequate diagnostic quality or is equivocal, invasive exercise testing is required.[11] Given the uncertainties with echocardiography, many clinicians proceed directly to invasive cardiopulmonary exercise testing (CPET) as the first step, but this practice may vary depending on local availability. A current and evidence-based diagnostic approach to HFpEF is shown in **Fig. 2**.[2,17]

Role of Noninvasive Cardiopulmonary Exercise Testing

Peak oxygen consumption (Vo_2) as measured by noninvasive CPET is the gold-standard assessment for aerobic capacity.[18–20] Reduced peak

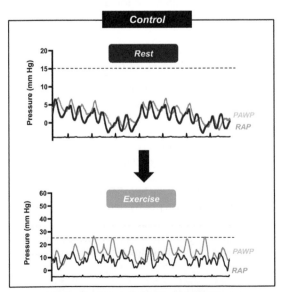
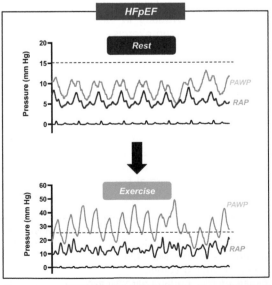

Fig. 1. Representative waveforms of pulmonary artery wedge pressure (PAWP) and right atrial pressure (RAP) in a control patient and a patient with HFpEF at rest and with exercise.

Patient with unexplained dyspnea

1. Assess non invasively: clinical, echo, natriuretic peptides

2. Determine pre test probability of HFpEF:

H₂FPEF Score			
Label	**Variable**	**Characteristics**	**Points**
H₂	Heavy	BMI >30 kg/m²	2
	Hypertension	≥2 BP meds	1
F	Atrial Fib	Persistent or Paroxysmal	3
P	Pulmonary Hypertension	RVSP >35 mm Hg on Echo	1
E	Old Age	Age >60 y	1
F	Filling Pressure	E/e' ratio >9 on Echo	1

HFA-PEFF Score				
	Functional	**Morphological**	**Biomarker (if in Sinus)**	**Biomarker (if in A. Fib)**
MAJOR (2 points each)	Septal e'<7 cm/s Lateral e'<10 cm/s or E/e' ≥15 or TRV >2.8 m/s (RVSP >35)	LAVI >34 ml/m² or LVMI ≥149/122 g/m² (M/W) and RWT >0.42	NT-proBNP > 220 pg/ml or BNP >80 pg/ml	NT-proBNP > 660 pg/ml or BNP >240 pg/ml
MINOR (1 point each)	E/e' 9-14 or GLS <16%	LAVI 29-34 ml/m² or LVMI >115/95 g/m2 (M/W) or RWT >0.42 or LV wall ≥12 mm	NT-proBNP > 125-220 pg/ml or BNP 35-80 pg/ml	NT-proBNP > 365-660 pg/ml or BNP 105-240 pg/ml

Probability of HFpEF		
Low	**Intermediate**	**High**
0-1	2-5	6-9

Probability of HFpEF (2 points per major criterion, 1 point per minor)		
Low	**Intermediate**	**High**
0-1	2-4	5-6

3. For intermediate cases, or when confirmation needed, consider:

- **Diastolic stress echocardiography**, or
- **Invasive Hemodynamic Testing**:

  Resting Conditions: PAWP ≥15 mm Hg or >18 mm Hg with saline or passive leg raise

  Exercise Conditions: PAWP ≥ 25 mm Hg (**Gold Standard**)

Fig. 2. The current Bayesian approach to the diagnosis of HFpEF. BMI, body mass index; BNP, brain natriuretic peptide; BP, blood pressure; GLS, global longitudinal strain; LAVI, left atrial volume index, LVMI, left ventricular mass index; PAWP, pulmonary artery wedge pressure; RVSP, right ventricular systolic pressure; RWT, relative wall thickness; TRV, tricuspid regurgitation velocity.

Vo_2 is commonly used as an end point for many clinical trials in HFpEF[21,22] and is known to be an important prognostic factor.[23,24] According to the Fick principle, Vo_2 is equal to the product of CO and arterial-venous O_2 content difference (AVO_2diff). Peak Vo_2 in patients with HFpEF and HFrEF may be limited by either or both components.[5,25,26] Earlier studies in HFrEF showed that low peak Vo_2 in HFrEF was related to reduced leg blood flow from poor CO,[27] but reduced peak Vo_2 cannot be assumed to reflect CO limitation because some patients display greater peripheral deficits.[7,25,26] Noninvasive CPET does not allow for measurement of CO or AVO_2diff, so the mechanism for impaired aerobic capacity cannot be ascertained. Another limitation of using CPET in isolation is that not all patients stop exercising due to limitations in convective O_2 delivery (CO) or peripheral O_2 uptake (AVO_2diff). For example, some patients may reach volitional fatigue earlier owing to elevation in pulmonary vascular pressures that leads them to cease exercise.

Despite these limitations, noninvasive CPET can play a role in the evaluation of HFpEF. Noninvasive CPET can be helpful to identify pulmonary disease. In addition to Vo_2, conventional CPET provides measures of Carbon dioxide production (Vco_2), tidal volume (V_T), minute ventilation (V_E), respiratory rate, and minute ventilation (V_E = $V_T \times$ respiratory rate) at rest and throughout the exercise. Objective effort is estimated by the respiratory exchange ratio (Vco_2/Vo_2), which ideally should exceed 1.10 at true peak exercise, but should nominally exceed 1.0. Ventilatory efficiency is assessed by the slope of expired volume per unit time ($\dot{V}_E$) to $\dot{V}CO_2$, which can be calculated from the slope of increase in $\dot{V}_E$ to $\dot{V}CO_2$ during exercise.[28] Pulmonary dead space (volume of dead space [V_D]) is the volume that does not participate in gas exchange, and the sum of anatomic dead space (conduit airways such as the mouth and trachea) and alveolar dead space. The degree of ventilation perfusion ratio $(\dot{V}/\dot{Q})$ mismatch can be estimated from the ratio of dead space ventilation to tidal volume (V_{DS}/V_T) determined from the modified alveolar gas equation (higher values indicate greater dead space ventilation and higher $\dot{V}/\dot{Q}$ mismatch).[29,30] Patients with lung disease may display arterial hypoxemia during exercise, as well as limitations in breathing reserve, which is defined by the ratio of peak exercise V_E to maximal voluntary ventilation (usually estimated as 35*FEV$_1$ [forced expiratory volume in the first second of expiration]). Patients with breathing reserve less than 20% likely display a ventilatory limitation to exercise indicating lung disease, whereas patients with HFpEF should display a preserved breathing reserve. Increases in V_E/V_{CO_2} slope as well as V_{DS}/V_T are commonly observed in both lung disease and HF and so are less useful to distinguish these two.[18,30] For example, elevation in left heart filling pressure with exercise in patients with HFpEF is correlated with greater ventilatory drive, more tachypneic breathing, impaired ventilation, and worse exercise capacity in HFpEF, leading to increases in V_{DS}/V_T.[30] Spirometry and sometimes lung diffusion can also be performed with modern CPET systems. Reduction in FEV$_1$/FVC (forced vital capacity) ratio should alert to the presence of obstructive lung disease. Balanced reductions in FEV$_1$ and FVC, with reduction in diffusing capacity of lung for carbon monoxide (D$_{LCO}$) can be seen with interstitial lung disease, but it is important to remember that modest restrictive deficits and impairments in lung gas diffusion are also commonly observed in patients with HF.[31]

In addition to distinguishing HF from lung disease, it is also necessary to discriminate HFpEF from NCD causes such as deconditioning. Here noninvasive CPET is somewhat helpful, but really only helpful at the extremes. Reddy and colleagues demonstrated that very low peak V_{O_2} (<14 mL/kg/min) by noninvasive CPET can discriminate HFpEF from NCD with excellent specificity (91%), whereas preserved peak V_{O_2} (>20 mL/kg/min) can exclude HFpEF with high sensitivity (90%) among patients with unexplained dyspnea and preserved EF. However, in the intermediate range (14<peak V_{O_2} < 20 mL/kg/min), which is where most evaluated patients fell, there was substantial and unacceptably high overlap between HFpEF and NCD.[32] For patients with this intermediate impairment in peak V_{O_2}, additional evaluation such as invasive hemodynamic exercise testing is needed, ideally paired with simultaneous CPET to provide maximal diagnostic insight.

PERFORMING AN INVASIVE EXERCISE HEMODYNAMICS
Protocol for Invasive Exercise Testing

Access is obtained most commonly in the internal jugular vein followed by placement of a 9F sheath, and in the radial artery using a 4F to 6F sheath under the supine position (depending on the requirement for coronary angiography or left heart catheterization during the same examination).[33] Solid-state pressure transducers are leveled at midaxillary in advance. Central venous pressure is transduced throughout the case through the sidearm of the 9F sheath. A 7F balloon-tipped catheter is advanced to the right atrium (RA) to demonstrate equalization with sidearm pressure. A 2F micromanometer is advanced to the tip of the balloon-tipped catheter and balanced to the mean fluid-filled catheter pressure. A micromanometer is preferred for high-fidelity exercise evaluations when possible given the poor frequency response of the fluid-filled catheter, which becomes limiting during exercise.

Right atrial pressure (RAP), pulmonary artery (PA) pressure (PAP), and pulmonary artery wedge pressure (PAWP) are measured at end expiration and also taking an average of at least 3 respiratory cycles, with both values included in the final report. PAWP position is confirmed via appearance on fluoroscopy, characteristic waveforms, and saturation at wedge position greater than or equal to 94%. Where possible, CO is optimally determined using the direct Fick method, which requires directly measured oxygen consumption (V_{O_2}) together with blood sampling to measure O_2 contents (=saturation $\times$ hemoglobin $\times$ 1.34) and P_{O_2} obtained from the radial artery and PA to calculate arterial venous O_2 difference (AVO$_2$-diff). If direct measures of V_{O_2} cannot be performed, CO is best determined using the thermodilution catheter, given the error in using assumed estimates of V_{O_2}.

After baseline data are acquired, the legs are placed in the binders of a supine cycle at a 90° angle, and the pressures are recorded with passive leg raise (PLR). Next, hemodynamic assessment and expired gas analysis are performed during exercise, starting at 20 W workload for 5 minutes (to allow imaging during submaximal exercise), and increasing by 20-W increments in 3-minute stages to volitional exhaustion. Symptoms of dyspnea and fatigue during exercise are rated by patients during each stage according to the Borg perceived dyspnea and fatigue scales. Simultaneous transthoracic echocardiography may be used with catheterization to evaluate for ventricular and atrial function, ventricular interdependence, valve disease, and lung congestion.[11,28,34,35] The protocol for the procedure is summarized in **Fig. 3**.

End Expiration Versus Respiratory Averaged Pressures

End expiration is closest to the true transmural vascular distending pressure because this is the point in the respiratory cycle when intrapleural pressure is closest to zero, lungs are at functional reserve capacity, and there is minimal airflow impacting intracardiac pressures. During exercise, some have advocated for use of pressures averaged over the entire respiratory cycle rather than end expiration. This approach may be advantageous in patients with obstructive airway disease in whom intrinsic positive end-expiratory pressure (auto-PEEP) develops. For such patients, in whom changes in intrathoracic pressure are dramatic and may contribute to elevated intravascular pressures, pressures averaged over the respiratory cycle may better account for the effect of intrathoracic pressure and auto-PEEP compared with end-expiratory pressure. However, for the vast majority of patients without these conditions, end-expiratory values can be readily obtained and would more accurately reflect the transmural hydrostatic pressure in the pulmonary veins and capillaries. In this majority of patients, using pressure averaged throughout the respiratory cycle underestimates transmural pressure due to the effect of inspiration falsely lowering measured pressures. Indeed, end expiration PAWP shows a stronger relationship with the development of exercise-induced lung congestion when compared with averaged PAWP over the respiratory cycle.[28]

Given differences in practice across laboratories, one reasonable solution is to report both sets of values, providing the referring physician with all data necessary for data interpretation.

Supine Versus Upright Exercise

Exercise right heart catheterization can be performed in either the supine or upright positions. In the authors' catheterization laboratories, supine exercise is preferred because venous return is maximized, increasing the sensitivity to detect diastolic reserve impairments. Normal ranges are also more familiar and well codified in the supine position. Although pressures are lower upright, prior studies have shown that the changes with exercise are similar in both positions, as are changes in the relationships between PAP and PAWP.[36,37] Pulmonary vascular resistance (PVR) decreases more with upright exercise owing to greater vascular recruitment, again due to changes associated with gravity. With upright exercise there may be greater ringing artifact and catheter whip, as well as greater variability in PAWP when measured in different West zones,[38] which is less relevant to supine exercise.[39]

NORMAL HEMODYNAMIC RANGES AT REST AND WITH EXERCISE

Normal ranges of resting and exercise hemodynamics are shown in **Table 1**. To interpret the data from an invasive hemodynamics, it is important to recognize the normal response to activity. PLR results in an acute increase in venous return to the heart as blood from the lower extremities is returned to the central circulation,[12] and therefore an increase in the PAWP with a PLR has

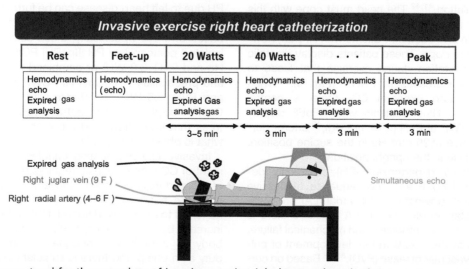

Fig. 3. The protocol for the procedure of invasive exercise right heart catheterization.

Table 1
Normal range of resting and exercise values

	Resting Values	Exercise Values	Comments
RAP (mm Hg)	0–6	<15 (supine)	Normal range with exercise not well defined
Pulmonary hypertension	Mean PAP≤20 (mm Hg)	Mean PAP<30 (mm Hg) with TPR<3 (WU)	N/A
Mean PAP/CO slope (mm Hg/L/min)	-	<3 (upright)	Less established for supine exercise
PAWP (mm Hg)	<15 (supine) <19 (with leg rise supine)	<25 (supine) <20 (upright)	Some references indicate normal resting values of <12 >20 during supine exercise may be abnormal in patients aged <50 y
PAWP/CO slope (mm Hg/L/min)	-	<2 (upright)	Less established for supine exercise
PVR (WU)	<2–3	<1.8	Exercise PVR increases with normal aging, similar to exercise PAWP
Forward flow	CI: 2.2–4.0 (L/min*m^2)	$\Delta CO>4.8 *\Delta V_{O_2}$ (L/min)	Expected increase in CO is 6 mL/min for each 1-mL/min increase in V_{O_2}
AVO$_2$diff (mL/dL)	-	>0.8 ×hemoglobin	Abnormalities may be seen in patients with and without HFpEF

CO is the cardiac output, TPR is total pulmonary resistance, defined by mean PAP divided by CO.
Abbreviations: CI, cardiac index; TPR, total pulmonary resistance.

been shown to provide good discrimination of HFpEF from NCD.[12,40] With the onset of exercise, there is further increase in venous return to the heart mediated by the combined actions of the skeletal muscle and respiratory pumps, together with sympathetic-mediated venoconstriction that shifts blood from the capacitance veins to the central circulation.[41,42] The heart must cope with this increase in venous return by enhancing diastolic relaxation and suction. Patients with HFpEF, however, fail to cope. These patients display diastolic reserve limitation during exercise that leads to excessive increases in PAWP (**Fig. 4**).[8] When venous return exceeds CO, there is central congestion. Thus, patients with HFpEF display higher PAWP at PLR (≥19 mm Hg),[40] and/or during exercise (≥25 mm Hg in the supine position, ≥20 mm Hg in the upright position).[11,12]

Pulmonary hypertension (PH) commonly develops in HFpEF as a consequence of passive elevation in downstream left atrial (LA) pressure. With sustained elevation in LA pressure there is progressive LA remodeling and mechanical failure, which is associated with the development of pulmonary vascular disease (PVD).[35,43] Based on current guidelines, PH is defined as mean PAP at rest (>20 mm Hg), with a PVR of 3 WU or more if the PH is precapillary. Definitions for exercise PH are less clear. Some have advocated for mean PAP during exercise (>30 mm Hg) provided that total pulmonary resistance (TPR) exceeds 3 WU.[44] Others consider exercise PH based on the increase in PA pressure relative to CO (see later discussion). PH due to left heart disease can be further categorized as those without or with concomitant PVD based on PVR. Specifically, these categories are isolated postcapillary PH ([IpcPH] PCWP≥15 mm Hg and PVR<3.0 WU) or combined postcapillary and precapillary PH ([CpcPH] PCWP≥15 mm Hg and PVR≥3.0 WU).[44] Patients with HFpEF with CpcPH display specific pathophysiological features that differ from and are more severe than what is observed in IpcPH.[9]

Invasive exercise testing enables the assessment of CO reserve, which requires measurement of CO and V_{O_2} in tandem. Convective O_2 delivery from the heart to the body (ie, CO) is closely matched to metabolic demand; that is, CO should increase by 6 mL for every 1-mL increase in whole-body V_{O_2} if the heart is adequately performing its duty as a pump and there is sufficient venous return (preload). For example, if V_{O_2} increases from

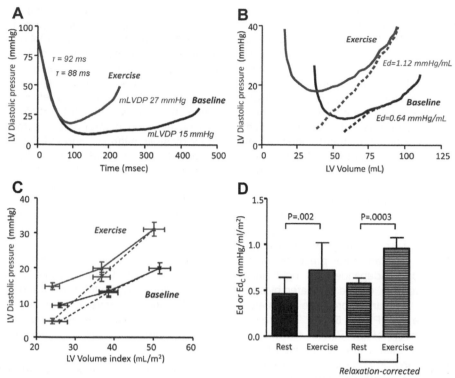

Fig. 4. Diastolic reserve limitations during exercise in patients with heart failure with preserved ejection fraction (HFpEF). (*A*) In a typical patient with HFpEF, there is dramatic elevation in mean left ventricular diastolic pressure (mLVDP) during exercise associated with limited hastening of isovolumic relaxation (reduction in the time constant of relaxation, τ). Inadequate relaxation reserve during exercise is coupled with an acute shift upward and to the left in the diastolic pressure-volume relationship, with an increase in operant diastolic elastance (Ed) as shown in an example patient (*B*) and in group data (*C, D*). The solid lines/bar graphs show raw unadjusted pressure-volume data and the dashed lines/hashed bar graphs show elastance data corrected for the effects of incomplete relaxation. (*From* Borlaug BA. Mechanisms of exercise intolerance in heart failure with preserved ejection fraction. Circ J. 2014;78(1):20-32.)

250 mL/min at rest to 1250 mL/min at peak exercise (1 L/min), a 6-L/min increase in CO is expected. By convention, peak CO values less than 80% of this level are considered to indicate impaired CO reserve, which is frequently observed in both HFrEF and HFpEF.[5,6,26,45] This concept can help pinpoint cardiac-specific exercise limitations in HFpEF. Although resting stroke volume (SV) and CO are generally normal in HFpEF, the ability to enhance those with exercise relative to metabolic needs is frequently (although not invariably) impaired. Subtle abnormalities in resting contractility in patients with HFpEF become more dramatic during stress because of the inability to enhance systolic function, which attenuates the increase in SV during exercise. This, in addition to limitations in chronotropic reserve, conspires to limit CO reserve in HFpEF.

Recent studies have shown added value for scaling pulmonary vascular pressures to increases in CO with exercise. Lewis and colleagues have shown that higher values of mean PAP/CO slope

(>3 mm Hg/l/min)[46] and PAWP/CO slope (>2 mm Hg/l/min)[47] during upright exercise were both associated with increased risk of adverse events, and the latter has also been proposed as an alternative diagnostic criterion for HFpEF (in addition to peak exercise PAWP≥25 mm Hg in the supine position). However, the upper limits of normal for these flow-normalized pressure changes with exercise have not been well established for patients in the supine position.

INTERPRETATION OF SPECIFIC HEMODYNAMIC SIGNATURES
Left-Sided Filling Pressures

Determination of left-sided filling pressures is crucially important because it allows estimation of pulmonary capillary pressure as it relates to dyspnea and PH, and also used clinically as an estimate of LV preload. Preload can be defined by the magnitude of distention or stretching of ventricular myocytes before the onset of contraction, which dictates the extent of myofiber shortening in the subsequent contraction according to Frank-Starling principle.[8] The PAWP or LV end-diastolic pressure (LVEDP) is a useful surrogate for preload and correlates with the LV end-diastolic volume (LVEDV), which determines end-diastolic myofiber stretch. Filling pressures for any preload (LVEDV) in the fully relaxed state are determined by both the compliance properties of the myocardium and extrinsic pericardial restraint mediated by the right heart and pericardium. PAWP reflects the LVEDV reasonably well at lower filling pressures. As PAWP increases, however, there is a weaker correlation between PAWP and preload, due to the impact of pericardial restraint increasing the PAWP through an external compressive contract force without contributing to end-diastolic myocyte stretch. LV transmural pressure, which reflects LV preload independent of right heart and pericardial restraint, can be estimated by subtracting extrinsic pericardial pressure (estimated by RAP) from the PAWP (**Fig. 5**).[11,48–51] Determination of how much of the PAWP elevation is due to pericardial interaction as opposed to LV filling is particularly important during exercise where pericardial interaction may play an increasingly important role due to the acute right heart dilation as venous return overwhelms the right ventricle, shifting the LV diastolic pressure volume relationship (**Fig. 6**).[51] Conversely, patients with isolated increases in PAWP with normal RAP have a more focal impairment in the left heart.

Right Atrial Pressure

Alternatively, when RAP and PAWP become elevated in tandem and equalize, this suggests that the heart has filled to the point at which the pericardium restrains further filling, and there is enhanced diastolic ventricular interaction (DVI) with the right heart and pericardium driving the PAWP elevation.[51] This is a distinct hemodynamic signature in patients with HF and a key reason for measuring RAP continuously throughout exercise testing. Patients with HFpEF and elevated RAP are more likely to develop lung congestion during exercise, due to the combined effects of increased fluid filtration caused by high PAWP and reduced pulmonary lymphatic drainage due to central venous hypertension.[28] Elevated RAP is associated with an increased risk of events and greater abnormalities in right ventricular-pulmonary arterial coupling.[52] The elastic pericardium exerts a compressive contact force on the surface of the myocardium that becomes more substantial when heart volume increases, as can occur in many forms of HF.[51]

Pericardial restraint plays an important role in determining hemodynamics, LV preload, and ventricular function. For example, total heart enlargement and cardiomegaly in HFpEF (in particular with right heart enlargement) creates the substrate for increased pericardial restraint and DVI, where the right heart influences the left in parallel.[44,53] When DVI is enhanced, left heart filling pressures can be elevated disproportionate to the degree of LV diastolic stiffness, and LVEDV is lower than expected (ie, LVEDP and LVEDV become uncoupled), resulting in failure to augment CO through failure of Frank-Starling reserve (see **Fig. 6**).[9,51] This phenomenon is commonly observed in patients with HF with acute on chronic volume overload severe tricuspid regurgitation, persistent atrial fibrillation, CpcPH, or obesity[9,34,35,48,53]—all situations in which exertional right heart filling pressure elevation may mediate decreases in left heart filling during exercise despite increases in left-sided filling pressures.[48] These instances are important examples where LV pressure does not equal volume.

Pulmonary and Systemic Vascular Loading Abnormalities

PH commonly develops in HFpEF as a consequence of passive elevation in downstream LA pressure,[35,54] but with sustained elevation in LA pressure there is progressive LA remodeling and mechanical failure, which is associated with the development of PVD. This more severe form of left heart disease PH, evidenced by an increase in PVR, is also termed *combined postcapillary and precapillary PH*.[35,43,55,56] These patients are more prone to developing severe impairments in pulmonary vascular-right heart coupling, greater ventricular interdependence, and more severe pulmonary limitations.[9,57–60] Despite the presence of an elevated PVR, these patients display greater lung congestion during exertion, which is coupled with increased dead space ventilation, lower alveolar ventilation, reduced lung diffusing capacity, abnormal ventilatory efficiency, and $\dot{V}/\dot{Q}$ mismatching leading to hypoxemia, which further limits O_2 delivery during stress.[53]

Systemic vascular resistance (SVR) is determined by dividing the mean arterial pressure minus central venous pressure by CO, converted to standard units. Pulsatile arterial load is assessed in a general way by the central aortic pulse pressure (PP = systolic blood pressure − diastolic blood pressure), effective arterial elastance (Ea), and total arterial compliance (TAC). Ea is a lumped measure of the total stiffness of the arterial system, which is assessed by end-

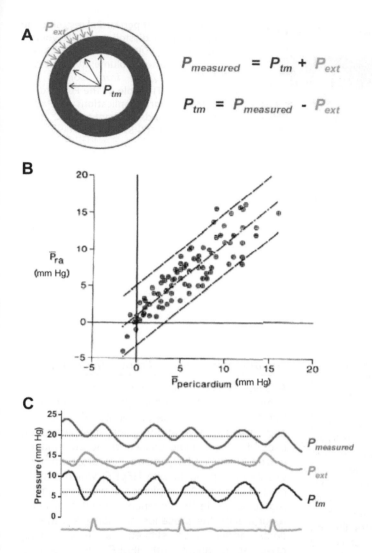

A

$$P_{measured} = P_{tm} + P_{ext}$$

$$P_{tm} = P_{measured} - P_{ext}$$

Fig. 5. Measured intracavitary and transmural pressures. (*A*) Pressure (P) measured is related as equal to the sum of the P_{tm} and the external pressure P_{ext} applied outside. (*B*) Pericardial pressure, a measure of P_{ext}, varies directly with $\bar{P}_{ra}$. (*C*) Example shows an estimation of LV P_{tm} as the difference between the measured pulmonary capillary wedge pressure (*red*) and the pericardial Pext, estimated by right atrial pressure (*green*). P_{ext} = external pressure; $\bar{P}_{ra}$ = right atrial pressure; P_{tm} = transmural pressure. (*From* Borlaug BA, Reddy YNV. The Role of the Pericardium in Heart Failure: Implications for Pathophysiology and Treatment. JACC Heart Fail. 2019 Jul;7(7):574-585.)

systolic central blood pressure/SV.[61] Ea is most strongly related to SVR and is also influenced by the heart rate. TAC approximates the linear portion of the pressure-volume relationship for the lumped arterial system. Although multiple methods exist to assess TAC, it is usually estimated as SV index/central PP in the catheterization laboratory.[62]

Ventricular and vascular stiffening increase with aging and comorbidity and are abnormally elevated in many patients with HFpEF. Acute afterload elevation in the setting of ventricular-arterial stiffening causes greater increase in blood pressure, which may then feedback to further impair diastolic relaxation, leading to dramatic increases in filling pressures during exercise.[63] Many patients with HFpEF manifest arterial reserve limitations only during exercise. Reddy and colleagues[64] compared indices of arterial stiffness and pulsatile hemodynamics at rest and during exercise in subjects with HFpEF and hypertensive control subjects to examine their relationships to cardiac hemodynamics. This study found that arterial load in HFpEF was similar to those in control subjects at rest, but during submaximal exercise, subjects with HFpEF displayed higher Ea index and reduced TAC index and at peak exercise there was greater reflected wave burden compared with control subjects. Importantly, these pulsatile arterial loads were directly correlated with higher LV filling pressures and depressed CO reserve.[64,65]

OTHER ASSESSMENTS
Peripheral Oxygen Utilization

According to the Fick principle, V_{O_2} is equal to the product of CO and AVO_2diff, and limitations in peak V_{O_2} may be explained by either component

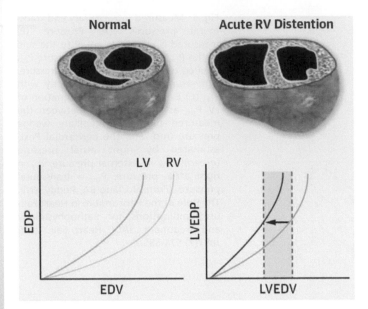

Fig. 6. Effects of pericardial restraint and unloading on diastolic pressure-volume relationships. EDP, end-diastolic pressure; EDV, end-diastolic volume; RV, right ventricular. (*Adapted from* Borlaug BA, Reddy YNV. The Role of the Pericardium in Heart Failure: Implications for Pathophysiology and Treatment. JACC Heart Fail. 2019 Jul;7(7):574-585.)

or both in tandem.[25,66] Acute enhancement in peripheral O_2 distribution, utilization, and extraction (ie, AVO_2diff reserve) during exercise plays a critical role because CO reserve is maximized during exercise. Although the heart increases its output during exercise, this enhanced flow needs to be distributed to tissues where perfusion is most needed, which is achieved by regional vasodilation in skeletal muscle and vasoconstriction in non-exercising regions such as the skin, splanchnic beds, and kidneys.[8] In many patients with HFpEF, there are substantial peripheral factors limiting aerobic capacity, manifest by an inability to augment AVO_2diff.[7,25] Other patients may display these peripheral impairments in the absence of HFpEF, and this peripheral reserve limitation is identified when the ratio of peak exercise AVO_2diff to hemoglobin is less than 0.8.[67] Distinguishing patients with predominant central limitations (due to blunted CO) from those with predominant peripheral limitations (due to AVO_2diff) may be important for clinical phenotyping. It must also be remembered that many patients with HF will stop exercising before the onset of lactic acidosis due to discomfort related to elevated PAWP, which may also be associated with a lower AVO_2diff in the absence of a true peripheral deficit. In other words, there may be an unwillingness to increase AVO_2diff rather than an inability to augment AVO_2diff. Scaling the latter to Vo_2 may better enable distinction of these 2 possibilities, akin to the $\Delta CO/\Delta Vo_2$ slope, but further study is required to establish normal ranges with supine and upright exercise.

Simultaneous Exercise Echocardiography

Addition of exercise echocardiography to invasive hemodynamic stress testing provides valuable information, including assessments of ventricular and valve structure and function. It is particularly useful to discriminate causes of the prominent V waves in the PAWP tracing that are commonly observed in patients with HFpEF, which may be related to poor LA compliance or worsening mitral regurgitation. In the absence of significant mitral regurgitation the presence of a large V wave reflects increased LA stiffness, as is commonly observed in patients with HFpEF.[68] Echocardiography with short axis imaging also allows determination of the degree of pericardial restraint with LV underfilling, which can be estimated from the degree of LV collapse and eccentricity index resulting in a more D-shaped LV and septum, yet another clinically relevant hemodynamic phenotype.[34,53,69] A higher eccentricity index and more collapsed LV for a given PAWP elevation reflects a greater degree of pericardial restraint. Another advantage of adding echocardiography is the ability to perform simultaneous lung ultrasonography, which enables evaluation of pulmonary congestion during exercise.[28,53]

Invasive Hemodynamic Phenotyping and Trial Eligibility

It is now widely accepted that HFpEF is a heterogeneous syndrome, and invasive hemodynamics provides robust data that can be used to subcategorize patients with HFpEF into specific pathophysiologic phenotypes.[70] As noted earlier, there may be important pathophysiologic and treatment differences between these patient phenogroups, including those with or without PVD, LA myopathy/stiffening, resting versus exercise-induced PAWP elevation, central versus peripheral limitations, and others, and this characterization may prove crucial to optimally individualize treatments targeting specific pathophysiologies. One example is the REDUCE LAP-HF II trial, which tested the safety and efficacy of an implantable device designed to lower PAWP by creating a therapeutic LA to RA shunt.[71] Overall, the trial was neutral, but in prespecified and posthoc analyses, it was found that patients with more severe PVD during exercise (defined by higher exercise PVR) had differential response to treatment, with evidence for harm in those with PVD and signal for benefit in patients without this form of latent exercise-induced PVD.[72] Invasive hemodynamics may also be helpful to ensure that true HFpEF is present. Plasma natriuretic peptide levels are most commonly used for this purpose in pharmaceutical trials, but it is notable that HF event rates in the REDCUE LAP-HF II trial greatly exceed those observed in pharmaceutical trials, despite the requirement for a much lower natriuretic peptide level for eligibility; this may be explained by the fact that patients were required to display hemodynamic proof of HFpEF to be eligible, based on resting and exercise PAWP.

Evaluation for Other Causes of Exertional Dyspnea

Several other causes of exertional dyspnea may be noted during invasive CPET in the patient under evaluation for suspected HFpEF. Some patients may display isolated peripheral limitations to exercise in the absence of HF, marked by AVO_2diff/hemoglobin ratio less than 0.8, with normal PAWP and PAP. One subgroup within this cohort includes patients with mitochondrial myopathies, who characteristically display higher-than-expected mixed venous O_2 saturation and thus low AVO_2diff, with an elevated $\Delta CO/\Delta Vo_2$ slope (often >1.2) but with marked increases in arterial lactate indicating anaerobic metabolism. Other patients may display blunted increases in CO ($\Delta CO/\Delta Vo_2 < 0.8$), but with no evidence of congestion (normal or low PAWP and RAP) and normal/hyperdynamic cardiac function, indicating isolated preload failure, or inability to augment venous return to the heart. Some patients may be identified to display resting or exercise-induced precapillary PH with elevated PAP but normal PAWP at rest and during exercise.

SUMMARY

Invasive CPET enables direct assessment of the hemodynamic abnormalities underlying HF and has now emerged as the gold-standard method to evaluate for the cause of unexplained dyspnea among patients with normal EF. In addition to its role for diagnosis of HFpEF, invasive exercise testing is useful to identify alternative causes of dyspnea due and may be useful to enhance patient phenotyping and to guide individualization of therapy and establish trial eligibility. With increasingly widespread use, the number of patients suffering from unexplained dyspnea has and will continue to contract, and accurate diagnosis of HFpEF will become more widespread, which is more important now than ever before given the emergence of highly effective therapies for patients with this form of HF.

CLINICS CARE POINTS

- HFpEF accounts for over one-half of all heart failure cases, and the incidence and prevalence are growing as the population ages and with an increasing prevalence of metabolic disorders including hypertension, diabetes and obesity. In contrast to HFrEF, few effective treatments for HFpEF have been identified, likely in large part because of marked heterogeneity in the phenotypes of HFpEF.

- HFpEF accounts for over one-half of all heart failure cases, and the incidence and prevalence are growing as the population ages and with an increasing prevalence of metabolic disorders including hypertension, diabetes and obesity. In contrast to HFrEF, few effective treatments for HFpEF have been identified, likely in large part because of marked heterogeneity in the phenotypes of HFpEF.

- The diagnosis of HFpEF is challenging because EF is preserved, echocardiography have low sensitivity to identify elevated filling pressure, and some patients with HFpEF display lower resting natriuretic peptide levels that often fall within the normal range.

- It is important to determine pre-test probability of HFpEF used by HFpEF scoring system (e.g. H_2FPEF Score or HFA-PEFF Score) for decision making to refer for invasive CPET in patients with unexplained dyspnea.

- Invasive CPET with echocardiography and blood gas sampling has emerged as the gold-standard method to evaluate for cause of dyspnea in patients with unexplained dyspnea and this method is useful for phenotyping patients into more mechanistically homogeneous groups that may enable more individualized treatment.

SOURCES OF FUNDING

B.A. Borlaug is supported by R01 HL128526 and U01 HL160226. S. Hsu is supported by K23 HL146889 and R01 HL114910. K. Omote is supported by Japan Heart Foundation/Bayer Yakuhin Research Grant Abroad, Japan and the JSPS Overseas Research Fellowships from the Japan Society for the Promotion of Science, Japan.

DISCLOSURES

None.

REFERENCES

1. Pfeffer MA, Shah AM, Borlaug BA. Heart failure with preserved ejection fraction in Perspective. Circ Res 2019;124:1598–617.

2.. Borlaug BA. Evaluation and management of heart failure with preserved ejection fraction. Nat Rev Cardiol 2020;17(9):559–73. https://doi.org/10.1038/s41569-020-0363-2.

3. Pieske B, Tschöpe C, de Boer RA, et al. How to diagnose heart failure with preserved ejection fraction: the HFA-PEFF diagnostic algorithm: a consensus recommendation from the Heart Failure Association (HFA) of the European Society of Cardiology (ESC). Eur Heart J 2019;40:3297–317.

4. Omote K, Verbrugge FH, Borlaug BA. Heart failure with preserved ejection fraction: Mechanisms and treatment Strategies. Annu Rev Med 2022;73: 321–37.

5. Abudiab MM, Redfield MM, Melenovsky V, et al. Cardiac output response to exercise in relation to metabolic demand in heart failure with preserved ejection fraction. Eur J Heart Fail 2013;15:776–85.

6. Borlaug BA, Kane GC, Melenovsky V, et al. Abnormal right ventricular-pulmonary artery coupling with exercise in heart failure with preserved ejection fraction. Eur Heart J 2016;37:3293–302.

7. Dhakal BP, Malhotra R, Murphy RM, et al. Mechanisms of exercise intolerance in heart failure with preserved ejection fraction: the role of abnormal peripheral oxygen extraction. Circ Heart Fail 2015;8: 286–94.

8. Borlaug BA. Mechanisms of exercise intolerance in heart failure with preserved ejection fraction. Circ J 2014;78:20–32.

9. Gorter TM, Obokata M, Reddy YNV, et al. Exercise unmasks distinct pathophysiologic features in heart failure with preserved ejection fraction and pulmonary vascular disease. Eur Heart J 2018;39: 2825–35.

10. Verbrugge FH, Omote K, Reddy YNV, et al. Heart failure with preserved ejection fraction in patients with normal natriuretic peptide levels is associated with increased morbidity and mortality. Eur Heart J 2022;43:1941–51.

11. Obokata M, Kane GC, Reddy YN, et al. Role of diastolic stress testing in the evaluation for heart failure with preserved ejection fraction: a simultaneous invasive-echocardiographic study. Circulation 2017;135:825–38.

12. Borlaug BA, Nishimura RA, Sorajja P, et al. Exercise hemodynamics enhance diagnosis of early heart failure with preserved ejection fraction. Circ Heart Fail 2010;3:588–95.

13. Reddy YNV, Carter RE, Obokata M, et al. A Simple, evidence-based approach to help guide diagnosis of heart failure with preserved ejection fraction. Circulation 2018;138:861–70.

14. Borlaug BA, Redfield MM. Diastolic and systolic heart failure are distinct phenotypes within the heart failure spectrum. Circulation 2011;123:2006–13; discussion 2014.

15. Sorimachi H, Verbrugge FH, Omote K, et al. Longitudinal Evolution of cardiac dysfunction in heart failure with normal natriuretic peptide levels. Circulation 2022;146(6):500–2.

16. Nauta JF, Hummel YM, van der Meer P, et al. Correlation with invasive left ventricular filling pressures and prognostic relevance of the echocardiographic diastolic parameters used in the 2016 ESC heart failure guidelines and in the 2016 ASE/EACVI recommendations: a systematic review in patients with heart failure with preserved ejection fraction. Eur J Heart Fail 2018;20:1303–11.

17. Hsu S, Fang JC, Borlaug BA. Hemodynamics for the heart failure clinician: a state-of-the-Art review. J Card Fail 2022;28:133–48.

18. Guazzi M, Adams V, Conraads V, et al. EACPR/AHA Scientific Statement. Clinical recommendations for cardiopulmonary exercise testing data assessment in specific patient populations. Circulation 2012; 126:2261–74.

19. Guazzi M, Arena R, Halle M, et al. Focused Update: clinical recommendations for cardiopulmonary exercise testing data assessment in specific patient populations. Circulation 2016;133:e694–711.

20. Malhotra R, Bakken K, D'Elia E, et al. Cardiopulmonary exercise testing in heart failure. JACC Heart Fail 2016;4:607–16.

21. Redfield MM, Chen HH, Borlaug BA, et al. Effect of phosphodiesterase-5 inhibition on exercise capacity and clinical status in heart failure with preserved

ejection fraction: a randomized clinical trial. Jama 2013;309:1268–77.

22. Borlaug BA, Anstrom KJ, Lewis GD, et al. Effect of Inorganic Nitrite vs Placebo on exercise capacity among patients with heart failure with preserved ejection fraction: the INDIE-HFpEF randomized clinical trial. Jama 2018;320:1764–73.

23. Guazzi M, Myers J, Arena R. Cardiopulmonary exercise testing in the clinical and prognostic assessment of diastolic heart failure. J Am Coll Cardiol 2005;46:1883–90.

24. Guazzi M, Labate V, Cahalin LP, et al. Cardiopulmonary exercise testing reflects similar pathophysiology and disease severity in heart failure patients with reduced and preserved ejection fraction. Eur J Prev Cardiol 2014;21:847–54.

25. Haykowsky MJ, Brubaker PH, John JM, et al. Determinants of exercise intolerance in elderly heart failure patients with preserved ejection fraction. J Am Coll Cardiol 2011;58:265–74.

26. Chomsky DB, Lang CC, Rayos GH, et al. Hemodynamic exercise testing. A valuable tool in the selection of cardiac transplantation candidates. Circulation 1996;94:3176–83.

27. Sullivan MJ, Knight JD, Higginbotham MB, et al. Relation between central and peripheral hemodynamics during exercise in patients with chronic heart failure. Muscle blood flow is reduced with maintenance of arterial perfusion pressure. Circulation 1989;80:769–81.

28. Reddy YNV, Obokata M, Wiley B, et al. Hemodynamic Correlates and Diagnostic Role of Cardiopulmonary Exercise Testing in Heart Failure with Preserved Ejection Fraction. JACC Heart Fail 2018;6(8):665–75.

29. Van Iterson EH, Johnson BD, Borlaug BA, et al. Physiological dead space and arterial carbon dioxide contributions to exercise ventilatory inefficiency in patients with reduced or preserved ejection fraction heart failure. Eur J Heart Fail 2017;19:1675–85.

30. Obokata M, Olson TP, Reddy YNV, et al. Haemodynamics, dyspnoea, and pulmonary reserve in heart failure with preserved ejection fraction. Eur Heart J 2018;39:2810–21.

31. Gehlbach BK, Geppert E. The pulmonary manifestations of left heart failure. Chest 2004;125:669–82.

32. Stavrakis S, Elkholey K, Morris L, et al. Neuromodulation of Inflammation to Treat heart failure with preserved ejection fraction: a Pilot randomized clinical trial. J Am Heart Assoc 2022;11:e023582.

33. Jain CC, Borlaug BA. Performance and interpretation of invasive hemodynamic exercise testing. Chest 2020;158:2119–29.

34. Obokata M, Reddy YNV, Pislaru SV, et al. Evidence supporting the existence of a distinct obese phenotype of heart failure with preserved ejection fraction. Circulation 2017;136:6–19.

35. Reddy YNV, Obokata M, Verbrugge FH, et al. Atrial dysfunction in patients with heart failure with preserved ejection fraction and atrial fibrillation. J Am Coll Cardiol 2020;76:1051–64.

36. Mizumi S, Goda A, Takeuchi K, et al. Effects of body position during cardiopulmonary exercise testing with right heart catheterization. Physiol Rep 2018;6: e13945.

37. Thadani U, Parker JO. Hemodynamics at rest and during supine and sitting bicycle exercise in normal subjects. Am J Cardiol 1978;41:52–9.

38. West JB, Dollery CT, Naimark A. Distribution of blood flow in isolated lung; relation to vascular and alveolar pressures. J Appl Phys 1964;19:713–24.

39. Stampfer M, Epstein SE, Beiser GD, et al. Exercise in patients with heart disease. Effects of body position and type and intensity of exercise. Am J Cardiol 1969;23:572–6.

40. van de Bovenkamp AA, Wijkstra N, Oosterveer FPT, et al. The Value of Passive Leg Raise During Right Heart Catheterization in Diagnosing Heart Failure With Preserved Ejection Fraction. Circulation Heart failure 2022;15:e008935.

41. Sorimachi H, Burkhoff D, Verbrugge FH, et al. Obesity, venous capacitance, and venous compliance in heart failure with preserved ejection fraction. Eur J Heart Fail 2021;23:1648–58.

42. Sorimachi H, Obokata M, Takahashi N, et al. Pathophysiologic importance of visceral adipose tissue in women with heart failure and preserved ejection fraction. Eur Heart J 2021;42:1595–605.

43. Omote K, Borlaug BA. Left atrial myopathy in heart failure with preserved ejection fraction. Circ J 2021. https://doi.org/10.1253/circj.CJ-21-0795. Online ahead of print.

44. Vachiery JL, Tedford RJ, Rosenkranz S, et al. Pulmonary hypertension due to left heart disease. Eur Respir J 2019;53.

45. Epstein SE, Beiser GD, Stampfer M, et al. Characterization of the circulatory response to maximal upright exercise in normal subjects and patients with heart disease. Circulation 1967;35:1049–62.

46. Ho JE, Zern EK, Lau ES, et al. Exercise pulmonary hypertension Predicts clinical Outcomes in patients with dyspnea on effort. J Am Coll Cardiol 2020;75: 17–26.

47. Eisman AS, Shah RV, Dhakal BP, et al. Pulmonary capillary wedge pressure patterns during exercise predict exercise capacity and incident heart failure. Circ Heart Fail 2018;11:e004750.

48. Andersen MJ, Nishimura RA, Borlaug BA. The hemodynamic basis of exercise intolerance in tricuspid regurgitation. Circ Heart Fail 2014;7: 911–7.

49. Belenkie I, Dani R, Smith ER, et al. Effects of volume loading during experimental acute pulmonary embolism. Circulation 1989;80:178–88.

50. Tyberg JV, Taichman GC, Smith ER, et al. The relationship between pericardial pressure and right atrial pressure: an intraoperative study. Circulation 1986;73:428–32.

51. Borlaug BA, Reddy YNV. The role of the pericardium in heart failure: implications for pathophysiology and treatment. JACC Heart Fail 2019;7:574–85.

52. Nagata R, Harada T, Omote K, et al. Right atrial pressure represents cumulative cardiac burden in heart failure with preserved ejection fraction. ESC Heart Fail 2022;9(2):1454–62. https://doi.org/10.1002/ehf2.13853.

53. Omote K, Sorimachi H, Obokata M, et al. Pulmonary Vascular Disease in Pulmonary Hypertension Due to Left Heart Disease: Pathophysiologic Implications. Eur Heart J 2022;7:ehac184. https://doi.org/10.1093/eurheartj/ehac184. Online ahead of print.

54. Omote K, Nagai T, Kamiya K, et al. Long-term prognostic significance of Admission tricuspid regurgitation pressure Gradient in Hospitalized patients with heart failure with preserved ejection fraction: a report from the Japanese Real-World Multicenter Registry. J Card Fail 2019;25:978–85.

55. Freed BH, Daruwalla V, Cheng JY, et al. Prognostic utility and clinical significance of cardiac Mechanics in heart failure with preserved ejection fraction: importance of left atrial strain. Circ Cardiovasc Imaging 2016;9.

56. Melenovsky V, Hwang SJ, Redfield MM, et al. Left atrial remodeling and function in advanced heart failure with preserved or reduced ejection fraction. Circ Heart Fail 2015;8:295–303.

57. Guazzi M, Dixon D, Labate V, et al. RV contractile function and its coupling to pulmonary circulation in heart failure with preserved ejection fraction: Stratification of clinical phenotypes and Outcomes. JACC Cardiovasc Imaging 2017;10:1211–21.

58. Melenovsky V, Hwang SJ, Lin G, et al. Right heart dysfunction in heart failure with preserved ejection fraction. Eur Heart J 2014;35:3452–62.

59. Obokata M, Reddy YNV, Melenovsky V, et al. Deterioration in right ventricular structure and function over time in patients with heart failure and preserved ejection fraction. Eur Heart J 2019;40:689–97.

60. Sugimoto T, Bandera F, Generati G, et al. Left atrial function Dynamics during exercise in heart failure: pathophysiological implications on the right heart and exercise ventilation inefficiency. JACC Cardiovasc Imaging 2017;10:1253–64.

61. Kelly RP, Ting CT, Yang TM, et al. Effective arterial elastance as index of arterial vascular load in humans. Circulation 1992;86:513–21.

62. Chemla D, Hébert JL, Coirault C, et al. Total arterial compliance estimated by stroke volume-to-aortic pulse pressure ratio in humans. Am J Phys 1998;274:H500–5.

63. Borlaug BA, Paulus WJ. Heart failure with preserved ejection fraction: pathophysiology, diagnosis, and treatment. Eur Heart J 2011;32:670–9.

64. Reddy YNV, Andersen MJ, Obokata M, et al. Arterial stiffening with exercise in patients with heart failure and preserved ejection fraction. J Am Coll Cardiol 2017;70:136–48.

65. Lau ES, Panah LG, Zern EK, et al. Arterial stiffness and vascular load in HFpEF: differences among women and men. J Card Fail 2022;28:202–11.

66. Houstis NE, Eisman AS, Pappagianopoulos PP, et al. Exercise intolerance in heart failure with preserved ejection fraction: diagnosing and Ranking its causes using Personalized O(2) Pathway analysis. Circulation 2018;137:148–61.

67. Melamed KH, Santos M, Oliveira RKF, et al. Unexplained exertional intolerance associated with impaired systemic oxygen extraction. Eur J Appl Physiol 2019;119:2375–89.

68. Reddy YNV, Obokata M, Egbe A, et al. Left atrial strain and compliance in the diagnostic evaluation of heart failure with preserved ejection fraction. Eur J Heart Fail 2019;21:891–900.

69. Koepp KE, Obokata M, Reddy YNV, et al. Hemodynamic and functional impact of Epicardial adipose tissue in heart failure with preserved ejection fraction. JACC Heart Fail 2020;8:657–66.

70. Sorimachi H, Omote K, Borlaug BA. Clinical phenogroups in heart failure with preserved ejection fraction. Heart Fail Clin 2021;17:483–98.

71. Shah SJ, Borlaug BA, Chung ES, et al. Atrial shunt device for heart failure with preserved and mildly reduced ejection fraction (REDUCE LAP-HF II): a randomised, multicentre, blinded, sham-controlled trial. Lancet 2022;399(10330):1130–40. https://doi.org/10.1016/S0140-6736(22)00016-2.

72. Borlaug BA, Blair J, Bergmann MW, et al. Latent Pulmonary Vascular Disease May Alter the Response to Therapeutic Atrial Shunt Device in Heart Failure. Circulation 2022;145(21):1592–604. https://doi.org/10.1161/CIRCULATIONAHA.122.059486.

Pharmacologic Therapy for Heart Failure with Preserved Ejection Fraction

Anthony E. Peters, MD, MS[a,b], Adam D. DeVore, MD, MHS[a,b],*

KEYWORDS

- Heart failure with preserved ejection fraction • Pharmacologic therapy • State-of-the-art

KEY POINTS

- An important aspect of high-quality heart failure with preserved ejection fraction (HFpEF) care is confirming the diagnosis and excluding mimickers.
- Symptom management is typically done with diuretics to manage dyspnea and volume overload.
- Optimization of comorbidities is also important.
- There are specific cardiovascular therapies—angiotensin II receptor type I blockers, mineralocorticoid receptor antagonists, angiotensin receptor–neprilysin inhibitors, and sodium–glucose cotransporter-2 inhibitors—with evidence to reduce HF hospitalizations that can be considered in select patients, particularly those on the lower end of the HFpEF spectrum (i.e., heart failure with mildly reduced ejection fraction).

INTRODUCTION

Heart failure with preserved ejection fraction (HFpEF) is a major public health problem, affecting greater than 3.1 million Americans and increasing in prevalence over time.[1–3] The pathophysiology of HFpEF is complex with multiple potential cardiac and noncardiac mechanisms (**Fig. 1**) along with growing evidence for the paradigm of comorbidity-driven systemic inflammation.[4,5] Patients living with HFpEF have a high burden of illness and poor outcomes. Compared with HF with reduced ejection fraction (HFrEF), symptom burden and health-related quality of life (HRQOL) is similarly severe in HFpEF,[6] and intermediate- and long-term survival is similar.[7] Although the impact of medical therapy on clinical outcomes in HFpEF has been modest in the setting of the complexity and heterogeneity of HFpEF, the field is rapidly evolving with much to consider for the practicing clinician in the management of symptoms and HF morbidity.

HFpEF Diagnosis and HFpEF Mimickers

An essential step in high-quality management of HFpEF is an accurate diagnosis, which can be challenging given its heterogeneity and overlap with other conditions. Diagnostic criteria are most clearly outlined in the European Society of Cardiology (ESC) guidelines, which describe three components for diagnosis: (1) signs and/or symptoms of HF, (2) preserved left ventricular ejection fraction [(LVEF) $\geq$50%], and (3) objective evidence of relevant structural and/or functional heart disease, consistent with the presence of LV diastolic dysfunction/raised LV filling pressures.[8] This third criterion is often assessed by cardiac imaging such as echocardiography (LV mass index, relative wall thickness, left atrial volume index, E/e', pulmonary artery (PA) systolic pressure, and resting tricuspid regurgitation velocity) or laboratory values (B-type natriuretic peptide [BNP]/ N-terminal [NT]-proB-type natriuretic peptide [NT-proBNP]), but can also be evaluated by

a Division of Cardiology, Duke University School of Medicine, Duke University Medical Center, 200 Trent Drive, 4th Floor, Orange Zone, Room #4225, Durham, NC 27710, USA; b Duke Clinical Research Institute, Duke University Medical Center, 200 Trent Drive, 4th Floor, Orange Zone, Room #4225, Durham, NC 27710, USA
* Corresponding author.
E-mail address: adam.devore@duke.edu

Cardiol Clin 40 (2022) 473–489
https://doi.org/10.1016/j.ccl.2022.06.004

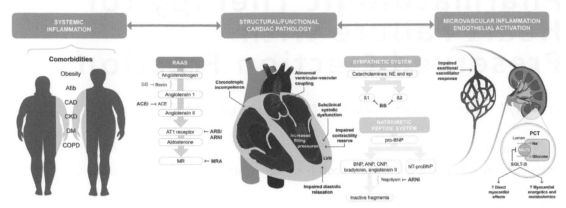

Fig. 1. Established and proposed pathophysiology of HFpEF and targets of currently available pharmacologic therapy. CKD, chronic kidney disease; CNP, C-type natriuretic peptide; COPD, chronic obstructive pulmonary disease; DM, diabetes mellitus; Epi, epinephrine; PCT, proximal convoluted tubule.

invasive hemodynamics. The American Heart Association/American College of Cardiology guidelines include similar diagnostic criteria.[9,10]

In challenging or borderline cases, the use of risk scores/algorithms, invasive hemodynamics with exercise, and exercise stress testing can be useful. Specifically, the H2FPEF score[11] and Heart Failure Association Pre-test assessment, Echocardiography and Natriuretic Peptide, Functional testing, Final etiology (HFA-PEFF) algorithm[12,13] are well-validated metrics to support the diagnostic process in HFpEF. The HFA-PEFF algorithm and the 2021 ESC updated guidelines (IIb recommendation) both specifically mention the use of invasive hemodynamics to confirm suspected HFpEF in select patients.[8,12] Over the past decade, exercise hemodynamics have been established as a reliable method to identify exercise-induced elevation in pulmonary capillary wedge pressure (PCWP) and PA systolic pressure and thereby diagnose a form of HFpEF in symptomatic patients with normal baseline pressures.[14] A representative approach from the Duke University Medical Center is shown in **Fig. 2**.[15] Exercise stress testing with imaging can also be used to elicit and measure abnormal hemodynamic responses to exercise, as referenced in the HFA-PEFF algorithm.[12]

Ruling out mimicking diseases in the diagnosis of HFpEF is also an important step. Prior HFpEF trials have likely been limited by including a broadly defined group of "HFpEF" patients with the inclusion of diagnosed and/or undiagnosed cardiomyopathies such as amyloidosis.[16] Identifying signs of HFpEF mimickers and sending timely workup before treating as typical HFpEF is critical to ensure patients with overlapping conditions, such as sarcoidosis, are able to receive targeted therapies such as immunosuppression

(**Table 1**, **Fig. 3**). For pharmacologic treatment of well-established cardiomyopathies with targeted therapies, we refer the reader to the following guidelines, society statements, and reviews— amyloidosis,[17,18] sarcoidosis,[19] and hypertrophic cardiomyopathy.[20]

Symptom Management

Loop diuretics remain the cornerstone of pharmacologic management of symptoms in HFpEF. While there are few dedicated trials of diuretics targeting morbidity/mortality outcomes in HF (especially in HFpEF or HFmrEF specifically), experience has been extended from subsets of HF studies such as the DOSE study as well as meta-analyses of diuretics in HF across the LVEF spectrum which demonstrate that diuretics likely improve exercise capacity.[21] Data from remote monitoring, for which the predominant response to abnormal data was diuretic changes, also provides indirect evidence that diuretics may reduce hospitalization risk in HFpEF.[22] The ROPA-DOP trial studied different diuretic strategies in patients with HFpEF specifically and found that dopamine did not affect renal function or any secondary outcomes, and that continuous loop diuretic use was associated with worse renal function but did not have a significant effect on clinical outcomes.[23] With this background, furosemide (oral, intravenous—intermittent, or continuous) remains the dominant, clinically utilized drug in HF overall and in HFpEF specifically. There is some evidence to support the unique benefits of torsemide over furosemide, including higher bioavailability, longer duration of effect, minor renal excretion, decreased potassium excretion in the urine, and enhanced natriuresis/diuresis.[24,25] Additionally, torsemide may have differential effects on renin–angiotensin–aldosterone

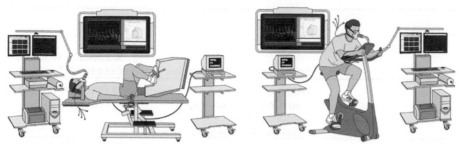

Fig. 2. Setup and protocol for invasive cardiopulmonary exercise testing with hemodynamics. The experimental setup in the catheterization laboratory is presented. All testing is performed in a fasting state. All invasive hemodynamic measurements are recorded in the supine position. Right heart catheterization through the internal jugular vein and a radial arterial catheterization are used to assess central hemodynamics, arterial pressures, and for blood gas analysis. Resting invasive measurements are obtained ~ 15 min after placement of central lines, sensors, and mask fitting (30–45 min), once steady state is achieved (legs down and up on the bike pedals). Following resting hemodynamics, patients undergoes supine cycle ergometry testing with simultaneous expired gas analysis. Patients are tested at a fixed workload of 20 W until patients reached a steady state of expired VO_2 or up to 7 min. After reaching steady state, patients are exercised to peak with a stepwise increase of 20 W every minute. Hemodynamic assessment during exercise is performed at 20 W and at peak exercise. Following exercise, recovery hemodynamics are assessed at 2 min and 5 min after peak exercise. Intracardiac pressures are taken as the average end-expiratory values across multiple respiratory cycles over a 10-s period. Breath-by-breath oxygen consumption is measured continuously throughout the study. Cardiac output is calculated via direct Fick method (VO_2, AVO_2-diff). Peak VO_2 values are determined by two readers independently. The Borg scale of perceived exertion (6–20) and assessments of leg fatigue (scale 0–10) and shortness of breath (scale 0–10) are obtained throughout the exercise phases at the same time intervals as the cardiac hemodynamic measurements. No general anesthetic agents are used during the study.

system (RAAS) and fibrosis regulation, although evidence is mixed.[26–28] Further, there is limited high-quality evidence on torsemide's association with HF hospitalizations and mortality.[29,30] In this setting, the ongoing TRANSFORM-HF trial, which compares torsemide to furosemide in hospitalized HF across the LVEF spectrum, should be informative to guide diuretic choice.[31] The trial is expected to complete enrollment in 2022.

Optimization of Comorbidities

Both cardiac and noncardiac comorbidities are influential in the outcomes of patients with HF and are particularly common and impactful in HFpEF.[32] Important cardiovascular (CV) comorbidities include hypertension (HTN), atrial fibrillation (AF), and coronary artery disease (CAD), and careful management of these conditions is the key to optimal HFpEF management. For HTN in patients with HFpEF, there are no definitive, first-line agents to achieve blood pressure (BP) control, but targeting a goal systolic BP of less than 130 mm Hg is recommended in the guidelines.[10] Other comorbidities and patient-specific factors (age, renal function, preferences, and so forth) typically drive antihypertensive choices. Angiotensin-converting enzyme inhibitors (ACEi)/angiotensin II receptor type I blockers (ARBs) may reduce left ventricular hypertrophy (LVH)/LV

mass, and therefore is a reasonable first-line agent for HTN in patients with HFpEF with LVH.[33] As discussed later, angiotensin receptor–neprilysin inhibitor (ARNI) therapy can also improve outcomes in patients with HFpEF and be considered for HTN control.

AF burden (and associated or distinct left atrial myopathy) can also be impactful in HFpEF, often resulting in a cyclical downward relationship between the pathologies of AF and HFpEF.[34–36] Anticoagulation is important as directed by guidelines and risk stratification. Several meta-analyses have indicated that mineralocorticoid receptor antagonist (MRA) therapy may reduce AF burden (first occurrence and recurrence) and recent finerenone data support this potential class effect.[37–39] Rate or rhythm control are both reasonable options, although there is early evidence that catheter ablation may improve LV diastolic function, symptom burden, and the New York Heart Association (NYHA) functional class in patients with HFpEF.[40,41] Distinguishing whether AF or HF is more responsible for driving patients' symptoms can be difficult; however, achieving predominant sinus rhythm and reassessing symptoms can be useful in this regard. Given these limited data and clinical context, it remains important to consider the risks/benefits of rhythm control, including ablation, in patients with AF and HFpEF.

Table 1
HFpEF mimickers

Mimicker	Select Signs and Symptoms	Additional Workup/ Diagnostic Testing to Consider
Amyloidosis	Prominent LVH, apical-sparing, low voltage, neuropathic/ gastrointestinal symptoms	Tc-PYP scan, light chains, CMR, TTR genotyping
Cardiac sarcoidosis	Arrythmias + conduction disease, syncope or aborted sudden cardiac death, signs of extracardiac sarcoidosis, unexplained dilated or restrictive cardiomyopathy	CMR or PET, extracardiac or endomyocardial biopsy
Hypertrophic cardiomyopathy	Variable ranging from asymptomatic to DOE, fatigue, chest pain, and exertional syncope; family history of HCM or unexplained LVH	Cardiac imaging led by echocardiography +/– CMR and exercise testing
Right ventricular myopathies (i.e., ARVC or RV infarct)	Presyncope/syncope, palpitations, arrhythmias; symptoms of RV failure	Echocardiography or CMR and/or hemodynamic cardiac catherization
Valvular disease	Murmur on exam; HF, angina, or syncope symptoms; predisposing condition (i.e., rheumatic disease, bicuspid aortic valve, aging)	Cardiac imaging +/– hemodynamic catherization
Pulmonary arterial HTN	Exertional dyspnea, fatigue; prominent P2 and RV heave on exam	Right heart catherization; autoimmune and HIV serologies, and liver/thyroid function tests
Constrictive pericarditis	Fluid overload, exertional dyspnea and fatigue; elevated JVP and Kussmaul sign	Echocardiography +/– hemodynamic cardiac catherization
High-output HF	Signs/symptoms of underlying disorder (i.e., obesity, liver disease, arteriovenous shunt, etc.), persistent tachycardia, typical signs/ symptoms of HF but warm and well-perfused extremities	Echocardiography +/– right heart cardiac catherization
Pulmonary embolism	(acute) Tachycardia, chest pain/cough in setting of exacerbating circumstance followed by (chronic) exertional dyspnea	CTPA, V/Q scan
Pulmonary disease (parenchymal or obstructive)	Predominant dyspnea symptoms with euvolemic exam	PFTs, pulmonary HRCT

Abbreviations: CMR, Cardiac magnetic resonance imaging; CTPA, computed tomography pulmonary angiogram; HIV, Human immunodeficiency virus; HRCT, High-resolution computed tomography; PFTs, Pulmonary function tests; Tc-PYP, Technetium phyrophosphate scintigraphy; TTR, transthyretin; V/Q, ventilation–perfusion.

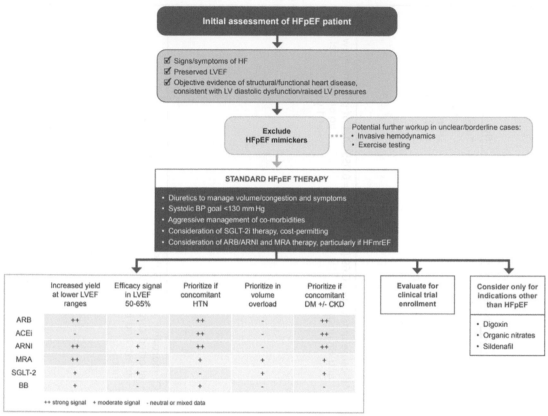

Fig. 3. Approach to diagnosis and pharmacologic management of patients with HFpEF. CKD, chronic kidney disease; DM, diabetes mellitus.

CAD in patients with HFpEF is another independent risk factor for poor outcomes and should also be aggressively investigated and managed; observational data have demonstrated that revascularization is associated with preservation of LVEF and lower mortality though higher-quality data are lacking.[42] Type II diabetes overlays with HFpEF phenotypes and should be managed as directed by established guidelines and scientific statements[43] with preference given to metformin and/or sodium–glucose cotransporter-2 inhibitors (SGLT2I) therapy when possible. Other common and impactful comorbidities including chronic obstructive pulmonary disease, anemia, sleep-disordered breathing, and obesity should be optimally treated as possible as part of complete HFpEF care.

Pharmacologic Therapy to Reduce HF Events

Clinical trials specific to pharmacologic treatment of HFpEF have traditionally fallen short of meeting primary outcomes of mortality/hospitalization (**Table 2**). While multiple clinical trials found that prior interventions, specifically ACEi/ARB and MRA, did not improve mortality, they did demonstrate a

signal of reduced risk of HF hospitalization in HFpEF. More recently, both ARNI and SGLT-2I have demonstrated the ability to significantly reduce HF hospitalization risk on top of established, standard therapy. In addition, the recent EMPEROR-PRESERVED trial was the first to definitively meet its primary composite outcome in an HFpEF-specific population. Before reviewing the primary trial data for each drug class, it is important to note that patients with HFpEF with recovered EF (i.e., previously with an LVEF < 40%) should generally receive continued HFrEF therapy. Additionally, the theme of differential effects across the spectrum of LVEF within HFpEF is a common finding in trials across drug classes and is supported by detailed analyses and recent ESC guidelines.

Angiotensin II Receptor Type I Blockers

ARBs inhibit the RAAS by blocking the angiotensin type I receptor on which angiotensin II acts, thereby leading to arterial and venous vasodilation, reduced BP, and decreased aldosterone secretion among other effects. ARBs clearly have a role in HFpEF as part of antihypertensive

Table 2
Selected HFpEF trial data and outcomes

Drugs	Trials	Populations	n	HFpEF Imaging Criteria	Primary Outcomes	Primary Outcomes HR/OR/RR[a]	Notes
ARB	CHARM-PRESERVED[44] (candesartan)	Age ≥18	3023	LVEF >40%	CV mortality and HF hosp	0.86 [0.74–1.00] P=0.051	Trend driven by HF hospitalizations Unadjusted HR =0.89 (0.77–1.03), P=0.12
	I-PRESERVE (irbesartan)	Age ≥60	4128	LVEF ≥45% Other potential echo criteria if no recent HF hospitalizations to qualify	All-cause mortality and CV hosp	0.95 [0.86–1.05] P=0.35	
ACEi	PEP-CHF[48] (perindopril)	Age ≥70	850	2 of 4 criteria among: • LVWMI of 1.4–1.6 • LAd >0.25 mm/m² BSA or >0.40 mm • IVS or PWT ≥12 mm • Evidence of impaired LV filling by at least one of:[b] • E/A ratio<0.5 • Deceleration time >280 ms from mitral inflow pattern • Isovolumic relaxation time >105 ms	All-cause mortality and HF hosp	0.69 [0.47–1.01] P=0.055	1/4 of pts withdrew to go on open label ACEI at 1 year
Spiro	TOPCAT[50,51]	Age ≥50	3445	LVEF ≥45%	CV mortality, aborted cardiac arrest, and HF hosp	Full cohort: 0.89 [0.77–1.04] P=0.14 Americas: 0.82 [0.69–0.98] P = 0.026	Full cohort: Reduced HF hospitalizations - HR 0.83 [0.69–0.99], P = 0.04 Americas: Reduced HF hospitalizations - HR, 0.82 [0.67–0.99], P = 0.04

Class	Trial	Age	N	LVEF	Primary Outcome	Result	Comments
BB	SENIORS[57] (nebivolol)	Age ≥70	2128	Any LVEF • Mean LVEF was 36% • 35% had LVEF >35%	All-cause mortality and CV hosp	0.86 [0.74–0.99] P = 0.039	Significant reduction in primary outcome in patients treated with >7.5 mg/day (n=58)
	J-DHF[60] (carvedilol)	Age ≥20	245	LVEF >40%	CV mortality and HF hosp	0.90 [0.55–1.49] P = 0.69	
ARNI	PARAGON-HF[54] (sacubitril/valsartan vs. valsartan)	Age ≥50	4822	LVEF ≥45% LA enlargement (LA diameter ≥ 3.8 cm, LA length ≥ 5 cm, LA area ≥ 20 cm^2, LA volume ≥ 55 mL, or LAVI ≥ 29 mL/m^2) OR LVH (IVST or PWT ≥ 1.1 cm)	CV mortality and HF hosp	0.87[a] [0.75–1.01] P = 0.06	Trends toward reduction in outcome of HF hospitalizations Significant improvement in NYHA class and nonsignificant improvement in KCCQ Significant reduction in risk of composite renal function worsening
SGLT-2	EMPEROR-PRESERVED[63] (empagliflozin)	Age ≥18	5988	LVEF >40%	CV mortality and HF hosp	0.79 [0.69–0.90] P<0.001	Effect driven primarily by HF hospitalizations
Digoxin	DIG-PRESERVED[67]	Age ≥21	988	LVEF >45%	HF mortality and HF hosp	0.82 [0.63–1.07] P = 0.14	Ancillary substudy within DIG trial Trend toward decreased HF hospitalizations (HR 0.79 [0.59–1.04], P = 0.09 Trend toward increased unstable angina hospitalizations

Abbreviations: IVS, intraventricular septum; LAd, left atrial diameter; LVEF, left ventricular ejection fraction; PWT, posterior wall thickness

[a] RR = rate ratio (all others are hazard ratios); note this RR is compared to valsartan control, as opposed to placebo control for other studies.

[b] Criteria recommended by the ESC Study Group on Diastolic Heart Failure.

regimens, but can also be considered for the separate indication of reducing CV events. While ARBs reduce systemic HTN, facilitate LV remodeling in HFpEF, and improve outcomes in HFrEF among other indications, there has not been definitive evidence for improvement in clinical outcomes in the *full spectrum* of patients with HFpEF. Still, evidence from the full, primary CHARM-Preserved trial demonstrated a trend toward a reduction in the primary outcome (reduced HF hospitalizations/CV mortality), driven by reduction in HF hospitalizations.[44] Further, post hoc analyses of the full CHARM Program[45] and recurrent hospitalizations in CHARM-Preserved[46] are encouraging for potential efficacy, particularly in HFmrEF and particularly when considering the full burden of rehospitalizations (instead of the first event alone). The I-PRESERVE trial also investigated the use of ARBs (irbesartan) in HFpEF; this trial was more clearly neutral and notably included a slighter higher LVEF cutoff (45% instead of 40%) and studied all-cause mortality and CV hospitalizations as its primary outcome (instead of HF-specific outcomes). ARB therapy has also been studied in patients with HTN and diastolic dysfunction in the VALsartan In Diastolic Dysfunction (VALIDD) trial; this study was neutral with diastolic relaxation velocity improving with lowering BP irrespective of the particular antihypertensive agent used.[47] Taken together, ARBs may be considered in patients with HFpEF to reduce *HF hospitalization risk*, especially if the patient has (1) a concomitant HTN indication, (2) demonstrates below normal LVEF, and (3) has some burden of HF hospitalization or potential risk as deemed by the provider.

Angiotensin-converting Enzyme Inhibitors

ACEi work by inhibiting ACE, and thereby reducing the conversion of angiotensin I to angiotensin II, leading to arterial and venous vasodilation, reduced BP, and decreased aldosterone secretion. ACEi and ARBs are used interchangeably in many conditions including HTN and HFrEF. In HFpEF, the data for ACE inhibitors are somewhat weaker than for ARBs. The Perindopril in Elderly People with Chronic Heart Failure (PEP-CHF) trial was the primary study to evaluate ACEi in this population and it was relatively underpowered due to low enrollment and event rates.[48] In this setting, the primary outcome of clinical morbidity/mortality was neutral. Still, the study demonstrated improved functional class and 6-min walk distance and reduced HF hospitalizations at 1 year along with trends toward reduction in the primary outcome at 1 year. Given these findings, ACEi can be considered in patients with HFpEF to

reduce *HF hospitalization risk* and improve *functional status*, especially if the patient has (1) a concomitant indication such as HTN and (2) has some burden of impaired functional status and HF hospitalization or potential risk as deemed by the provider. There is insufficient evidence to compare ACEi and ARBs in HFpEF or to use them interchangeably.

Mineralocorticoid Receptor Antagonists

MRAs bind to the mineralocorticoid receptor, thereby inhibiting the action of aldosterone, leading to increased natriuresis, decreased kaliuresis, and reduced BP among other effects. There is substantial mechanistic evidence that MRAs, namely spironolactone, improve pathophysiology in HFpEF from the Aldo-DHF trial, which demonstrated an improvement in E/e′ ratio and a decrease in LVH and NT-proBNP levels.[49] Evidence of clinical outcomes comes largely from the Treatment of Preserved Cardiac Function Heart Failure with an Aldosterone Antagonist (TOPCAT) trial.[50] Overall results from the primary analysis of the TOPCAT trial were neutral, but there are several secondary, post hoc, and subgroup analyses that support the benefit of spironolactone in HFpEF. First, the secondary outcome of HF hospitalizations (hazard ratio [HR] 0.83 [0.69–0.99], $P = .04$) was reduced in the full cohort analysis. Second, post hoc analysis of the Americas subgroup demonstrated significant improvement in primary outcome (HR 0.82 [0.69–0.98], $P = .026$).[51] This subgroup analysis was initiated due to an "unusually large (~fourfold) difference" in placebo group primary event rate in patients from Russia/Georgia compared to those from the Americas and demonstrated distinct baseline differences, outcomes, and potential treatment effects (renal, hyperkalemia, and BP) in the population enrolled from Russia/Georgia, raising concern for whether these patients had "true HFpEF" and reliability of delivery of spironolactone in the intervention arm.[51,52] Additionally, post hoc analysis of the influence of LVEF on outcomes demonstrated a significant treatment modification effect for the primary outcome and HF hospitalizations with stronger benefit in patients with LVEF less than 50%.[53] It is reasonable to consider spironolactone in patients with HFpEF with appropriate renal function and potassium (estimated glomerular filtration rate >30 mL/min and potassium <5.0 mEq/L) reduce *HF hospitalization risk*, especially if the patient has (1) some burden of HF hospitalization or potential risk as deemed by the provider, (2) has additional relative indication/benefit of use including volume control, hypokalemia, or HTN, and/or (3) demonstrates below normal LVEF.

Angiotensin Receptor–Neprilysin Inhibitors

ARNI therapy combines the prodrug sacubitril with ARB therapy, thereby adding the effect of a neprilysin inhibitor, preventing the breakdown of natriuretic peptides and leading to prolonged effects of peptides including natriuresis and vasodilation among other pleiotropic effects. The pivotal trial of ARNI therapy in HFpEF was the Prospective Comparison of ARNI with ARB Global Outcomes in HF with Preserved Ejection Fraction (PARAGON-HF) trial.[54] In this trial, the primary outcome of CV mortality and HF hospitalizations was neutral with a trend toward reduced risk (rate ratio 0.87 [0.75–1.01], $P = .06$). There were further encouraging findings with a significant improvement in NYHA class and in the renal composite outcome with ARNI therapy. Prespecified subgroup analyses also suggested a higher degree of benefit in women and patients with median LVEF ≤57% and the intervention arm also demonstrated a lower incidence of hyperkalemia. Further post hoc analyses underscored these interaction effects of sex and LVEF, particularly with regards to HF hospitalization and demonstrating a higher LVEF cutoff for statistically significant effect among women (LVEF 65%–70%) versus men (LVEF 55%–60%).[55] In the setting of the borderline outcome of PARAGON-HF and phase 2 evidence for a reduction in NT-proBNP through sacubitril/valsartan use, another large, phase 3 trial was pursued to assess NT-proBNP levels, exercise capacity, and quality of life: the Prospective Comparison of ARNI versus Comorbidity-Associated Conventional Therapy on Quality of Life and Exercise Capacity (PARALLAX) trial.[56] While this trial redemonstrated a significant reduction in NT-proBNP levels in the intervention arm, there was no significant difference in 6-min walk distance, KCCQ clinical summary score, or NYHA class. Given this evidence base to date, ARNI therapy can be considered in patients with HFpEF to reduce *HF hospitalization risk*, especially if the patient has (1) some burden of HF hospitalization or potential risk as deemed by the provider, (2) demonstrates below normal EF if male (or any LVEF <65%–70% if female), (3) has some hyperkalemia history or elevated risk, and/or (4) has insurance coverage or financial means to support cost above generic therapy options (MRA and ARB).

Beta Blockers

Beta-adrenergic blocking (BB) agents bind and block B1 and B2 receptors (with variable specificity) and result in reduced chronotropy and inotropy, decreased renin release, and, for nonselective BBs, peripheral vasodilation. BBs are often utilized in patients with HFpEF, but this is predominantly driven by other indications: AF, angina/CAD, and HTN, among others. Several studies and meta-analyses have investigated use of BB in HF across the EF spectrum (HFrEF + HFpEF) with encouraging results. Specifically, the Study of the Effects of Nebivolol Intervention on Outcomes and Rehospitalisation in Seniors with Heart Failure (SENIORS) found a positive primary outcome of all-cause mortality and CV hospitalization in a large, elderly HF population.[57] Interaction analysis of this study has demonstrated no interaction effects by the LVEF group, but notably, only 35% had LVEF greater than 35%, and few had LVEF greater than 50%. Therefore, one should exercise caution in extrapolating this finding to the full spectrum of patients with HFpEF.[58] Additionally, a large meta-analysis of BBs according to LVEF demonstrated that the beneficial effects of BBs in HFrEF with respect to mortality and hospitalization may extend to LVEF 40% to 49% but not for LVEF ≥ 50%.[59] The Japanese Diastolic Heart Failure Study (J-DHF) is one of the few studies to examine the use of BBs specifically in patients with HFpEF and found neutral results for the primary outcome of CV mortality and HF hospitalizations, although there was some evidence of a significant reduction in this outcome in a small subgroup at closer to the target dose (carvedilol > 7.5 mg/d; target = 20 mg/d).[60] Lastly, there is growing evidence that HR-limited exercise intolerance (symptomatic chronotropic incompetence) may play a significant role in HFpEF, and this evidence base now includes a recent randomized, controlled trial demonstrating that BB *withdrawal* improves peak V$_{O_2}$ in patients with HFpEF.[61] Taken together, these studies support the select use of BBs in patients with HFpEF to reduce *HF mortality and hospitalization risk,* only if the patient (1) demonstrates below normal EF, (2) has additional relative indication/benefit of use including AF or HTN, and/or (3) is not HR-limited in exertion (recommend maintaining a low threshold for exercise testing and/or reassessment of symptoms on/off BB).

Sodium–Glucose Cotransporter-2 Inhibitors

SGLT-2I block sodium–glucose cotransporter-2 in the proximal convoluted tubule, thereby reducing glucose and sodium reabsorption as well as reducing BP and increasing diuresis by several potential mechanisms. Early encouraging data for the efficacy of SGLT-2I in HFpEF came from prespecified subgroup analysis (LVEF <50% and ≥50%) of the SOLOIST trial, which demonstrated a consistent reduction in primary outcome without heterogeneity.[62] Still, there were relatively few patients with HFpEF (n = 256) in the study, and the trial was terminated early due to loss of funding from the sponsor; so, conclusions of efficacy in HFpEF were limited. This was followed by the landmark EMPEROR-preserved trial, which focused exclusively on patients with HFpEF and showed a robust reduction in the primary outcome of CV mortality and HF hospitalizations.[63] Subgroup and post hoc pooled analyses demonstrated a wide range of similar, clinically meaningful effects up to LVEF 65% and attenuation of efficacy as EF rises above this threshold.[63,64] Further, SGLT-2I therapy improves HRQOL as measured by the Kansas City Cardiomyopathy Questionnaire (KCCQ) by 12 weeks postinitiation of therapy and sustained through at least 1 year.[65,66] Given this data, SGLT-2I therapy can be considered in patients with HFpEF to reduce *HF hospitalization risk and improve HRQOL*, especially if the patient has (1) some burden of low HRQOL and/or HF hospitalization or potential risk as deemed by the provider, (2) demonstrates below LVEF less than 65%, and/or (3) has insurance coverage or financial means to support cost above generic therapy options (MRA and ARB).

Other Pharmacologic Agents

Several other pharmacologic agents have been studied in HFpEF with neutral results. The primary digoxin study included a sub-study, DIG-PRESERVED, which focused on HFpEF and found neutral results for the primary outcome of HF mortality/hospitalization.[67] The study did indicate a trend toward decreased HF hospitalizations but also a trend toward increased unstable angina hospitalizations. Phosphodiesterase-5 inhibitors such as sildenafil have been studied in the Phosphodiesterase-5 Inhibition to Improve Clinical Status and Exercise Capacity in Heart Failure with Preserved Ejection Fraction (RELAX) trial without evidence of improvement in peak oxygen consumption (at 24 weeks) or in secondary outcomes such as 6-min walk distance.[68] Organic nitrates (ie, isosorbide mononitrate and dinitrate) and inorganic nitrite have also been studied in the Nitrate's Effect on Activity Tolerance in Heart Failure with Preserved Ejection Fraction (NEAT-HFpEF) and Inorganic Nitrite Delivery to Improve Exercise Capacity in Heart Failure With Preserved Ejection Fraction (INDIE-HFpEF) trials.[69,70] In the NEAT-HFpEF trial, treatment with isosorbide mononitrate

was associated with decreased activity level (significant in hours per day and in accelerometer units when assessed across all dose regimens) and did not affect 6-min walk distance, QOL scores, or NT-proBNP levels.[69] However, INDIE-HFpEF demonstrated no significant differences in peak oxygen consumption, daily activity levels, QOL, functional class, E/e' ratio, or NT-proBNP levels.[70] Overall, there is no strong evidence to support the use of these medications (digoxin, sildenafil, organic, or inorganic nitrates/nitrites) in patients with HFpEF at this time outside of ongoing clinical trials or alternative indications.

Considerations for HFmrEF Subset

As referenced earlier and in **Fig. 3**, almost all pharmacologic therapies in HFpEF have some degree of heterogeneity in reducing HF events across the HFpEF LVEF spectrum (EF 40%–65%). Within this spectrum, HFmrEF (EF 41%–49%) is an increasingly recognized and emphasized entity including earning a distinct treatment recommendations section in the recent 2021 ESC guidelines.[8] Theory and evidence on HFmrEF as a distinct entity or transition between HFrEF and HFpEF are mixed,[71] but the syndrome seems to carry some similarities to HFrEF in terms of HF etiology, outcomes, and response to therapy. While there are no substantial, prospective trials of pharmacologic therapy in HFpEF,[8] subgroup and interaction analyses from HFpEF trials as well as meta-analyses support the consideration of ARB,[45,46] MRA,[53] BB,[59] ARNI,[54,55] and SGLT-2i[63,64] therapies, particularly in HFmrEF.

Nonpharmacologic Therapy

Nonpharmacologic therapy has demonstrated some promise in HFpEF and is described in detail in other reviews.[72,73] Briefly, both exercise training and caloric restriction (independently and additive) have been shown to improve peak oxygen consumption through the Study of the Effect of Caloric Restriction and Exercise Training in Patients With Heart Failure and a Normal Ejection Fraction (SECRET) and Exercise training in Diastolic Heart Failure (Ex-DHF) trial, while the recent Rehabilitation Therapy in Older Acute Heart Failure Patients (REHAB-HF) study (including over half of the HFpEF patients) showed improvement in physical function, frailty, quality of life, and depression.[74–76] Left atrial shunt devices (interatrial shunt devices, [IASD]) demonstrated reduced PCWP during exercise in HFpEF and a strong 1-year safety profile, but initial results from REDUCE-LAP HF II were neutral.[77–80] Meanwhile, the HFpEF subset of the CHAMPION trial and the prepandemic sensitivity

Table 3
Selected phase III/IV ongoing pharmacologic trials in HFpEF

Acronym (Identifier)	Intervention	Projected Enrollment	LVEF (%)	Age (years)	NYHA class II–IV	Elevated BNP/NT-proBNP	Other	Primary Outcome
					Select Population Criteria			
DELIVER (NCT03619213)	Dapagliflozin (SGLT2i)	6263	> 40	≥ 40	✓	✓		Composite: CV mortality, HF hospitalization, and urgent HF visit
SPIRRIT (NCT02901184)	Spironolactone (MRA)	Original target 3200	≥ 40	≥ 50	✓	✓	On regular loop diuretic dose	Composite: CV mortality and HF hospitalization
SPIRIT-HF (NCT04727073)	Spironolactone (MRA)	Estimated 1300	≥ 40	≥ 50	✓	✓		Composite: CV mortality and HF hospitalization
FINEARTS-HF (NCT04435626)	Finerenone (MRA)	Estimated 5500	≥ 40	≥ 40	✓	✓	On diuretic therapy	
PARAGLIDE-HF (NCT03988634)	Sacubitril/ valsartan (ARNI)	Original target 800; revised 450	>40	≥ 18	-	✓	Within 30 days of worsening HF event[a]	Change in NT-proBNP
ENDEAVOR (NCT04986202)	AZD4831 (MPO inhibitor)	Estimated 1485	> 40	40–85	✓	✓		Change in KCCQ total symptom score; 6MWD
STEP HFpEF DM (NCT04916470)	Semaglutide (GLP-1)	Estimated 610	≥ 45	≥ 18	✓	-		Change in KCCQ clinical summary score
SUMMIT (NCT04847557)	Tirzepatide (GIP and GLP-1)	Estimated 700	≥ 50	≥ 40	✓	✓		Composite: All-cause mortality, HF events, 6MWD, KCCQ clinical summary score; Change in 6MWD

(continued on next page)

Table 3
(continued)

Acronym (Identifier)	Intervention	Projected Enrollment	LVEF (%)	Age (years)	NYHA class II-IV	Elevated BNP/NT-proBNP	Other	Primary Outcome
					Select Population Criteria			
BLOCK HFpEF (NCT04434664)	Amlodipine vs Metoprolol Succinate (crossover)	Estimated 50	> 50	18–90	-	~✓[b]	Echo/clinical criteria[b]	Change in SBP

Abbreviations: 6MWD, 6 min walk distance; KCCQ, Kansas City Cardiomyopathy Questionnaire; GIP, glucose-dependent insulinotropic polypeptide; GLP-1, glucagon-like peptide-1 analogue; SBP, systolic blood pressure.

[a] Worsening HF event defined as hospitalization, emergency department visit or out-of-hospital urgent HF visit, all requiring IV diuretics.

[b] Elevated filling pressures defined by at least one of the following criteria: (A) Mitral E/e' ratio (lateral or septal) >8 with low e' velocity (septal e' <7 cm/s or lateral e' <10 cm/s) and at least one of the following: (a) Enlarged left atrium (LA volume index >34 mL/m²); (b) Chronic loop diuretic use for management of symptoms; c. Elevated natriuretic peptides (BNP levels >100 ng/L or NT-proBNP levels >300 ng/L); (B) Mitral E/e' ratio (lateral or septal) >14; (C) Previously elevated invasively determined filling pressures based on one of the following criteria: (a) Resting LVEDP >16 mmHg; (b) Mean PCWP >12 mmHg; (c) PCWP or LVEDP ≥25 mmHg with exercise; and (D) Previous acutely decompensated heart failure requiring IV diuretics.

analysis of GUIDE-HF (full analysis was neutral) both showed a reduction in HF hospitalizations through PA pressure monitoring and medication adjustments based on hemodynamics.[22,81] In summary, exercise interventions, caloric restriction, and left atrial shunt devices have all been shown to improve physiologic parameters in patients with HFpEF, while hemodynamic-guided therapy with PA pressure monitoring devices has shown to reduce HF hospitalizations by some analyses.

Future Directions

Moving forward in the field of pharmacologic therapy, several areas of investigation will be important. First, trial enrollment remains an enormous challenge in HFpEF. Despite the prevalence of HFpEF, enrollment in trials specific to HFpEF has commonly been difficult, slow, and inefficient. Additionally, patients enrolled in HFpEF trials differ substantially from patients commonly encountered in routine practice with HFpEF.[82] Second, several studies have shown that well-established, effective therapies in HFrEF are utilized well below optimal targets for prescription and dosing.[83–85] This is likely to be a challenge in HFpEF as well and underscores the need to study the implementation of therapies in HFpEF. Third, several trials including SPIRRIT, SPIRIT-HF, and FINEARTS-HF should better define the role of MRA therapy in HFpEF, while continued investigation of ideal BP control and effects of heart rate lowering agents (such as in BLOCK HFpEF) should help the field to optimize HFpEF pharmacologic therapy (**Table 3**). Several ongoing studies including the PARAGLIDE and DELIVER trials will further inform the efficacy of ARNI and SGLT-2I therapy in HFpEF (see **Table 3**).[86] Lastly, several emerging therapies (some established in other fields and some novel) have the potential to contribute to future pharmacologic regimens for HFpEF. Inorganic nitrites remain one of these emerging therapies despite the neutral results of the INDIE-HFpEF trials given the mechanistic evidence base (inorganic nitrite's conversion/activity during hypoxia and acidosis; and lack of tolerance/tachyphylaxis) and several encouraging clinical studies[70,87–90]; given this background, there are, at least, three phase II trials actively studying potassium nitrate or sodium nitrite therapy (KNO3CK OUT HFPEF, PH-HFpEF, and INABLE-Training), targeting the nitric oxide-soluble guanylate cyclase enzyme-cyclic guanosine monophosphate (cGMP)-cGMP-dependent protein kinase G pathway. Additionally, IV iron therapy (FAIR-HFpEF trial), traditional diabetic/obesity drugs

such as GLP-1 agonists, and novel mechanisms such as MPO inhibition are under ongoing investigation in HFpEF (see **Table 3**). As described briefly earlier, device therapy has shown promise in HFpEF; in addition to left atrial/ IASD and invasive PA pressure monitoring, the procedural fields of baroreflex activation therapy/vagus nerve stimulation, splanchnic nerve modulation, and LV reconstruction/expanders, among others, have the potential to target the pathophysiology of HFpEF.[91,92] For many of these future directions of research, the continued evolution of imaging techniques such as global longitudinal strain will be important to further stratify and phenotype patients with HFpEF.[93]

SUMMARY

The pharmacologic management of HFpEF is an evolving field. Symptomatic management with diuretics and optimization of comorbidities remain important components of therapy. Therapies such as ARB, ACEi, ARNI, MRA, and SGLT-2I have been shown to reduce HF hospitalization risk, particularly in lower ranges of LVEF within HFpEF. Ongoing trials and investigations of emerging agents have the potential to further inform the optimal medical regimen for patients with HFpEF.

CLINICS CARE POINTS

- Confirmation of the HFpEF diagnosis and exclusion of mimicking diseases is a key first step in the care of patients with symptoms of HFpEF.

- In challenging or borderline cases, the use of risk scores/algorithms, invasive hemodynamics with exercise, and exercise stress testing can be useful.

- Diuretic therapy remains critical to symptom and volume management, while their effect on hospitalization and mortality should be informed by the ongoing TRANSFORM-HF trial.

- Optimization of comorbidities including AF, CAD, hypertension, obesity, and diabetes is also a key component of HFpEF management.

- Specific therapies including ARB/ARNI, MRA, and SGLT-2i should be utilized to reduce the risk of HF hospitalization, particularly in patients with EF on the lower end of the HFpEF/HFmrEF spectrum.

DISCLOSURE

Dr. A. E. Peters is supported by the National Heart Lung and Blood Institute (T32HL069749). Dr. A. D. DeVore reports research funding through his institution from the American Heart Association, Amgen, Biofourmis, Bodyport, Cytokinetics, American Regent, Inc, The National Heart, Lung, and Blood Institute, and Novartis. He also provides consulting services for and/or receives honoraria from Abiomed, Amgen, AstraZeneca, Cardionomic, InnaMed, LivaNova, Natera, Novartis, Procyrion, Story Health, Vifor, and Zoll.

FUNDING STATEMENT

Dr. Peters is supported by the National Heart Lung and Blood Institute (T32HL069749).

ACKNOWLEDGMENTS

We thank Kim Best for her development of graphical figures for this article.

REFERENCES

1. Oktay AA, Rich JD, Shah SJ. The emerging epidemic of heart failure with preserved ejection fraction. Curr Heart Fail Rep 2013;10(4):401–10.
2. Steinberg BA, Zhao X, Heidenreich PA, et al. Trends in patients hospitalized with heart failure and preserved left ventricular ejection fraction: prevalence, therapies, and outcomes. Circulation 2012;126(1):65–75.
3. Virani SS, Alonso A, Aparicio HJ, et al. Heart disease and Stroke Statistics—2021 update: a report from the American Heart Association. Circulation 2021. https://doi.org/10.1161/cir.0000000000000950.
4. Paulus WJ, Tschöpe C. A novel paradigm for heart failure with preserved ejection fraction: comorbidities drive myocardial dysfunction and remodeling through coronary microvascular endothelial inflammation. J Am Coll Cardiol 2013;62(4):263–71.
5. Paulus WJ, Zile MR. From systemic inflammation to myocardial fibrosis: the heart failure with preserved ejection fraction paradigm Revisited. Circ Res Published Online 2021;1451–67.
6. Lewis EF, Lamas GA, O' Meara E, et al. Characterization of health-related quality of life in heart failure patients with preserved versus low ejection fraction in CHARM. Eur J Heart Fail 2007;9(1):83–91.
7. Shah KS, Xu H, Matsouaka RA, et al. Heart Failure With Preserved, Borderline, and Reduced Ejection Fraction: 5-Year Outcomes. J Am Coll Cardiol 2017;70(20):2476–86.
8. McDonagh TA, Metra M, Adamo M, et al. 2021 ESC Guidelines for the diagnosis and treatment of acute and chronic heart failure. Eur Heart J 2021;42(36): 3599–726.
9. Yancy CW, Jessup M, Bozkurt B, et al. 2013 ACCF/AHA guideline for the management of heart failure: A report of the American college of cardiology foundation/american heart association task force on practice guidelines. J Am Coll Cardiol 2013;62(16): e147–239.
10. Yancy CW, Jessup M, Bozkurt B, et al. 2017 ACC/AHA/HFSA Focused Update of the 2013 ACCF/AHA Guideline for the Management of Heart Failure: A Report of the American College of Cardiology/American Heart Association Task Force on Clinical Practice Guidelines and the Heart Failure Society of Amer. Circulation 2017;136(6):e137–61.
11. Reddy YNV, Carter RE, Obokata M, Redfield MM, Borlaug BA. A simple, evidence-based approach to help guide diagnosis of heart failure with preserved ejection fraction. Circulation 2018;138(9): 861–70.
12. Pieske B, Tschöpe C, de Boer RA, et al. How to diagnose heart failure with preserved ejection fraction: the HFA–PEFF diagnostic algorithm: a consensus recommendation from the Heart Failure Association (HFA) of the European Society of Cardiology (ESC). Eur J Heart Fail 2020;22(3):391–412.
13. Barandiarán Aizpurua A, Sanders-van Wijk S, Brunner-La Rocca HP, et al. Validation of the HFA-PEFF score for the diagnosis of heart failure with preserved ejection fraction. Eur J Heart Fail 2020; 22(3):413–21.
14. Borlaug BA, Nishimura RA, Sorajja P, Lam CSP, Redfield MM. Exercise hemodynamics enhance diagnosis of early heart failure with preserved ejection fraction. Circ Hear Fail 2010;3(5):588–95.
15. Rao VN, Kelsey MD, Blazing MA, Pagidipati NJ, Fortin T, Fudim M. Unexplained Dyspnea on Exertion: The Difference the Right Test Can Make. Circ Heart Fail 2022;1–4.
16. Oghina S, Bougouin W, Bézard M, et al. The Impact of Patients With Cardiac Amyloidosis in HFpEF Trials. JACC Hear Fail 2021;9(3):169–78.
17. Garcia-Pavia P, Rapezzi C, Adler Y, et al. Diagnosis and treatment of cardiac amyloidosis: a position statement of the ESC Working Group on Myocardial and Pericardial Diseases. Eur Heart J 2021;42(16): 1554–68.
18. Kittleson MM, Maurer MS, Ambardekar A V., et al. Cardiac Amyloidosis: Evolving Diagnosis and Management: A Scientific Statement from the American Heart Association. Circulation. Published online 2020:E7-E22. doi:10.1161/CIR.0000000000000792
19. Gilotra N, Okada D, Sharma A, Chrispin J. Management of cardiac sarcoidosis in 2020. Arrhythmia Electrophysiol Rev 2021;9(4):182–8.
20. Ommen SR, Mital S, Burke MA, et al. 2020 AHA/ACC Guideline for the Diagnosis and Treatment of Patients With Hypertrophic Cardiomyopathy. Circulation 2020;142.

21. Faris R, Flather M, Purcell H, Henein M, Poole-Wilson P, Coats A. Current evidence supporting the role of diuretics in heart failure: A meta analysis of randomised controlled trials. Int J Cardiol 2002; 82(2):149–58.

22. Adamson PB, Abraham WT, Bourge RC, et al. Wireless pulmonary artery pressure monitoring guides management to reduce decompensation in heart failure with preserved ejection fraction. Circ Hear Fail 2014;7(6):935–44.

23. Sharma K, Vaishnav J, Kalathiya R, et al. Randomized Evaluation of Heart Failure With Preserved Ejection Fraction Patients With Acute Heart Failure and Dopamine: The ROPA-DOP Trial. JACC Hear Fail 2018;6(10):859–70.

24. Dinicolantonio JJ. Should torsemide be the loop diuretic of choice in systolic heart failure? Future Cardiol 2012;8(5):707–28.

25. Knauf H, Mutschler E. Clinical Pharmacokinetics and Pharmacodynamics of Torasemide. Clin Pharmacokinet 1998;34(1):1–24.

26. Tsutamoto T, Sakai H, Wada A, et al. Torasemide inhibits transcardiac extraction of aldosterone in patients with congestive heart failure [3]. J Am Coll Cardiol 2004;44(11):2252–3.

27. Yamato M, Sasaki T, Honda K, et al. Effects of torasemide on left ventricular function and neurohumoral factors in patients with chronic heart failure. Circ J 2003;67(5):384–90.

28. Gravez B, Tarjus A, Jimenez-Canino R, et al. The Diuretic Torasemide Does Not Prevent Aldosterone-Mediated Mineralocorticoid Receptor Activation in Cardiomyocytes. PLoS One 2013;8(9). https://doi.org/10.1371/journal.pone.0073737.

29. Miles JA, Hanumanthu BK, Patel K, Chen M, Siegel RM, Kokkinidis DG. Torsemide versus furosemide and intermediate-term outcomes in patients with heart failure: An updated meta-analysis. J Cardiovasc Med 2019;20(6):379–88.

30. Abraham B, Megaly M, Sous M, et al. Meta-Analysis Comparing Torsemide Versus Furosemide in Patients With Heart Failure. Am J Cardiol 2020; 125(1):92–9.

31. Greene SJ, Velazquez EJ, Anstrom KJ, et al. Pragmatic Design of Randomized Clinical Trials for Heart Failure: Rationale and Design of the TRANSFORM-HF Trial. JACC Hear Fail 2021;9(5):325–35.

32. Mentz RJ, Kelly JP, Von Lueder TG, et al. Noncardiac comorbidities in heart failure with reduced versus preserved ejection fraction. J Am Coll Cardiol 2014;64(21):2281–93.

33. Fagard RH, Celis H, Thijs L, Wouters S. Regression of left ventricular mass by antihypertensive treatment: A meta-analysis of randomized comparative studies. Hypertension 2009;54(5):1084–91.

34. Reddy YNV, Obokata M, Verbrugge FH, Lin G, Borlaug BA. Atrial Dysfunction in Patients With Heart Failure With Preserved Ejection Fraction and Atrial Fibrillation. J Am Coll Cardiol 2020;76(9):1051–64.

35. Kotecha D, Lam CSP, Van Veldhuisen DJ, Van Gelder IC, Voors AA, Rienstra M. Heart Failure With Preserved Ejection Fraction and Atrial Fibrillation: Vicious Twins. J Am Coll Cardiol 2016;68(20): 2217–28.

36. Carlisle MA, Fudim M, DeVore AD, Piccini JP. Heart Failure and Atrial Fibrillation, Like Fire and Fury. JACC Hear Fail 2019;7(6):447–56.

37. Alexandre J, Dolladille C, Douesnel L, et al. Effects of Mineralocorticoid Receptor Antagonists on Atrial Fibrillation Occurrence: A Systematic Review, Meta-Analysis, and Meta-Regression to Identify Modifying Factors. J Am Heart Assoc 2019;8(22). https://doi.org/10.1161/JAHA.119.013267.

38. Liu T, Korantzopoulos P, Shao Q, Zhang Z, Letsas KP, Li G. Mineralocorticoid receptor antagonists and atrial fibrillation: A meta-analysis. Europace 2016;18(5):672–8.

39. Filippatos G, Bakris GL, Pitt B, et al. Finerenone Reduces New-Onset Atrial Fibrillation in Patients With Chronic Kidney Disease and Type 2 Diabetes. J Am Coll Cardiol 2021;78(2):142–52.

40. Cha YM, Wokhlu A, Asirvatham SJ, et al. Success of ablation for atrial fibrillation in isolated left ventricular diastolic dysfunction: A comparison to systolic dysfunction and normal ventricular function. Circ Arrhythmia Electrophysiol 2011;4(5):724–32.

41. Black-Maier E, Ren X, Steinberg BA, et al. Catheter ablation of atrial fibrillation in patients with heart failure and preserved ejection fraction. Hear Rhythm 2018;15(5):651–7.

42. Hwang SJ, Melenovsky V, Borlaug BA. Implications of coronary artery disease in heart failure with preserved ejection fraction. J Am Coll Cardiol 2014; 63(25):2817–27.

43. Dunlay SM, Givertz MM, Aguilar D, et al. Type 2 Diabetes Mellitus and Heart Failure a Scientific Statement from the American Heart Association and the Heart Failure Society of America. Circulation 2019; 140. https://doi.org/10.1161/CIR.0000000000000691.

44. Yusuf S, Pfeffer MA, Swedberg K, et al. Effects of candesartan in patients with chronic heart failure and preserved left-ventricular ejection fraction: the CHARM-Preserved Trial. Lancet 2003;362(9386): 777–81.

45. Lund LH, Claggett B, Liu J, et al. Heart failure with mid-range ejection fraction in CHARM: characteristics, outcomes and effect of candesartan across the entire ejection fraction spectrum. Eur J Heart Fail 2018;20(8):1230–9.

46. Rogers JK, Pocock SJ, McMurray JJV, et al. Corrigendum to "Analysing recurrent hospitalizations in heart failure: A review of statistical methodology, with application to CHARM-Preserved" [Eur J Heart Fail 2014;16:33-40]. Eur J Heart Fail 2014;16(5):592.

47. Solomon SD, Janardhanan R, Verma A, et al. Effect of angiotensin receptor blockade and antihypertensive drugs on diastolic function in patients with hypertension and diastolic dysfunction: a randomised trial. Lancet 2007;369(9579):2079–87.

48. Cleland JGF, Tendera M, Adamus J, Freemantle N, Polonski L, Taylor J. The perindopril in elderly people with chronic heart failure (PEP-CHF) study. Eur Heart J 2006;27(19):2338–45.

49. Edelmann F. Effect of spironolactone on diastolic function in hypertensive left ventricular hypertrophy. JAMA. Published online 2013. https://doi.org/10.1038/jhh.2014.83.

50. Pitt B. Spironolactone in heart failure with preserved ejection fraction. N Engl J Med 2014;258(1774):10.

51. Pfeffer MA, Claggett B, Assmann SF, et al. Regional variation in patients and outcomes in the treatment of preserved cardiac function heart failure with an aldosterone antagonist (TOPCAT) trial. Circulation 2015;131(1):34–42.

52. Pfeffer MA, Braunwald E. Treatment of heart failure with preserved ejection fraction: Reflections on its treatment with an aldosterone antagonist. JAMA Cardiol 2016;1(1):7–8.

53. Solomon SD, Claggett B, Lewis EF, et al. Influence of ejection fraction on outcomes and efficacy of spironolactone in patients with heart failure with preserved ejection fraction. Eur Heart J 2016;37(5):455–62.

54. Solomon SD, McMurray JJV, Anand IS, et al. Angiotensin–Neprilysin Inhibition in Heart Failure with Preserved Ejection Fraction. N Engl J Med 2019;381(17):1609–20.

55. Solomon SD, Vaduganathan M, Claggett B L, et al. Sacubitril/Valsartan across the Spectrum of Ejection Fraction in Heart Failure. Circulation. Published online 2020;352–61.

56. Pieske B. Effect of Sacubitril/Valsartan vs Standard Medical Therapies on Plasma NT-proBNP Concentration and Submaximal Exercise Capacity in Patients With Heart Failure and Preserved Ejection Fraction The PARALLAX Randomized Clinical Trial. JAMA 2021;1919–29. https://doi.org/10.1001/jama.2021.18463.

57. Flather MD, Shibata MC, Coats AJS, et al. FAST-TRACK Randomized trial to determine the effect of nebivolol on mortality and cardiovascular hospital admission in elderly patients with heart failure (SENIORS). Eur Heart J 2005;26(3):215–25.

58. van Veldhuisen DJ, Cohen-Solal A, Böhm M, et al. Beta-Blockade With Nebivolol in Elderly Heart Failure Patients With Impaired and Preserved Left Ventricular Ejection Fraction. Data From SENIORS (Study of Effects of Nebivolol Intervention on Outcomes and Rehospitalization in Seniors With Heart Failure). J Am Coll Cardiol 2009;53(23):2150–8.

59. Cleland JGF, Bunting KV, Flather MD, et al. Beta-blockers for heart failure with reduced, mid-range, and preserved ejection fraction: An individual patient-level analysis of double-blind randomized trials. Eur Heart J 2018;39(1):26–35.

60. Yamamoto K, Origasa H, Hori M. Effects of carvedilol on heart failure with preserved ejection fraction: The Japanese Diastolic Heart Failure Study (J-DHF). Eur J Heart Fail 2013;15(1):110–8.

61. Palau P, Seller J, Domínguez E, et al. Effect of β-Blocker Withdrawal on Functional Capacity in Heart Failure and Preserved Ejection Fraction. J Am Coll Cardiol 2021;78(21):2042–56.

62. Bhatt DL, Szarek M, Steg PG, et al. Sotagliflozin in Patients with Diabetes and Recent Worsening Heart Failure. N Engl J Med 2021;384(2):117–28.

63. Anker SD, Butler J, Filippatos G, et al. Empagliflozin in Heart Failure with a Preserved Ejection Fraction. N Engl J Med 2021;385(16):1451–61.

64. Butler J, Packer M, Filippatos G, et al. Effect of empagliflozin in patients with heart failure across the spectrum of left ventricular ejection fraction. Eur Heart J 2021;1–11. Available at: https://academic.oup.com/eurheartj/advance-article/doi/10.1093/eurheartj/ehab798/6455932.

65. Butler J, Filippatos G, Siddiqi TJ, et al. Empagliflozin , Health Status , and Quality of Life in Patients with Heart Failure and Preserved Ejection Fraction : The EMPEROR-Preserved Trial.

66. Nassif ME, Windsor SL, Borlaug BA, et al. The SGLT2 inhibitor dapagliflozin in heart failure with preserved ejection fraction: a multicenter randomized trial. Nat Med 2021;27(11):1954–60.

67. Ahmed A, Rich MW, Fleg JL, et al. Effects of digoxin on morbidity and mortality in diastolic heart failure: The ancillary digitalis investigation group trial. Circulation 2006;114(5):397–403.

68. Redfield MM, Chen HH, Borlaug BA, et al. Effect of phosphodiesterase-5 inhibition on exercise capacity and clinical status in heart failure with preserved ejection fraction: A randomized clinical trial. JAMA 2013;309(12):1268–77.

69. Redfield MM, Anstrom KJ, Levine JA, et al. Isosorbide Mononitrate in Heart Failure with Preserved Ejection Fraction. N Engl J Med 2015;373(24):2314–24.

70. Borlaug BA, Anstrom KJ, Lewis GD, et al. Effect of Inorganic Nitrite vs Placebo on Exercise Capacity among Patients with Heart Failure with Preserved Ejection Fraction: The INDIE-HFpEF Randomized Clinical Trial. JAMA 2018;320(17):1764–73.

71. Lam CSP, Solomon SD. Fussing over the middle child. Circulation 2017;135(14):1279–80.

72. Vaishnav J, Sharma K. A Stepwise Guide to the Diagnosis and Treatment of Heart Failure with Preserved Ejection Fraction. J Card Fail 2021. https://doi.org/10.1016/j.cardfail.2021.12.013.

73. Wintrich J, Kindermann I, Ukena C, et al. Therapeutic approaches in heart failure with preserved

ejection fraction: past, present, and future. Clin Res Cardiol 2020;109(9):1079–98.

74. Kitzman DW, Brubaker P, Morgan T, et al. Effect of caloric restriction or aerobic exercise training on peak oxygen consumption and quality of life in obese older patients with heart failure with preserved ejection fraction: A randomized clinical trial. JAMA - J Am Med Assoc. 2016;315(1):36–46.

75. Mentz RJ, Whellan DJ, Reeves GR, et al. Rehabilitation Intervention in Older Patients With Acute Heart Failure With Preserved Versus Reduced Ejection Fraction. JACC Hear Fail 2021;9(10):747–57.

76. Edelmann F, Gelbrich G, Dngen HD, et al. Exercise training improves exercise capacity and diastolic function in patients with heart failure with preserved ejection fraction: Results of the Ex-DHF (exercise training in diastolic heart failure) pilot study. J Am Coll Cardiol 2011;58(17):1780–91.

77. Feldman T, Mauri L, Kahwash R, et al. Transcatheter Interatrial Shunt Device for the Treatment of Heart Failure with Preserved Ejection Fraction (REDUCE LAP-HF i [Reduce Elevated Left Atrial Pressure in Patients with Heart Failure]): A Phase 2, Randomized, Sham-Controlled Trial. Circulation 2018;137(4):364–75.

78. Shah SJ, Feldman T, Ricciardi MJ, et al. One-Year Safety and Clinical Outcomes of a Transcatheter Interatrial Shunt Device for the Treatment of Heart Failure with Preserved Ejection Fraction in the Reduce Elevated Left Atrial Pressure in Patients with Heart Failure (REDUCE LAP-HF I) Trial: A Ran. JAMA Cardiol 2018;3(10):968–77.

79. Berry N, Mauri L, Feldman T, et al. Transcatheter InterAtrial Shunt Device for the treatment of heart failure: Rationale and design of the pivotal randomized trial to REDUCE Elevated Left Atrial Pressure in Patients with Heart Failure II (REDUCE LAP-HF II): Rationale and design of REDUCE LA. Am Heart J 2020;226:222–31.

80. Shah SJ, Borlaug BA, Chung ES, et al. Atrial shunt device for heart failure with preserved and mildly reduced ejection fraction (REDUCE LAP-HF II): a randomised, multicentre, blinded, sham-controlled trial. Lancet 2022;6736(22):1–11.

81. Lindenfeld JA, Zile MR, Desai AS, et al. Haemodynamic-guided management of heart failure (GUIDE-HF): a randomised controlled trial. Lancet 2021;398(10304):991–1001.

82. Greene SJ, DeVore AD, Sheng S, et al. Representativeness of a Heart Failure Trial by Race and Sex: Results From ASCEND-HF and GWTG-HF. JACC Hear Fail 2019;7(11):980–92.

83. Greene SJ, Butler J, Albert NM, et al. Medical Therapy for Heart Failure With Reduced Ejection Fraction: The CHAMP-HF Registry. J Am Coll Cardiol 2018;72(4):351–66.

84. Greene SJ, Fonarow GC, DeVore AD, et al. Titration of Medical Therapy for Heart Failure With Reduced Ejection Fraction. J Am Coll Cardiol 2019;73(19):2365–83.

85. Brunner-La Rocca HP, Linssen GC, Smeele FJ, et al. Contemporary Drug Treatment of Chronic Heart Failure With Reduced Ejection Fraction: The CHECK-HF Registry. JACC Hear Fail 2019;7(1):13–21.

86. Solomon SD, de Boer RA, DeMets D, et al. Dapagliflozin in heart failure with preserved and mildly reduced ejection fraction: rationale and design of the DELIVER trial. Eur J Heart Fail 2021;23(7):1217–25.

87. Zamani P, Rawat D, Shiva-Kumar P, et al. Effect of inorganic nitrate on exercise capacity in heart failure with preserved ejection fraction. Circulation 2015;131(4):371–80.

88. Borlaug BA, Koepp KE, Melenovsky V. Sodium Nitrite Improves Exercise Hemodynamics and Ventricular Performance in Heart Failure with Preserved Ejection Fraction. J Am Coll Cardiol 2015;66(15):1672–82.

89. Borlaug BA, Melenovsky V, Koepp KE. Inhaled Sodium Nitrite Improves Rest and Exercise Hemodynamics in Heart Failure with Preserved Ejection Fraction. Circ Res 2016;119(7):880–6.

90. Eggebeen J, Kim-Shapiro DB, Haykowsky M, et al. One Week of Daily Dosing With Beetroot Juice Improves Submaximal Endurance and Blood Pressure in Older Patients With Heart Failure and Preserved Ejection Fraction. JACC Hear Fail 2016;4(6):428–37.

91. Fudim M, Abraham WT, von Bardeleben RS, et al. Device Therapy in Chronic Heart Failure: JACC State-of-the-Art Review. J Am Coll Cardiol 2021;78(9):931–56.

92. Rosalia L, Ozturk C, Shoar S, et al. Device-Based Solutions to Improve Cardiac Physiology and Hemodynamics in Heart Failure With Preserved Ejection Fraction. JACC Basic to Transl Sci 2021;6(9-10):772–95.

93. DeVore AD, McNulty S, Alenezi F, et al. Impaired left ventricular global longitudinal strain in patients with heart failure with preserved ejection fraction: insights from the RELAX trial. Eur J Heart Fail 2017;19(7):893–900.

Nonpharmacological Strategies in Heart Failure with Preserved Ejection Fraction

Natalie J. Bohmke, MS, EP-C[a,b,1], Hayley E. Billingsley, MS, RD, CEP[a,b,1],
Danielle L. Kirkman, PhD, MS, RCEP[a,b,*],
Salvatore Carbone, PhD, MS, FHFSA[a,b,*]

KEYWORDS

- HFpEF • Exercise • HIIT training • Dietary pattern • Caloric restriction • Sodium restriction
- Malnutrition • Obesity

KEY POINTS

- Patients with heart failure with preserved ejection fraction (HFpEF) have reduced cardiorespiratory fitness (CRF) which has a detrimental impact on survival and quality of life.
- Both moderate-intensity and high-intensity exercise training result in beneficial increases in CRF and quality of life in patients with HFpEF.
- Exercise training adaptations resulting in improved CRF are more likely peripheral than cardiac in nature in patients with HFpEF.
- Caloric restriction-induced weight loss and exercise training, both alone and in combination, produce increases in CRF and quality of life that are proportional to weight loss.
- Personalized nutrition interventions result in decreases in mortality post-hospitalization for patients with heart failure (HF); however, future investigation should be performed specifically in patients with HFpEF.
- Dietary patterns may be instrumental in primary and secondary prevention of HFpEF, large, randomized control trials are urgently needed.

INTRODUCTION

Heart failure (HF) with preserved ejection fraction (HFpEF) is associated with poor prognosis, reduced cardiorespiratory fitness (CRF), and quality of life (QoL).[1] Pharmaceutical therapies for HFpEF are limited, making HFpEF one of the greatest unmet medical needs in cardiovascular medicine.[1] Nonpharmacological therapies, particularly exercise training (ET) and dietary interventions, are attractive strategies to improve CRF, QoL and clinical outcomes in this population. The aim of this narrative review is to characterize the effects of nonpharmacological therapies in patients with HFpEF, with a focus on ET and dietary interventions.

REDUCED CARDIORESPIRATORY FITNESS IN PATIENTS WITH HEART FAILURE WITH PRESERVED EJECTION FRACTION

Exercise intolerance, characterized by exertional fatigue and dyspnea on exertion, is a hallmark symptom of HFpEF.[2] Patients with HFpEF have

---

[a] Department of Kinesiology & Health Sciences, College of Humanities & Sciences, Virginia Commonwealth University, 500 Academic Centre, Room 113C 1020 W Grace Street, Richmond, VA 23220, USA; [b] Division of Cardiology, Department of Internal Medicine, VCU Pauley Heart Center, Virginia Commonwealth University, West Hospital 6th Floor, North Wing Box, 980036 Richmond, VA 23298, USA
[1] equal contribution.
* Corresponding authors.
E-mail addresses: dlkirkman@vcu.edu (D.L.K.); scarbone@vcu.edu (S.C.)

Cardiol Clin 40 (2022) 491–506
https://doi.org/10.1016/j.ccl.2022.06.003

low CRF, defined as peak oxygen consumption ($VO_{2\ peak}$) compared to age-matched individuals without HFpEF.[3–6] This results in patients working at high percentages of their maximal capacity even when completing typical activities of daily living. Ultimately, this has detrimental consequences on their QoL. The Fick equation defines $VO_{2\ peak}$ as the product of cardiac output (heart rate [HR] • stroke volume [SV]) and arterio-venous oxygen (a-vO$_2$) difference.[3–8] Although central cardiac limitations significantly contribute to reduced $VO_{2\ peak}$,[9] a-vO$_2$ difference[6,7] is also significantly lower in HFpEF. This poses a paradigm shift away from the heart, and rather implicates peripheral limitations as a key contributor to the markedly reduced CRF in this population. These peripheral limitations have been proposed to result from a low skeletal muscle capillary to muscle fiber ratio,[3] a higher percentage of type II glycolytic muscle fibers,[3] as well as lower oxidative phosphorylation rates and a greater reliance on anaerobic glycolysis during activity.[5] Citrate synthase activity and porin protein expression in the skeletal muscle, markers of mitochondrial function and content, are lower in HFpEF compared to healthy controls which may further contribute to altered oxygen utilization and reduced $VO_{2\ peak}$.[4] Finally, patients with HFpEF have an increased intermuscular fat/skeletal muscle mass ratio, which could shunt blood flow away from the muscle thus reducing oxygen delivery and utilization.[4]

EXERCISE TRAINING

Despite the lack of data on the effects of exercise training (ET) in HFpEF on hard clinical outcomes such as mortality and hospitalizations, ET consistently improves CRF in this population through both cardiac[10] and peripheral adaptations.[11,12] However, among different ET studies, there is often inconsistency related to the modality and/or intensity of ET implemented, making it difficult to identify the most effective exercise prescription. We will, therefore, discuss the role of different forms of ET with a particular focus on QoL, CRF, and its physiological determinants.

Moderate Continuous Training

Moderate-intensity, continuous exercise training (MCT) is a traditional form of exercise prescription that typically involves prolonged bouts (30–60 minutes) of sustained moderate-intensity aerobic exercise. In HFpEF, MCT interventions have varied in mode and duration.

In a 16-week randomized controlled trial in 52 patients with HFpEF, MCT involving walking and cycling three times a week for a duration of 60 minutes per session, with intensity progressively increased from 40% to 70% heart rate reserve (HRR), was compared with an attention control group that received telephone calls every two weeks from study staff focused on retention, reminders of upcoming study visits and new medical events without discussing exercise.[13] In this study, MCT resulted in superior improvements in $VO_{2\ peak}$ compared to the attention control group (MCT + 2.7 mL•kg^{-1}•min^{-1} vs. Control − 0.3 mL•kg^{-1}•min^{-1}).[13] MCT also led to significant increases in power output, exercise time, peak HR, HRR, oxygen pulse, ventilatory anaerobic threshold, and 6-minute walk test (6MWT) distance compared to the control group.[13] In this trial, a subset analysis of 40 patients with adequate echocardiographic images during upright rest and maximal cycle exercise showed no differences between groups in cardiac function parameters,[14] suggesting that the improvements in CRF resulted from peripheral adaptations.

The Study of the Effect of Caloric Restriction and Exercise Training in Patients With Heart Failure and a Normal Ejection Fraction (SECRET) trial utilized a factorial randomized controlled approach to explore the effects of MCT, caloric restriction (CR), both, or usual care control on coprimary outcomes of $VO_{2\ peak}$ and self-reported QoL assessed via Minnesota Living with Heart Failure Questionnaire (MLHFQ) in 100 patients with obesity and HFpEF.[15] The MCT intervention consisted of 1-hour supervised aerobic ET 3 times weekly, usually walking, based on individualized prescription with the intensity increased as tolerated.[15] The effects of CR in this trial will be discussed in greater detail later in this review. After 20 weeks, those assigned to MCT lost ~3% of their body weight and increased $VO_{2\ peak}$ by 1.2 mL•kg^{-1}•min^{-1}.[15] No changes in cardiac function, assessed by echocardiography and cardiac magnetic resonance imaging, were observed with MCT, thus providing further support for peripherally mediated training adaptations. Self-reported QoL did not improve in the MCT group.[15]

Recently, the Heart Failure Exercise and Resistance Training (HEART) Camp trial included 204 patients with HF randomized to HEART Camp training or enhanced usual care (EUC) for 18 months.[16] All patients were provided with a free membership to an exercise facility with professional exercise staff. Study staff assisted patients with equipment and provided safety advice; however, only the intervention group received ongoing individualized instruction and goal setting with a trained exercise professional. Fifty-nine patients in the original trial had HFpEF, with 25 randomized to ET and 34 randomized to

EUC. There was a significant improvement in functional capacity reported as 6MWT distance in ET compared to EUC at 18 months (ET +63.25 meters vs. Control +13.16 meters).[17]

Although there is evidence to support that MCT can increase VO_{2peak} in patients with HFpEF, the mechanisms of improvement require further elucidation. Although improvements in both systolic and diastolic function have been reported following ET,[18] most studies suggest that the improvements in CRF are largely due to noncardiac peripheral adaptations.[13,14,19,20] The reduced a-vO_2 characteristic of patients with HFpEF,[6,7] illustrating reduced oxygen delivery, extraction and utilization at the level of the skeletal muscle (SM), can be improved with MCT.[14] The exact mechanisms responsible for the exercise-related improvements in a-vO_2 differences are not fully understood. In a salt-sensitive murine model of HFpEF, ET preserved SM capillary density, maintained mitochondrial function and citrate synthase activity, and induced fiber type shifts to more fatigue-resistant type I fibers.[21] In contrast, another study has shown that ET in rats with obesity and HFpEF was unable to reverse impaired SM functionality apart from attenuated lactate dehydrogenase activity.[22] Further mechanistic work is needed in animal models of HFpEF, in addition to patients with HFpEF, on SM and mitochondrial adaptations to examine their contribution to exercise intolerance and potential improvement following ET.

High-intensity Interval Training

High-intensity interval training (HIIT) consists of a series of vigorous-intensity bouts of exercise separated by low-intensity, active recovery. In comparison to MCT, this mode of aerobic training is attractive due to shorter exercise duration and higher enjoyment levels in the general population.[23] HIIT elicits superior metabolic adaptations including a greater reduction in blood pressure, waist circumference, triglycerides, cholesterol, and fasting glucose in both the general population and untrained individuals with overweight or obesity.[24,25] To date, 2 trials have compared treadmill-based HIIT and MCT in patients with HFpEF.[26,27]

In a small pilot trial, 15 patients were randomized to four weeks of MCT or HIIT. The MCT intervention included a progressive increase in duration from 15 to 30 minutes of exercise, increasing from 60 to 70% maximum heart rate (MHR). HIIT training progressively increased to 4, 4-minute intervals at 85–90% MHR separated by 3 minutes at 50% MHR. Cardiorespiratory adaptations were observed in the HIIT group ($VO_{2\ peak}$ +1.8 mL•kg^{-1}•min^{-1}) with no changes following the MCT intervention ($VO_{2\ peak}$ −0.1 mL•kg^{-1}•min^{-1}).[26] In contrast, another study with a longer duration of ET (12 weeks) comparing MCT with HIIT found that both modalities of ET were efficacious at improving VO_{2peak}. However, increases in VO_{2peak} were substantially higher following HIIT (HIIT +3.5 mL•kg^{-1}•min^{-1}; MCT + 1.9 mL•kg^{-1}•min^{-1}).[27] Additionally, in both MCT and HIIT over the 12-week training period, peak oxygen pulse, oxygen uptake efficiency slope, and maximal ventilation increased, and minute ventilation divided by carbon dioxide production (V_E/VCO_2) (a major predictor of prognosis in HF) decreased similarly. Both MCT and HIIT significantly improved QoL measured by the MLHFQ.[27]

The Optimizing Exercise Training in Prevention and Treatment of Diastolic Heart Failure (OPTI-MEX-CLIN) trial randomized 180 patients to HIIT, MCT, or guideline-directed control with 3 months of in-person exercise followed by nine months of supervised, virtual training.[20] The HIIT intervention was 3, 38-minute sessions with a 10-minute warmup, 4, 4-minute intervals at 80–90% HRR and three minutes of active recovery; MCT consisted of 5, 40-minute sessions a week at 35–50% HRR; the guideline control received advice at the start of the study based on German physical activity guidelines with counseling to achieve 30 minutes of walking most days of the week. Both HIIT and MCT groups had significant improvements in VO_{2peak} at three months compared to the control group (HIIT +1.1 mL•kg^{-1}•min^{-11}; MCT +1.1 mL•kg^{-1}•min^{-1}; control −0.6 mL•kg^{-1}•min^{-1}) though there were no significant differences between groups at 12 months (HIIT +0.9 mL•kg^{-1}•min^{-1}; MCT +0.0 mL•kg^{-1}•min^{-1}; control −0.6 mL•kg^{-1}•min^{-1}).[20] Despite the improvements in VO_{2peak} at 3 months, there were no changes in V_E/VCO_2 slope or workload performed at the ventilatory threshold (VT).[20]

The physiological mechanisms driving the potential benefits of HIIT are unclear; specifically, whether HIIT may affect cardiac central vs peripheral limitations to reduce CRF has been explored only in a few studies. In a four-week trial investigating the effects of HIIT vs MCT in HFpEF on cardiac function, HIIT demonstrated significant improvements in diastolic dysfunction grade, with a reduction in E wave and increased deceleration time. No cardiac changes were reported after MCT.[26] In contrast, 12 weeks of HIIT and MCT equally decreased E/e', a measure of left ventricular (LV) filling pressure with no other changes in cardiac function.[27] Adding greater variability to the literature, OPTIMEX-CLIN demonstrated no differences between groups in cardiac function at any time point along with no changes in N-terminal probrain natriuretic peptide (NT-proBNP).[20] Studies of HIIT and MCT support that peripheral, rather than central, adaptations underlie the improvements in VO_{2peak} following ET in patients with HFpEF.

Vascular dysfunction in HFpEF may play a role in HFpEF-related exercise intolerance by hampering oxygen delivery to skeletal muscle.[28,29] In addition, arterial stiffness in HFpEF can contribute to exercise intolerance by altering the arterial hemodynamics and subsequently increasing the late systolic left ventricular pulsatile load.[30–32] Despite improving CRF, MCT and HIIT have not been associated with improved vascular function, measured by brachial artery flow-mediated dilation and carotid arterial stiffness and distensibility, following interventions ranging from 4 to 16 weeks.[3,26] These lack of improvements in macro-vascular function following training, suggest that the adaptations observed following training in HFpEF may rather be due to changes within the microvasculature or in peripheral SM O_2 utilization (**Fig. 1**).

Combined Resistance and Aerobic Exercise Training

To date, resistance exercise training in HFpEF has only been conducted in 2 published trials in combination with aerobic exercise training.[18] The Exercise Training in Diastolic Heart Failure (EX-DHF) study implemented a 12-week combined aerobic and resistance training intervention that resulted in a significant improvement in $VO_{2\ peak}$ (+2.6 mL•kg^{-1}•min^{-1}) and 6MWT distance.[18] The combined aerobic and resistance exercise training improved left atrial volume index, but no other cardiac parameters.[18] ET also improved self-reported physical function as assessed by both the Short Form-36 and MLHFQ.[18] A 12-month randomized controlled trial that compared MCT, HIIT, and resistance training progressively increased intensity throughout the program. Participants completed 30–60 minute sessions of walking, cycling, or swimming with a combination of maximal steady state (MSS), base pace, and interval training in the program.[33] MSS was determined from VT and lactate threshold, base pace was 1–20 beats below MSS, intervals were >95% HR peak, and recovery was less than base pace.[33] ET progressively increased to include 3 MSS sessions a month, 4 × 4 intervals twice a week, and 1–2 days of resistance training per week.[33] The control group received a combination of yoga, balance and strength training 3 times a week for a year.[33] There was a significant improvement in VO_{2peak} in the ET group and no change in the control group (ET +5.3 mL•kg^{-1}•min^{-1}; control −0.5 mL•kg^{-1}•min^{-1}).[33] Following ET, left ventricular end-systolic volume and stroke volume significantly increased and myocardial

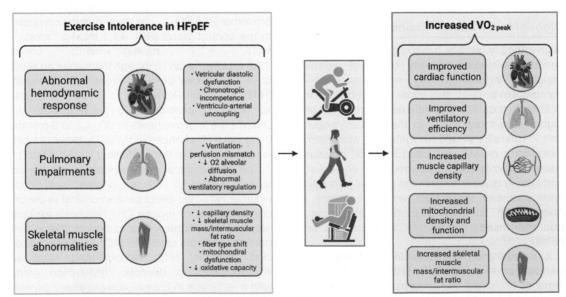

Fig. 1. *Determinants of reduced cardiorespiratory fitness and the role of exercise training in HFpEF.* Patients with heart failure with preserved ejection fraction (HFpEF) have exercise intolerance, which can be assessed as a reduction of cardiorespiratory fitness. This may result from cardiorespiratory impairments and skeletal muscle abnormalities. Exercise training in HFpEF improves central and peripheral factors to increase exercise capacity. Created with BioRender.com.

stiffness decreased, compared to no significant changes observed in the control group.[33]

Lastly, results from SECRET-II (NCT02636439), which compared resistance exercise, MCT and CR to MCT and CR with no resistance exercise in 88 patients with HFpEF and obesity over 20 weeks have not yet been made available, in addition to other ongoing clinical trials specifically testing the efficacy of different forms of ET in HFpEF (**Table 1**). Considering the fact that patients with HFpEF present an elevated risk for sarcopenia (i.e., reduced muscular strength, SM, and its functionality) and sarcopenic obesity (i.e., sarcopenia in presence of obesity),[34–36] resistance ET may be beneficial by increasing SM and muscular strength; however, additional trials that investigate changes in body composition are needed.[37–39]

Inspiratory Muscle Training

Inspiratory Muscle Training (IMT) utilizes a threshold inspiratory muscle trainer with patients breathing at a set resistance and rate of breathing. In other disease populations such as chronic obstructive pulmonary disease, IMT improves the metabolic efficiency of inspiratory muscles, in addition to increasing inspiratory muscle strength and endurance.[40] IMT also improves cardiac autonomic modulation, assessed by heart rate variability.[41] In HF, patients have an exaggerated ventilatory response to exercise that increases the metabolic demand of the inspiratory muscle and subsequently shunts blood flow away from the locomotor muscles culminating in earlier onset of fatigue.[42] Therefore, it is plausible that the previously reported beneficial adaptations to IMT in COPD may also improve exercise capacity in HFpEF. Two IMT trials have been conducted in HFpEF. In a randomized crossover trial, IMT was conducted with 20 minutes of IMT twice a day for 12 weeks. Resistance of IMT was set at 25–30% maximal inspiratory mouth pressure (% MIP) which was adjusted following weekly testing. At 12 weeks, there was a significant improvement in VO_{2peak} following IMT (IMT: + 2.9 mL•kg^{-1}•min^{-1}; control −1.0 mL•kg^{-1}•min^{-1}), V_E/VCO_2 slope, and 6 MWT distance.[43] In addition, IMT improved QoL assessed by the MLFHQ.[43] There were no significant changes in echocardiographic parameters or NT-proBNP following the 12 weeks of IMT.[43] Another pilot study randomized 20 patients with HFpEF to IMT or usual care. IMT included 20 minutes of at-home training once a day, for 24 weeks, at 30% of MIP, assessed monthly.[44] On multivariate analysis, IMT was significantly associated with the increase in AT (estimated treatment effect: 2.866 ± 1.161, $p = 0.02$) and associated with the improvement in % MIP (estimated treatment effect: 31.997 ± 13.981, $p = 0.03$).[44] No additional CRF variables were significantly associated with the treatment, and echocardiography and QoL data were not included. IMT is a promising intervention for patients with low levels of CRF or mobility impairments; however, additional work is needed to understand the impact of IMT on HFpEF.

Dietary Interventions in Heart Failure with Preserved Ejection Fraction

In addition to ET, dietary interventions can also improve $VO_{2\ peak}$ and QoL in patients with HFpEF.[15,45] Moreover, multiple ongoing dietary intervention trials in HFpEF have appointed measures of CRF as the primary or a secondary outcome (see **Table 1**). Here, we present information solely on changes to diet, rather than the addition of nutraceuticals, but we have previously explored the latter topic in patients with HF.[46,47]

Caloric Restriction and Intentional Weight Loss

Obesity, defined as excess fat mass (FM) that impairs health, substantially increases the risk for HF.[48] This relationship between obesity and HF is heavily mediated by the reduced CRF[49] and glycemic abnormalities[50] related to obesity. Importantly, up to 80% of patients with HFpEF also have comorbid overweight or obesity,[51] to the extent that an obese HFpEF phenotype has been proposed.[52] Of particular concern, obesity exacerbates declines in VO_{2peak} in patients with HFpEF,[53,54] contributing to a worsened prognosis and QoL.[6,55] With these considerations, it seems appropriate to investigate weight loss as a therapeutic modality in patients with the obese HFpEF phenotype. The effect of weight loss in the setting of established HF is, however, controversial. In this respect, there is an obesity paradox[48] whereby weight loss has been associated with increased all-cause and cardiovascular mortality regardless of left ventricular ejection fraction (LVEF) and body mass index (BMI) in HF.[56,57] In an observational cohort of patients with HFpEF weight loss was significantly associated with a 5-fold and 3-fold increased risk for all-cause mortality and HF readmission, respectively, in patients with a BMI≤25.0 kg/m^2, but not in patients with a BMI≥25.0 kg/m^2, suggesting that adverse outcomes associated with weight loss may be particularly pronounced in those individuals who are

Table 1
Ongoing and anticipated nonpharmacological trials in patients with HFpEF

NCT/PI	Trial Type	Targeted Population	N	Intervention	Primary Outcome
Exercise Training					
NCT03465072 Benjamin Lavine	Single-Arm, Open Label	HFpEF	22	8 Weeks ET 3x per week, 30–40 minutes per Session	Change in Muscle Sympathetic Nerve Activity Change in $VO_{2\,peak}$
NCT05162859 Isabel Fegers-Wustrow and Stephan Mueller	Observational Retrospective Study	HFpEF	100	Long-term follow-up (4.6–9.1 years) of patients that were recruited for OptimEX-Clin (control, HIIT, or MCT) or Ex-DHF (usual care or MCT and resistance training)	Change in $VO_{2\,peak}$
NCT05002075 Ambarish Pandey	Randomized Controlled Trial	HFpEF	20	24 weeks of home-based ET through m-heath cardiac rehab application vs SOC	Change in standard physical performance battery score
NCT03184311 Arno Schmidt-Trucksäss	Randomized Controlled Trial	HFpEF	86	HIIT vs. MCT, 12 weeks of supervised cycle ergometry ET 3 times a week, HIIT: 4, 4-minute intervals at 85–95% peak HR with 3 min active recovery at 60–80% peak HR; MCT: 47 minutes at 60–70% peak HR	Change in $VO_{2\,peak}$
NCT05115890 Kanokwen Bunsawat	Single-Arm, Open Label	HFpEF	35	Two-legged, knee extensor exercise training, 3 days per week for 8 weeks. Exercise intensity will range between 40% and 90% of maximal work rate, reassessed every 2 weeks	Change in 6MWT distance Change in muscle blood flow
NCT05255172 Katarina Steding-Ehrenborg and Håkan Arheden	Randomized Controlled Trial	HFpEF	120	ET vs SOC; 12 weeks of aerobic exercise, 3 sessions of cycling a week, 2 supervised sessions with 20 minutes cycling below AT, and 1 unsupervised session of 30 minutes of "somewhat hard" walking or cycling	Change in $VO_{2\,peak}$

(continued on next page)

Table 1
(continued)

NCT/PI	Trial Type	Targeted Population	N	Intervention	Primary Outcome
NCT02762825 Steven J. Keteyian	Randomized Controlled Trial	HFpEF	66	HIIT vs MCT, HIIT: 4 mins 90% HRR with 3 min recovery 60–70% HRR, resistance training performed once a week, MCT: 30 mins, 3 times a week, 60–80% HRR	Change in VO$_{2\ peak}$
NCT03924479 Thomas P. Olson	Randomized Controlled Trial	HFpEF	30	Breathing muscle training vs sham, 8 weeks of 30 minutes of breathing training ~ 15 times each minute once a day, intervention resistance at 40% maximal breathing strength, sham resistance at 2% maximal breathing strength	Change in breathing muscle oxygen cost Change in respiratory muscle blood flow Change in systolic and diastolic blood pressure

Combined Dietary Intervention and Exercise Training

NCT/PI	Trial Type	Targeted Population	N	Intervention	Primary Outcome
NCT05236413 Siddartha Angadi	Randomized Controlled Trial	HFpEF	36	HIIT training vs. DASH diet vs. HIIT training and DASH diet, exercise supervised, all meals provided to participants, for 4 weeks	Change in VO$_{2\ peak}$
NCT02636439 Dalane Kitzman	Randomized Controlled Trial	HFpEF, Obesity	88	Resistance training, CR and MCT vs. CR and MCT for 20 weeks in patients with HFpEF and obesity	Change in VO$_{2\ peak}$

Dietary Intervention

NCT/PI	Trial Type	Targeted Population	N	Intervention	Primary Outcome
NCT04173117 Grace Walters and Emer Brady	Single-Arm, Open Label	HFpEF and T2DM	20	Low-calorie meal replacement program (~810 kcals/day) for 12 weeks or once 50% excess body weight is lost, whichever comes first	Recruitment and retention rate

(continued on next page)

Table 1
(continued)

NCT/PI	Trial Type	Targeted Population	N	Intervention	Primary Outcome
NCT04235699 Sitaramesh Emani	Randomized Controlled Trial	HFpEF	24	Hypocaloric ketogenic diet vs. hypocaloric low-fat diet, all meals provided to participants, for 4 weeks	Change in VO$_{2\ peak}$
NCT04942548 Darlene Kim	Not Specified	HFpEF, HFpEF and PAH	25	Ketogenic diet, not provided - dietary counseling given to participants to follow the diet over 6 months	Change in MLHFQ (HFpEF), Change in PAH-SYMPACT (HFpEF and PAH)
NCT05117086 Francene Steinberg	Single-Arm, Open Label	HF	25	Dietary counseling to follow the DASH dietary pattern for 6 months	Dietary Intake, DASH Diet Score, systolic and diastolic blood pressure at baseline, 3, and 6 months
NCT03966755 Salvatore Carbone	Randomized Controlled Crossover Trial	HFpEF, Obesity	30	Unsaturated fatty acid supplementation vs. SOC (dietary sodium and saturated fat restriction), each phase 12 weeks, 6-week washout period in-between	Change in 24-hour dietary recall, change in biomarkers of UFA intake
NCT02892747 Véronique Bendedyga	Randomized Controlled Trial	HF	295	Personalized dietary counseling aimed at preventing malnutrition and reducing sodium intake vs. control (no personalized counseling) for 6 months	Number, duration, and reasons for hospitalization

Abbreviations: 6MWT, six-minute walk test; AT, anaerobic threshold; CR, caloric restriction; DASH, Dietary Approaches to Stop Hypertension; ET, exercise training; HF, heart failure; HIIT, high-intensity interval training; HR, heart rate; HRR, heart rate reserve; MCT, moderate continuous training; m-health, mobile health; MLHFQ, Minnesota Living with Heart Failure Questionnaire; PAH, Pulmonary Arterial Hypertension; PAH-SYMPACT, Pulmonary Arterial Hypertension Symptoms, and Impact questionnaire; SOC, standard of care; VO$_{2\ peak}$, peak oxygen consumption.

already lean.[57] In both of the above analyses, intentionality of the weight loss was not known.[56,57] Unintentional weight loss observed in HF may be due to cachexia-catabolism of SM and adipose tissue associated with severe disease.[36] Thus, poor outcomes observed with weight loss may be the result of a marker of increasing disease severity rather than a consequence of weight loss itself.

Outside of its relationship with weight loss, inadequate caloric intake may be independently associated with poor outcomes in patients with HF, even if they have concomitant obesity,[58,59] indicating that caution is warranted when pursuing weight loss through CR in patients with HF.

Only 2 trials of intentional weight loss in HFpEF have been completed to date. The SECRET trial described previously, utilized a factorial randomized control trial to explore the effects of CR with all meals and snacks, except for breakfast, provided by the research team and energy and nutrient requirements calculated by a research dietitian, MCT, both, or usual care control on coprimary outcomes of $VO_{2\ peak}$ and MLHFQ.[15] After 20 weeks, patients assigned to CR lost ~7% of their body weight and $VO_{2\ peak}$ was increased by CR (+1.3 mL•kg^{-1}•min^{-1}).[15] CR did not increase one of the coprimary endpoints of QoL measured as the changes in MLHFQ; however, CR increased the secondary endpoint of QoL assessed via the KCCQ. Notably, outside a decrease in LV mass and relative wall thickness with CR, no changes were noted in cardiac parameters for CR, suggesting that the changes in $VO_{2\ peak}$ were driven by peripheral changes.[15] This is illustrated by an inverse association between increases in $VO_{2\ peak}$ and reductions in FM, as well as a positive association between increases in $VO_{2\ peak}$ and thigh SM to intermuscular fat ratio.[15]

Another recent trial assigned 60 patients with HFpEF and obesity to combined CR and exercise training for 15 weeks, assessing a coprimary outcome of QoL assessed by MLHFQ and 6MWT distance.[60] The authors suggested that the format utilized, offering meal replacement bars and shakes for 2 daily meals as well as an exercise prescription without supervision, more closely mirrored a typical clinical setting than SECRET, which provided supervised exercise training and daily meals and snacks to participants.[60] It should be noted that participants did have weekly in-person follow-up alternating between dietitians, exercise specialists, and behavioral specialists for the duration of the trial.[60] At 15 weeks, there was a significant increase in 6MWT distance (223 to 281 meters) as well as an improvement in MLHFQ (37% score decrease).[60] Patients lost 6.7% of their body weight at the 15 week mark- some weight regain occurred by 26 weeks, but a 5.3% total decrease from baseline was maintained.[60] There was a significant association between weight change and MLHFQ score and inverse association with 6MWT distance, suggesting that a greater decrease in weight would result in a greater improvement in both parameters.[60] Lastly, changes in echocardiography were measured and the only significant change was a decrease in E/e' at 26, but not 15 weeks.[60] Most notably, there was 32% attrition rate- 19 of the 60 patients enrolled did not reach the 15 week mark and were excluded from analysis. This, along with the nonrandomized intervention, likely favorably biased the results of the study.[60] Only 8% attrition was observed in SECRET[15]; it is possible that SECRET's more frequent in-person

interaction encouraged participants to complete the program.

Intentional weight loss appears to improve CRF and QoL in patients with HFpEF and obesity. An analysis that included patients who initially participated in SECRET, however, underlined that weight regain is likely to occur post-intervention, most of which is FM,[61] potentially increasing the risk for sarcopenia and sarcopenic obesity. Taken together, low adherence to the intervention and high risk for weight regain clearly highlight the limitations of CR and emphasize the potential need for regular, long-term follow-up with a multidisciplinary team to maintain weight loss.

Malnutrition-targeted Interventions

Protein-energy malnutrition describes inadequate caloric and protein intake to support health. In a clinical setting, however, the term malnutrition is often used to encompass lean mass abnormalities that may be better defined as sarcopenia, sarcopenic obesity (Fig. 2) or cachexia.[36] Malnutrition has long been a concern in patients with HF,[62] and has been linked to higher risk of mortality in patients with HFpEF.[63]

While no studies have conducted malnutrition interventions specifically on patients with HFpEF, the PICNIC trial (Nutritional Intervention Program in Hospitalized Patients with Heart Failure who are Malnourished) established a diagnosis of malnutrition based on the Mini-Nutritional Assessment (MNA) score in 120 patients hospitalized for decompensated HF (LVEF 49 ± 17%).[64] Individualized intervention focusing on diet optimization and supplements as needed began while patients were still hospitalized and continued for 6 months. At 12 months, the composite endpoint of all-cause mortality or readmission for HF occurred in 61% of the control group and 27% of those assigned to individualized nutrition care (HR: 0.45, 95% CI 0.19–0.62).[64] At 24 months, 47% of the intervention group and 73% of the control group had met the primary endpoint (HR: 0.53, 95% CI 0.31–0.89), demonstrating the long-term clinical benefit of the intervention. The point estimate for benefit was similar in HFpEF and in participants with LVEF <50%.[65]

A subgroup analysis of the EFFORT trial (Effect of Early Nutritional Support on Frailty, Functional Outcomes, and Recovery of Malnourished Medical Inpatients) included 645 inpatients based on a Nutritional Risk Screening 2002 (NRS) score at admission and documented HF regardless of LVEF.[66] Nutrition support was individualized to the patient and focused on meeting caloric, protein, and micronutrient intake goals while

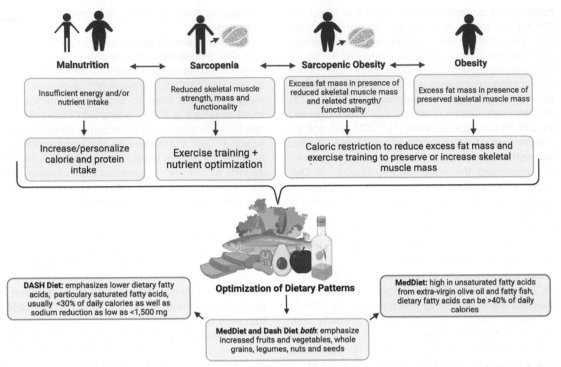

Fig. 2. *Nutrition status abnormalities in HFpEF and targeted interventions in HFpEF.* Patients with heart failure with preserved ejection fraction (HFpEF) have a high risk and high prevalence of nutrition status abnormalities including malnutrition, sarcopenia, sarcopenic obesity, and obesity alone. There is a high likelihood of patients with HFpEF transitioning between these states, therefore, care should be taken to reevaluate patients on a regular basis and personalize nutrition care for the early identification of nutrition status abnormalities. Created with BioRender.com.

inpatient.[66] Patients assigned to control consumed standard inpatient diet without nutrition consultation.[66] At 30 days, 14.8% of control participants had died from any cause compared to only 8.4% of intervention participants (adjusted OR: 0.44, 95% CI: 0.26–0.75).[66] Although subgroups, including HFpEF, were investigated, sample sizes were small and there was no evidence of effect heterogeneity among subgroups.[66]

Although malnutrition worsens outcomes in HF, little is known about the incidence and treatment of malnutrition specifically in HFpEF. Malnutrition is likely under-recognized in this population due to high rates of comorbid overweight and obesity which may mask unintended weight loss, body composition changes, and inadequate intake. Further work should be conducted to examine the effects of nutrition interventions such as personalized nutrition support across the BMI spectrum in patients with HFpEF on CRF and clinical outcomes.

Sodium

While sodium restriction is perhaps the most widely utilized clinical nutrition therapy for HF, there is inadequate evidence to support beneficence.[46] Across international guidelines, recommended restriction varies from <1500 mg to <3000 mg/day, reflecting a lack of consensus on what level of restriction, if any, may produce physiologic benefit.[67] Few sodium restriction interventions have included patients with HFpEF[68,69] with only one trial to date has focused on patients with HFpEF.[70]

In a randomized study of 65 patients with HF regardless of LVEF either received nutrition counseling on adhering to sodium (2000–2400 mg/day) and fluid restriction (1.5 L/day) or control, which consisted of generalized advice to reduce sodium and fluid intake over 6 months.[68] The intervention group significantly reduced 24-hour urinary sodium, a marker of intake, by ~8% (2070 ± 727 mg/L to 1670 ± 487 mg/L), while urinary sodium increased in the control group by 29%. QoL, on the customized questionnaire, significantly increased and self-reported symptoms of HF decreased with intervention versus control.

The SODIUM-HF (Study of Dietary Intervention Under 100 mmol in Heart Failure) pilot trial randomized 38 patients with HF regardless of LVEF to either 6 months of low (1500 mg/day) or moderate (2300 mg/day) sodium intake for 6 months. A dietitian counseled both groups on following the recommended levels of sodium restriction and maintaining a usual diet outside of this. At 6 months, both groups significantly decreased self-reported sodium intake with no differences between the 2 groups (low sodium: 2137 to 1398 vs. moderate sodium: 2678 to 1461). QoL on the KCCQ improved in low sodium and trended toward an increase in the moderate sodium group without differences between groups. No significant changes occurred in self-reported HF symptoms. The multi-center SODIUM-HF trial (NCT02012179) randomized 806 outpatients with HF (mean LVEF ~36%, mean BMI ~30 kg/m²) to either low sodium (1500 mg/day) or control.[71] The dietitian-guided strategy successfully reduced reported sodium intake by ~25% (from 2,268 to 1,658 mg/day). The open-label intervention did not meet the primary composite endpoint of cardiovascular-related hospitalization, cardiovascular-related emergency department visit, or all-cause death (adjusted HR: 0.99, 95% CI 0.66–1.47), nor the individual components of the composite endpoint taken individually. Moreover, the intervention was not associated with improved 6MWT distance, while it was associated with improved QoL and reduction in NYHA class. Considering the open-label nature of the study and the lack of improvements in the primary endpoint, these potential improvements in QoL and NYHA classes should be considered exploratory. Of note, enrolled participants had relatively low sodium intake at the start of the trial, which remained low throughout the duration of the study (from 2,119 to 2,073 mg/day), and a lower-than-expected event rate, which could have attenuated potential benefits.[71]

Only one trial has investigated the effects of sodium restriction on patients with HFpEF specifically.[70] While admitted for decompensated HF, 53 patients with HFpEF were randomized to sodium (800 mg/day) and fluid (800 mL/day) restriction or standard of care (4000 mg sodium and unlimited fluid).[70] No difference was observed in the primary outcome of weight loss at discharge between groups (intervention −1.6 ± 2.2 kg vs. control: −1.8 ± 2.1 kg) nor was any difference detected between groups in clinical congestion score.[70] Importantly, caloric intake during admission was lower in the intervention group than the control (intervention: 1159 ± 238 kcals vs. control: 1471 ± 265 kcals),[70] a common, and concerning, observation in sodium restriction trials.[47,68,72]

Currently, there is inadequate evidence to recommend sodium restriction for the management of HF signs and symptoms in the inpatient and outpatient settings. Large trials adequately powered to examine outcomes in HFpEF patients specifically are necessary. Moreover, future work should focus on isocaloric sodium restriction interventions to avoid unintended weight loss and inadequate intake in a population at elevated risk for malnutrition.

Dietary Patterns and Time of Eating

The dietary patterns best investigated for their effects on HF primary and secondary prevention remain the Mediterranean diet (MedDiet) and the Dietary Approaches to Stop Hypertension (DASH) diet. Still, limited work, especially randomized control trials, has been performed in this area. and even less has focused specifically on HFpEF.

Greater adherence to the MedDiet has been associated with a lower risk for HF,[73] and favorable outcomes in those with established HF, particularly acute decompensated HF.[74,75] However, little is known about the effects of MedDiet in patients with HFpEF.[76] Though it is not clear which feature of the MedDiet may contribute to improved outcomes in HF, including HFpEF, the role of unsaturated fatty acids (UFA), including foods such as mixed nuts and EVOO, typical foods of the MedDiet, warrants discussion. In a cross-sectional analysis of 23 patients with obesity and HFpEF, greater intake of UFA was significantly associated with favorable VO_{2peak} as well as measures of cardiac function and body composition.[77] Recently, in the UFA-Preserved study we have shown that UFA-rich foods supplementation, without CR, can be achieved with dietary counseling in 9 patients with HFpEF and obesity for 12 weeks, with monthly in-person visits and weekly phone calls conducted by the research dietitian.[45] Our ongoing UFA-Preserved 2 trial is further investigating the feasibility of the intervention of daily supplementation of UFA versus standard of care nutrition consisting of sodium and saturated fatty acids control following the Dietary Guidelines for Americans in 30 patients with both obesity and HFpEF in a randomized controlled cross-over study (NCT03966755).

Plasma levels of a specific type of UFA, N-3 polyunsaturated fatty acids (PUFA), have been associated with lower all-cause mortality in patients with HFpEF as well as more favorable CRF and body composition.[78,79] No randomized control trial has been performed to investigate the effects of N-3 PUFA and clinical outcomes in HFpEF.

Excellent adherence to the DASH diet is also associated with a lower risk for HF.[80] However, in patients with HFpEF, the DASH diet has been only investigated in a few studies. In inpatients admitted for decompensated HF regardless of LVEF, the GOURMET-HF trial randomized at the time of discharge 66 patients to 4 weeks of home-delivered DASH, sodium-restricted meals (<1500 mg/day), or usual care post-hospitalization.[81] At 4 weeks, the primary outcome of QoL assessed via KCCQ increased in both groups without in-between group difference (DASH/sodium restriction:+13 vs. control:+10).[81] However, HF readmissions at 4 weeks trended lower in the intervention group (DASH/sodium restriction: 11% vs. control: 27%, $P = 0.06$).[81] No analysis by type (HFpEF vs. HFrEF) was available, but earlier work demonstrated that 3 weeks of a sodium-restricted DASH diet reduced systolic and diastolic blood pressure and improved diastolic function and ventricular-arterial coupling in patients with HFpEF.[82,83]

Outside of dietary patterns, time of eating may also represent a modifiable and impactful factor in patients with HF. In our recent cross-sectional analysis of 12 patients with HFpEF and obesity, patients that ate the last evening meal after the meantime of the sample, 7:25 pm, had a greater $VO_{2\ peak}$ and exercise time than those who ate prior to 7:25pm,[84] with a positive association between increasing lateness of meal and greater CRF.[84]

Although MedDiet and DASH patterns have been associated with reduced risk for HF and related complications, larger randomized control trials, specifically in HFpEF, are required to demonstrate the efficacy of these dietary patterns on CRF, QoL, and ultimately clinical outcomes. Randomized control trials are also warranted to investigate the effects of alterations in time of eating in patients with HFpEF.

SUMMARY

Despite a paucity of pharmaceutical therapies proven to improve outcomes in HFpEF, nonpharmaceutical therapies through exercise and dietary interventions have demonstrated promising effects on CRF, QoL, and potentially clinical outcomes, particularly in patients with abnormal nutritional status (see **Figs. 1** and **2**). Future directions of exploration should include resistance training exercises as well as large, randomized control trials of dietary interventions specifically in patients with HFpEF. Moreover, understanding the mechanisms responsible for the potential improvements warrant further study.

CLINICS CARE POINTS

- Consider prescribing either moderate-intensity or high-intensity exercise training to patients with HFpEF, as exercise training is associated with beneficial increases in cardiorespiratory fitness (CRF) and quality of life

- In patients with obesity and HFpEF, caloric restriction-induced weight loss and exercise training, both alone and in combination, can produce increases in CRF and quality of life proportional to the weight loss achieved

- For hospitalized patients with HF, personalized nutrition interventions should be considered as decreases in mortality post-hospitalization have been observed

- Consider counseling patients to shift to a healthier dietary pattern, such as the Mediterranean or DASH diet which may be instrumental in primary and secondary prevention of HFpEF, although randomized control trials are urgently needed

DISCLOSURES

Supported by Career Development Awards 19CDA34740002 (DK), 19CDA34660318 (SC) from the American Heart Association, and Clinical and Translational Science Awards Program UL1TR002649 from National Institutes of Health to Virginia Commonwealth University (DK and SC).

REFERENCES

1. Del Buono MG, Iannaccone G, Scacciavillani R, et al. Heart failure with preserved ejection fraction diagnosis and treatment: an updated review of the evidence. Prog Cardiovasc Dis 2020;63(5):570–84.

2. Obokata M, Olson TP, Reddy YNV, et al. Haemodynamics, dyspnoea, and pulmonary reserve in heart failure with preserved ejection fraction. Eur Heart J 2018;39(30):2810–21.

3. Kitzman DW, Brubaker PH, Herrington DM, et al. Effect of endurance exercise training on endothelial function and arterial stiffness in older patients with heart failure and preserved ejection fraction: a randomized, controlled, single-blind trial. J Am Coll Cardiol 2013;62(7):584–92.

4. Molina AJ, Bharadwaj MS, Van Horn C, et al. Skeletal muscle mitochondrial content, oxidative capacity, and Mfn2 expression are reduced in older patients with heart failure and preserved ejection fraction

and are related to exercise intolerance. JACC Heart Fail 2016;4(8):636–45.

5. Bhella PS, Prasad A, Heinicke K, et al. Abnormal haemodynamic response to exercise in heart failure with preserved ejection fraction. Eur J Heart Fail 2011;13(12):1296–304.

6. Zamani P, Proto EA, Mazurek JA, et al. Peripheral determinants of oxygen utilization in heart failure with preserved ejection fraction: central role of adiposity. JACC BTS 2020;5(3):211–25.

7. Wolsk E, Kaye D, Komtebedde J, et al. Central and peripheral determinants of exercise capacity in heart failure patients with preserved ejection fraction. JACC Heart Fail 2019;7(4):321–32.

8. Haykowsky MJ, Kouba EJ, Brubaker PH, et al. Skeletal muscle composition and its relation to exercise intolerance in older patients with heart failure and preserved ejection fraction. Am J Cardiol 2014; 113(7):1211–6.

9. Trankle C, Canada JM, Buckley L, et al. Impaired myocardial relaxation with exercise determines peak aerobic exercise capacity in heart failure with preserved ejection fraction. ESC Heart Fail 2017; 4(3):351–5.

10. Wagner PD. Central and peripheral aspects of oxygen transport and adaptations with exercise. Sports Med 1991;11(3):133–42.

11. Haykowsky MJ, Brubaker PH, John JM, et al. Determinants of exercise intolerance in elderly heart failure patients with preserved ejection fraction. J Am Coll Cardiol 2011;58(3):265–74.

12. Lavie CJ, Ozemek C, Carbone S, et al. Sedentary behavior, exercise, and cardiovascular health. Circ Res 2019;124(5):799–815.

13. Kitzman DW, Brubaker PH, Morgan TM, et al. Exercise training in older patients with heart failure and preserved ejection fraction: a randomized, controlled, single-blind trial. Circ Heart Fail 2010;3(6):659–67.

14. Haykowsky MJ, Brubaker PH, Stewart KP, et al. Effect of endurance training on the determinants of peak exercise oxygen consumption in elderly patients with stable compensated heart failure and preserved ejection fraction. J Am Coll Cardiol 2012;60(2):120–8.

15. Kitzman DW, Brubaker P, Morgan T, et al. Effect of caloric restriction or aerobic exercise training on peak oxygen consumption and quality of life in obese older patients with heart failure with preserved ejection fraction: a randomized clinical trial. JAMA 2016;315(1):36–46.

16. Norman JF, Kupzyk KA, Artinian NT, et al. The influence of the HEART Camp intervention on physical function, health-related quality of life, depression, anxiety and fatigue in patients with heart failure. Eur J Cardiovasc Nurs 2020;19(1):64–73.

17. Alonso WW, Kupzyk KA, Norman JF, et al. The HEART camp exercise intervention improves exercise adherence, physical function, and patient-reported outcomes in adults with preserved ejection fraction heart failure. J Card Fail 2022;28(3):431–42.

18. Edelmann F, Gelbrich G, Dungen HD, et al. Exercise training improves exercise capacity and diastolic function in patients with heart failure with preserved ejection fraction: results of the Ex-DHF (Exercise training in Diastolic Heart Failure) pilot study. J Am Coll Cardiol 2011;58(17):1780–91.

19. Fujimoto N, Prasad A Fau - Hastings JL, Hastings Jl Fau - Bhella PS, et al. Cardiovascular effects of 1 year of progressive endurance exercise training in patients with heart failure with preserved ejection fraction. Am Heart J 2012;164(6):869–77.

20. Mueller S, Winzer EB, Duvinage A, et al. Effect of high-intensity interval training, moderate continuous training, or guideline-based physical activity advice on peak oxygen consumption in patients with heart failure with preserved ejection fraction: a randomized clinical trial. JAMA 2021;325(6):542–51.

21. Bowen TS, Rolim NP, Fischer T, et al. Heart failure with preserved ejection fraction induces molecular, mitochondrial, histological, and functional alterations in rat respiratory and limb skeletal muscle. Eur J Heart Fail 2015;17(3):263–72.

22. Bowen TS, Herz C, Rolim NPL, et al. Effects of endurance training on detrimental structural, cellular, and functional alterations in skeletal muscles of heart failure with preserved ejection fraction. J Card Fail 2018;24(9):603–13.

23. Thum JS, Parsons G, Whittle T, et al. High-intensity interval training elicits higher enjoyment than moderate intensity continuous exercise. pLOS ONE 2017; 12(1):e0166299.

24.. Gripp F, Nava RC, Cassilhas RC, et al. HIIT is superior than MICT on cardiometabolic health during training and detraining. Eur J Appl Physiol 2021; 121(1):159–72.

25. Cuddy TF, Ramos JS, Dalleck LC. Reduced exertion high-intensity interval training is more effective at improving cardiorespiratory fitness and cardiometabolic health than traditional moderate-intensity continuous training. Int J Environ Res Public Health 2019;16(3):483.

26. Angadi SS, Mookadam F, Lee CD, et al. High-intensity interval training vs. moderate-intensity continuous exercise training in heart failure with preserved ejection fraction: a pilot study. J Appl Physiol 2015;119(6):753–8.

27. Donelli da Silveira A, Beust de Lima J, da Silva Piardi D, et al. High-intensity interval training is effective and superior to moderate continuous training in patients with heart failure with preserved ejection fraction: a randomized clinical trial. Eur J Prev Cardiol 2020;27(16):1733–43.

28. Dipla K, Triantafyllou A, Koletsos N, et al. Impaired muscle oxygenation and elevated exercise blood

pressure in hypertensive patients. Hypertension 2017;70(2):444–51.

29. Drexler H. Changes in the peripheral circulation in heart failure. Curr Opin Cardiol 1995;10(3): 268–73.

30. Hundley WG, Kitzman Dw Fau - Morgan TM, Morgan Tm Fau - Hamilton CA, et al. Cardiac cycle-dependent changes in aortic area and distensibility are reduced in older patients with isolated diastolic heart failure and correlate with exercise intolerance. J Am Coll Cardiol 2001;38(3):796–802.

31. Tartière-Kesri L, Tartière Jm Fau - Logeart D, Logeart D Fau - Beauvais F, Beauvais F Fau - Cohen Solal A, Cohen Solal A. Increased proximal arterial stiffness and cardiac response with moderate exercise in patients with heart failure and preserved ejection fraction. J Am Coll Cardiol 2012;59(5):455-61

32. Kitzman DW, Herrington DM, Brubaker PH, et al. Carotid arterial stiffness and its relationship to exercise intolerance in older patients with heart failure and preserved ejection fraction. Hypertension 2013; 61(1):112–9.

33. Hieda MA-O, Sarma SA-O, Hearon CMJA -O, et al. One-year committed exercise training reverses abnormal left ventricular myocardial stiffness in patients with stage b heart failure with preserved ejection fraction. Circulation 2021;144(12):934–46.

34. Carbone S, Popovic D, Lavie CJ, et al. Obesity, body composition and cardiorespiratory fitness in heart failure with preserved ejection fraction. Future Cardiol 2017;13(5):451–63.

35. Kirkman DL, Bohmke N, Billingsley HE, et al. Sarcopenic obesity in heart failure with preserved ejection fraction. Front Endocrinol (Lausanne) 2020;11: 558271.

36. Carbone S, Billingsley HE, Rodriguez-Miguelez P, et al. Lean mass abnormalities in heart failure: the role of sarcopenia, sarcopenic obesity, and cachexia. Curr Probl Cardiol 2020;45(11):100417.

37. Lavie CJ, Carbone S, Neeland IJ. Prevention and treatment of heart failure: we want to pump you up. JACC Cardiovasc Imaging 2021;14(1):216–8.

38. Kirkman DL, Lee D-C, Carbone S. Resistance exercise for cardiac rehabilitation. Prog Cardiovasc Dis 2022. In Press. Jan-Feb 2022;70:66-72.

39. Carbone S, Kirkman DL, Garten RS, et al. Muscular strength and cardiovascular disease: an updated state-of-the-art narrative review. J Cardiopulm Rehabil Prev 2020;40(5):302–9.

40. Langer D, Ciavaglia C, Faisal A, et al. Inspiratory muscle training reduces diaphragm activation and dyspnea during exercise in COPD. J Appl Physiol 1985;125:381–92.

41. Cutrim ALC, Duarte AAM, Silva-Filho AC, et al. Inspiratory muscle training improves autonomic modulation and exercise tolerance in chronic obstructive pulmonary disease subjects: a randomized-controlled trial. Respir Physiolo Neurobiol 2019; 263:31–7.

42. Del Buono MG, Arena R, Borlaug BA, et al. Exercise intolerance in patients with heart failure: JACC state-of-the-art review. J Am Coll Cardiol 2019;73(17): 2209–25.

43. Palau P, Domínguez E, Núñez E, et al. Effects of inspiratory muscle training in patients with heart failure with preserved ejection fraction. Eur J Prev Cardiol 2014;21(12):1465–73.

44. Kinugasa Y, Sota T, Ishiga N, et al. Home-based inspiratory muscle training in patients with heart failure and preserved ejection fraction: a preliminary study. J Card Fail 2020;26(11):1022–3.

45. Carbone S, Billingsley Hayley E, Canada Justin M, et al. Unsaturated fatty acids to improve cardiorespiratory fitness in patients with obesity and HFpEF. JACC Basic Transl Sci 2019;4(4):563–5.

46. Billingsley HE, Hummel SL, Carbone S. The role of diet and nutrition in heart failure: a state-of-the-art narrative review. Prog Cardiovasc Dis 2020;63(5): 538–51.

47. Allen KE, Billingsley HE, Carbone S. Nutrition, heart failure, and quality of life: beyond dietary sodium. JACC Heart Fail 2020;8(9):765–9.

48. Carbone S, Lavie CJ, Elagizi A, et al. The impact of obesity in heart failure. Heart Fail Clin 2020;16(1): 71–80.

49. Kokkinos P, Faselis C, Franklin B, et al. Cardiorespiratory fitness, body mass index and heart failure incidence. Eur J Heart Fail 2019;21(4):436–44.

50. Patel KV, Segar MW, Lavie CJ, et al. Diabetes status modifies the association between different measures of obesity and heart failure risk among older adults: a pooled analysis of community-based NHLBI cohorts. Circulation 2022;145(4):268–78.

51. Pandey A, LaMonte M, Klein L, et al. Relationship between physical activity, body mass index, and risk of heart failure. J Am Coll Cardiol 2017;69(9): 1129–42.

52. Obokata M, Reddy YNV, Pislaru SV, et al. Evidence supporting the existence of a distinct obese phenotype of heart failure with preserved ejection fraction. Circulation 2017;136(1):6–19.

53. Carbone S, Canada JM, Buckley LF, et al. Obesity contributes to exercise intolerance in heart failure with preserved ejection fraction. J Am Coll Cardiol 2016;68(22):2487–8.

54. Van Tassell B, Canada J, Buckley L, et al. Interleukin-1 blockade in heart failure with preserved ejection fraction: the diastolic heart failure anakinra response trial 2 (DHART2). Circulation 2017; 136(Suppl 1). https://pubmed.ncbi.nlm.nih.gov/30354558/.

55. Reddy YNV, Rikhi A, Obokata M, et al. Quality of life in heart failure with preserved ejection fraction: importance of obesity, functional capacity, and

physical inactivity. Eur J Heart Fail 2020;22(6): 1009–18.

56. Pocock SJ, McMurray JJV, Dobson J, et al. Weight loss and mortality risk in patients with chronic heart failure in the candesartan in heart failure: assessment of reduction in mortality and morbidity (CHARM) programme. Eur Heart J 2008;29(21): 2641–50.

57. Kamisaka K, Kamiya K, Iwatsu K, et al. Impact of weight loss in patients with heart failure with preserved ejection fraction: results from the FLAGSHIP study. ESC Heart Fail 2021;8(6):5293–303.

58. Bilgen F, Chen P, Poggi A, et al. Insufficient calorie intake worsens post-discharge quality of life and increases readmission burden in heart failure. JACC: Heart Fail 2020;8(9):756–64.

59. Katano S, Yano T, Kouzu H, et al. Energy intake during hospital stay predicts all-cause mortality after discharge independently of nutritional status in elderly heart failure patients. Clin Res Cardiol 2021;110(8):1202–20.

60. El Hajj EC, El Hajj MC, Sykes B, et al. Pragmatic weight management program for patients with obesity and heart failure with preserved ejection fraction. J Am Heart Assoc 2021;10(21):e022930.

61. Houston DK, Miller ME, Kitzman DW, et al. Long-term effects of randomization to a weight loss intervention in older adults: a pilot study. J Nutr Gerontol Geriatr 2019;38(1):83–99.

62. Carr JG, Stevenson LW, Walden JA, et al. Prevalence and hemodynamic correlates of malnutrition in severe congestive heart failure secondary to ischemic or idiopathic dilated cardiomyopathy. Am J Cardiol 1989;63(11):709–13.

63. Minamisawa M, Seidelmann SB, Claggett B, et al. Impact of malnutrition using geriatric nutritional risk index in heart failure with preserved ejection fraction. JACC Heart Fail 2019;7(8):664–75.

64. Bonilla-Palomas JL, Gámez-López AL, Castillo-Domínguez JC, et al. Nutritional intervention in malnourished hospitalized patients with heart failure. Arch Med Res 2016;47(7):535–40.

65. Bonilla-Palomas JL, Gámez-López AL, Castillo-Domínguez JC, et al. Does nutritional intervention maintain its prognostic benefit in the long term for malnourished patients hospitalised for heart failure? Revista Clínica Española 2018;218(2):58–60.

66. Hersberger L, Dietz A, Bürgler H, et al. Individualized nutritional support for hospitalized patients with chronic heart failure. J Am Coll Cardiol 2021; 77(18):2307–19.

67. Vest AR, Chan M, Deswal A, et al. Nutrition, obesity, and cachexia in patients with heart failure: a consensus statement from the heart failure society of America scientific statements committee. J Card Fail 2019;25(5):380–400.

68. Colín RE, Castillo ML, Orea TA, et al. Effects of a nutritional intervention on body composition, clinical status, and quality of life in patients with heart failure. Nutrition 2004;20(10):890–5.

69. Colin-Ramirez E, McAlister FA, Zheng Y, et al. The long-term effects of dietary sodium restriction on clinical outcomes in patients with heart failure. The SODIUM-HF (Study of Dietary Intervention under 100 mmol in Heart Failure): a pilot study. Am Heart J 2015;169(2):274–281 e271.

70. Machado dA KS, Rabelo-Silva ER, Souza GC, et al. Aggressive fluid and sodium restriction in decompensated heart failure with preserved ejection fraction: results from a randomized clinical trial. Nutrition 2018;54:111–7.

71. Ezekowitz JA, Colin-Ramirez E, Ross H, et al. Reduction of dietary sodium to less than 100 mmol in heart failure (SODIUM-HF): an international, open-label, randomised, controlled trial. The Lancet 2022;399(10333):1391–400.

72. Jefferson K, Ahmed M, Choleva M, et al. Effect of a sodium-restricted diet on intake of other nutrients in heart failure: implications for research and clinical practice. J Card Fail 2015;21(12):959–62.

73. Levitan EB, Lewis CE, Tinker LF, et al. Mediterranean and DASH diet scores and mortality in women with heart failure. Circ Heart Fail 2013;6(6):1116–23.

74. Miró O, Estruch R, Martín-Sánchez Francisco J, et al. Adherence to mediterranean diet and all-cause mortality after an episode of acute heart failure. JACC: Heart Fail 2018;6(1):52–62.

75. Carbone S, Billingsley HE, Abbate A. The mediterranean diet to treat heart failure: a potentially powerful tool in the hands of providers. JACC Heart Fail 2018; 6(3):264.

76. Billingsley H, Rodriguez-Miguelez P, Del Buono MG, et al. Lifestyle interventions with a focus on nutritional strategies to increase cardiorespiratory fitness in chronic obstructive pulmonary disease, heart failure, obesity, sarcopenia, and frailty. Nutrients 2019; 11(12):2849.

77. Carbone S, Canada JM, Buckley LF, et al. Dietary fat, sugar consumption, and cardiorespiratory fitness in patients with heart failure with preserved ejection fraction. JACC Basic Transl Sci 2017;2(5): 513–25.

78. Lechner K, Scherr J, Lorenz E, et al. Omega-3 fatty acid blood levels are inversely associated with cardiometabolic risk factors in HFpEF patients: the Aldo-DHF randomized controlled trial. Clin Res Cardiol 2021 2022;111(3):308–21. In Press.

79. Matsuo N, Miyoshi T, Takaishi A, et al. High plasma docosahexaenoic acid associated to better prognoses of patients with acute decompensated heart failure with preserved ejection fraction. Nutrients 2021; 13(2):371.

80. Goyal P, Balkan L, Ringel JB, et al. The dietary approaches to stop hypertension (DASH) diet pattern and incident heart failure. J Card Fail 2021;27(5): 512–21.

81. Hummel SL, Karmally W, Gillespie BW, et al. Home-delivered meals postdischarge from heart failure hospitalization. Circ Heart Fail 2018;11(8):e004886.

82. Hummel SL, Seymour EM, Brook RD, et al. Low-sodium dietary approaches to stop hypertension diet reduces blood pressure, arterial stiffness, and oxidative stress in hypertensive heart failure with preserved ejection fraction. Hypertension 2012; 60(5):1200–6.

83. Hummel SL, Seymour EM, Brook RD, et al. Low-sodium DASH diet improves diastolic function and ventricular–arterial coupling in hypertensive heart failure with preserved ejection fraction. Circ Heart Fail 2013;6(6):1165–71.

84. Billingsley HE, Dixon DL, Canada JM, et al. Time of eating and cardiorespiratory fitness in patients with heart failure with preserved ejection fraction and obesity. Nutr Metab Cardiovasc Dis 2021;31(8):2471–3.

Device Therapy for Heart Failure with Preserved Ejection Fraction

Husam M. Salah, MD[a], Allison P. Levin, MD[b], Marat Fudim, MD, MHS[c],*

KEYWORDS

- Device therapy • HFpEF • Interatrial shunt • Atrial shunt • Baroreflex activation therapy
- Cardiac contractility modulation • Splanchnic nerve modulation • Phrenic nerve stimulation

KEY POINTS

- Owing to its heterogeneity, heart failure with preserved ejection fraction (HFpEF) has limited effective pharmacologic therapies.
- Device therapy for HFpEF primarily targets structural and neurohormonal abnormalities that would not be amenable to pharmacologic approaches.
- Current device therapies being investigated for HFpEF include left atrial unloading (eg, left-to-right atrial shunts), cardiac contractility modulation, autonomic modulation, and respiratory modulation.

INTRODUCTION

Heart failure with preserved ejection fraction (HFpEF) is a heterogeneous clinical syndrome with several phenotypes that are driven by diverse causes and complex underlying pathophysiologic factors.[1] HFpEF is generally characterized by atrial dysfunction, abnormalities in diastolic and systolic reserve, preload reserve failure, elevated intracardiac filling pressures, pulmonary hypertension, chronotropic incompetence, and endothelial dysfunction.[1–4] Despite many shared clinical characteristics, the mechanistic heterogeneity of this syndrome has resulted in a dearth of effective pharmacologic treatment options. The first positive large-scale medication-based trial, EMPEROR-Preserved (Empagliflozin Outcome Trial in Patients with Chronic Heart Failure with Preserved Ejection Fraction), was only recently published. This trial demonstrated a reduction in the composite risk of cardiovascular death and heart failure (HF) hospitalization in patients with HFpEF with empagliflozin.[5] No other pharmacologic treatment to date has shown meaningful clinical benefits in HFpEF, and successful strategies have been limited to the management of its common comorbidities.

Device therapy has emerged as an alternative approach to address certain structural and neurohormonal abnormalities in patients with HFpEF that are not amenable to pharmacologic interventions. The unmet clinical need for effective symptomatic and hemodynamic improvement in HFpEF and major changes in the regulatory environment for the investigation and approval of devices over the past decade have accelerated development, trial-based evaluation, and patient access to device therapy for HF (**Fig. 1**).[6] This review summarizes the current landscape of device therapy in patients with HFpEF.

Structural Interventions: Left-To-Right Atrial Shunts

Elevated left atrial filling pressures during exercise is one of the hallmarks of HFpEF and is inversely correlated with peak VO$_2$ (oxygen consumption)

a Department of Medicine, University of Arkansas for Medical Sciences, 4301 West Markham Street, Little Rock, AR 72205, USA; b Department of Medicine, Harvard Medical School, Massachusetts General Hospital, 55 Fruit Street, Boston, MA 02114, USA; c Division of Cardiology, Duke University School of Medicine, Duke Clinical Research Institute, 2301 Erwin Road, Durham, NC, 27710, USA
* Corresponding author.
E-mail address: marat.fudim@gmail.com

Cardiol Clin 40 (2022) 507–515
https://doi.org/10.1016/j.ccl.2022.06.005
0733-8651/22/© 2022 Elsevier Inc. All rights reserved.

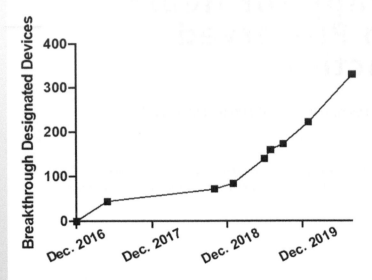

Fig. 1. The approval of breakthrough designation therapies by the US Food and Drug Administration in a 5-year span. From Fudim M, Abraham WT, von Bardeleben RS, Lindenfeld J, Ponikowski PP, Salah HM, Khan MS, Sievert H, Stone GW, Anker SD, Butler J. Device Therapy in Chronic Heart Failure: JACC State-of-the-Art Review. J Am Coll Cardiol. 2021 Aug 31;78(9):931–56.

during exercise.[7,8] Alleviation of increased left atrial pressure by decompressing the left atrium via an iatrogenic shunt (left-to-right atrial or left atrium-to-coronary sinus shunt) was proposed as a possible therapeutic intervention in patients with HFpEF. Several left-to-right atrial shunt devices have been under investigation in patients with HFpEF. Three devices with the most mature clinical program to date are presented.

InterAtrial Shunt Device System

The InterAtrial Shunt Device (IASD) is a self-expanding, percutaneously deployed, bare metal stent with a double-disc shape and a central opening that is implanted via a transseptal puncture at the mid fossa ovalis to create an interatrial conduit.[9] Phase 1 and 2 trials of the IASD in patients with HFpEF had promising results. In REDUCE LAP-HF (Reduce Elevated Left Atrial Pressure in Patients with Heart Failure), a phase 1, open-label, single-arm trial in 68 patients with HFpEF, IASD use reduced exercise pulmonary capillary wedge pressure (PCWP) in 58% of participants at 6 months, with no periprocedural or device-related complications.[10] Subsequently, the phase 2, randomized, sham-controlled REDUCE LAP-HF I trial (n = 94) showed a greater reduction in PCWP during all stages of exercise in patients treated with the IASD compared with sham with no complications at 1-month follow-up (P = 0.028, **Fig. 2**).[11] In light of these positive results, the phase 3 REDUCE LAP-HF II study was conducted to investigate the impact of IASD versus sham procedure on a composite outcome of (1) cardiovascular mortality or nonfatal ischemic stroke at 12 months, (2) HF events at 24 months, and (3) change in Kansas City Cardiomyopathy

Questionnaire (KCCQ) overall summary score at 12 months. This randomized, sham-controlled trial in patients with symptomatic HFpEF (left ventricular ejection fraction [LVEF] of ≥ 40%) with a PCWP of 25 mm Hg or more during exercise did not find any difference in the primary composite outcome.[12] In a posthoc analysis, patients with a peak exercise pulmonary vascular resistance (PVR) of less than 1.74 Wood units had benefit from the IASD with a win ratio of 1.28 (P = 0.032). Those with a peak exercise PVR greater than or equal to 1.74 Wood units who were treated with the IASD experienced worse outcomes, with increased incident rate ratio for HF events and worsening of the KCCQ overall summary score.[12] The results of this posthoc analysis highlight a potential difference in the response to the IASD based on PVR, which warrants further investigations.

V-Wave shunt device

The V-Wave shunt device is a percutaneously implanted, hourglass-shaped IASD that allows unidirectional flow from the left atrium to the right atrium. This device was the first IASD to be evaluated in patients with heart failure with reduced ejection fraction (HFrEF). In a proof-of-principal cohort study in patients with HFrEF (n = 10), the V-Wave shunt device resulted in an improvement in New York Heart Association (NYHA) functional class, quality of life, and PCWP at 3 months in 80% of participants.[13]

Subsequently, in a single-arm, open-label study of 38 patients on optimal medical therapy with NYHA functional class III and IV regardless of ejection fraction (30 patients with HFrEF and 8 with HFpEF), implantation of the V-Wave shunt device

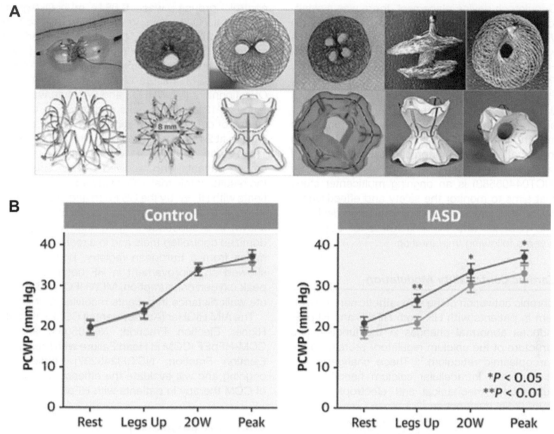

Fig. 2. (*A*) Different forms of interatrial shunt devices. (*B*) Creating a left-to-right atrial shunt in a state of elevated left atrial pressure results in a reduction of this abnormally increased pressure. (*From* Fudim M, Abraham WT, von Bardeleben RS, Lindenfeld J, Ponikowski PP, Salah HM, Khan MS, Sievert H, Stone GW, Anker SD, Butler J. Device Therapy in Chronic Heart Failure: JACC State-of-the-Art Review. J Am Coll Cardiol. 2021 Aug 31;78(9):931–56.) (*From* T. Feldman, L. Mauri, R. Kahwash et al., Transcatheter Interatrial Shunt Device for the Treatment of Heart Failure With Preserved Ejection Fraction (REDUCE LAP-HF I [Reduce Elevated Left Atrial Pressure in Patients With Heart Failure]), Circulation, 137(4), 2018, pp. 364-375.)

resulted in improvement in NYHA functional class, quality of life, and 6-minute walk distance at 3 and 12 months.[14] Although 36% of the shunts' valves were stenotic at 12 months, those with patent shunts had lower long-term mortality and HF hospitalizations as well as larger reductions in PCWP.[14]

Following adjustments in the initial device design, the RELIEVE-HF (Reducing Lung Congestion Symptoms in Advanced Heart Failure; NCT03499236) study was launched to evaluate the efficacy and safety of the V-Wave shunt device in patients with NYHA functional class III and IV regardless of LVEF. Recruitment is ongoing.

Occlutech atrial flow regulator
The Occlutech atrial flow regulator is a percutaneously implanted, self-expandable, double-disc wire mesh that allows bidirectional interatrial

flow.[15] In a study that included 12 patients with severe pulmonary hypertension who experienced syncope due to right-sided HF,[16] implantation of the Occlutech atrial flow regulator resulted in relief of syncopal episodes in all patients and improvement in 6-minute walk distance (from 377.3 ± 33.2 to 423 ± 31.32 m), systemic oxygen transport (from 367.5 ± 75.5 to 428.0 ± 67.1 mL/min/m^2), and cardiac index (from 2.36 ± 0.52 to 2.89 ± 0.56 L/min/m^2).[16] At a median follow-up of 189 days, the device was patent in all patients.[16]

The PRELIEVE (Pilot Study to Assess Safety and Efficacy of a Novel Atrial Flow Regulator in Heart Failure Patients) study was a prospective, nonrandomized study that included 53 symptomatic patients with HF (HFrEF = 24 patients, HFpEF = 29 patients) and PCWP greater than or equal to 15 mm Hg at rest or greater than or equal to 25 mm Hg during exercise.[17] At 3 months after

Occulotech device placement, there was a significant decrease in PCWP by 5 mm Hg (*P* = 0.0003) for the whole cohort; this decrease was more pronounced in HFpEF compared with HFrEF (PCWP decrease in HFrEF: 4 mm Hg, *P* = 0.1 vs PCWP decrease in HFpEF: 5 mm Hg, *P* = 0.0004).[17] The device was patent in 92% of the patients at 12 months.[17] There were 2 major adverse events, which were device embolization into the left atrium requiring surgical intervention in 1 patient and postprocedural bleeding and syncope in another.[17] The AFteR registry (NCT04405583) is an ongoing multicenter study that aims to monitor the safety and effectiveness of the Occlutech atrial flow regulator device in 100 patients with HF (regardless of LVEF) for 3 years following implantation.

Cardiac Contractility Modulation

Chronic activation of the sympathetic nervous system in patients with HF (both HFrEF and HFpEF) induces abnormal changes in the function and structure of the calcium regulatory proteins in the sarcoplasmic reticulum.[18] These changes result in abnormal intracellular calcium handling with subsequent mechanical and electrophysiologic myocardial dysfunction.[18]

Cardiac contractility modulation (CCM) therapy using the OPTIMIZER System delivers a biphasic, high-voltage ($\sim$7.5 V), long-duration ($\sim$20 milliseconds) electrical stimulation to the right ventricular septum during the absolute refractory period of the action potential.[19] Because the electrical stimulation is delivered during the refractory period, it does not trigger myocardial contraction, but it results in an amplification of the intracellular calcium signal within the cardiomyocyte due to an increase in calcium influx and calcium-induced calcium release from the sarcoplasmic reticulum.[19,20] The chronic amplification of intracellular calcium signal subsequently leads to molecular, structural, and functional changes in the myocardium that enhances contractility and decreases LV volume (**Fig. 3**).[19]

The current evidence, which is based on the FIX-HF-5C trial (Evaluate Safety and Efficacy of the OPTIMIZER System in Subjects with Moderate-to-Severe Heart Failure), supports the use of CCM in patients with HFrEF. Ongoing studies are evaluating the use of this therapy in patients with HFpEF. The FIX-HF-5C trial randomized 160 patients with HFrEF (LVEF 25%–45%) with NYHA functional class III to IV and QRS duration less than 130 milliseconds to CCM or medical therapy.[19] At 24 weeks, the mean difference in peak oxygen consumption between the CCM and control groups was 0.084 mL O_2/kg/min (15.04 mL O_2/kg/min vs 14.20 mL O_2/kg/min) with a 98.9% probability that CCM is superior to control.[19] Compared with control, patients with CCM also had greater improvement in NYHA functional class, Minnesota Living with Heart Failure Questionnaire (MLWHFQ), and 6-minute walk distance at 12 and 24 weeks and fewer composite events of cardiovascular mortality or HF hospitalizations at 24 weeks (2.9% vs 10.8%; *P* = 0.028).[19] There was an 89.7% complication-free rate among patients who received CCM.[19] Based on the results of this trial, CCM was approved for patients with HFrEF by the US Food and Drug Administration (FDA) in 2019.[6] The benefits were also shown in a subsequent meta-analysis of 4 randomized controlled trials and in a real-world experience from a European registry, both of which showed an improvement in HF hospitalizations, peak oxygen consumption, MLWHFQ, and 6-minute walk distance in patients receiving CCM.[21,22]

The AIM HIGHer (Assessment of CCM in HF with Higher Ejection Fraction; NCT05064709) and CCM-HFpEF (CCM in Heart Failure with Preserved Ejection Fraction; NCT03240237) studies are ongoing and will evaluate the efficacy and safety of CCM therapy in patients with HFpEF.

Autonomic Modulation

Baroreflex activation therapy

Baroreflex dysfunction and autonomic dysregulation are closely associated with the development and progression of LV dysfunction. A growing body of evidence supports the presence of diminished vagal control of heart rate and activation of the sympathetic nervous system in patients with HFpEF.[23,24] The afferent limb of the baroreflex originates from receptors in the carotid sinus and aortic arch that are stimulated in response to arterial distention.[6] The efferent inputs to the sympathetic and parasympathetic fibers originate from the rostral ventrolateral medulla and nucleus ambiguous.[6] Baroreflex activation therapy (BAT) generates electrical impulses from an implanted pulse generator in the pectoral region that stimulate the carotid baroreceptors.[6] Stimulation of the carotid baroreceptors results in a centrally mediated decrease in sympathetic activity and an activation of the parasympathetic pathway, thus counteracting the sympathetic activation and the parasympathetic withdrawal associated with HF[6]; this induces arterial and venodilation with a resultant reduction in stressed blood volume and improved renal salt and water handling.[25]

BAT was initially studied in patients with HFrEF in the randomized, phase 2 HOPE4HF trial

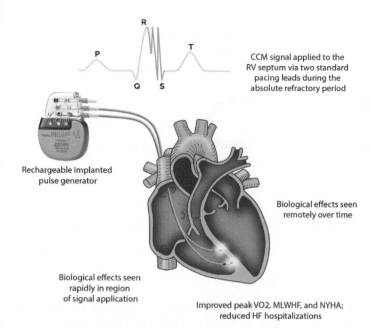

CCM signal applied to the RV septum via two standard pacing leads during the absolute refractory period

Rechargeable implanted pulse generator

Biological effects seen remotely over time

Biological effects seen rapidly in region of signal application

Improved peak VO2, MLWHF, and NYHA; reduced HF hospitalizations

Fig. 3. Cardiac contractility modulation using the OPTIMIZER system delivers an electrical signal to the right ventricular septum during the absolute refractory period resulting in amplification of intracellular calcium with subsequent changes that enhance myocardial contractility. Abbreviations: CCM, cardiac contractility modulation; RV, right ventricle, VO2, oxygen consumption; MLWHFQ, Minnesota Living with Heart failure Questionnaire; NYHA, New York Heart Association. *(Courtesy of OPTIMIZER® SMART, Impulse Dynamics, Marlton, NJ. with permission.)*

(Barostim Hope of Heart Failure Study), which included 146 patients with NYHA functional class III and LVEF less than or equal to 35%.[26] Compared with control, BAT with the Barostim Neo system resulted in a significantly greater improvement in 6-minute walk distance (59.6 ± 14 m vs 1.5 ± 13.2 m; $P = 0.004$), quality of life as assessed by the MLWHFQ with a between-group difference of −19.5 ± 4.2 points favoring BAT ($P < 0.001$), and NYHA functional class with 55% vs 24% achieving greater than or equal to 1 class improvement for the BAT and control groups, respectively ($P = 0.002$).[26] The 6-month freedom from major adverse neurologic and cardiovascular events was 97.2%.[26] Subsequently, the pivotal BeAT-HF (Baroreflex Activation Therapy for Heart Failure) trial randomized 408 patients with HFrEF (LVEF ≤35%) with NYHA functional class II to III to either BAT combined with medical therapy or medical therapy alone. BeAT-HF confirmed the efficacy and safety of BAT therapy by demonstrating improvement in quality of life, 6-minute walk distance, and NT-proB-type natriuretic peptide (NT-proBNP) along with a 97% free rate of major adverse neurologic, cardiovascular, or procedure-related events.[27] At present, BAT with the Barostim Neo system is FDA approved for patients with symptomatic HF with NYHA functional class III, LVEF less than or equal to 35%, and NT-proBNP less than 1600 pg/mL who are not candidates for cardiac resynchronization therapy (**Fig. 4**).[6] Although BAT's efficacy in patients with HFpEF has not been evaluated yet, BAT may be a

promising therapy for this population given that baroreflex dysfunction is a shared pathophysiology between most HF phenotypes (regardless of LVEF) and is closely associated with LV dysfunction.[28,29] The BAROSTIM THERAPY In Heart Failure With Preserved Ejection Fraction (NCT02876042) is an ongoing study that aims to evaluate the efficacy of BAT in patients with concurrent resistant hypertension and HFpEF.

Splanchnic nerve modulation

Disturbance of volume distribution, in the absence of a true increase in total body volume, can result in elevation of intracardiac filling pressures and HF exacerbation.[30,31] The splanchnic vascular compartment is the largest reservoir for intravascular blood volume and plays a key role in regulating volume redistribution.[32] Sympathetic fibers originating from splanchnic nerves are the main regulator of the venous and arterial vascular tone of the splanchnic vascular compartment.[33] Activation of the splanchnic nerves results in vasoconstriction of the splanchnic vasculatures with subsequent reduction in splanchnic capacitance. This central recruitment of blood volume can overwhelm the failing heart.[34] Therefore, splanchnic nerve modulation has been suggested as a potential therapy to address disturbance of volume distribution in patients with HF (see **Fig. 4**).[35–38]

The concept of splanchnic nerve blockade as a therapeutic approach in HF was initially studied in patients with acute advanced HFrEF, in whom bilateral splanchnic nerve block with 1% lidocaine resulted in a temporary reduction of intracardiac

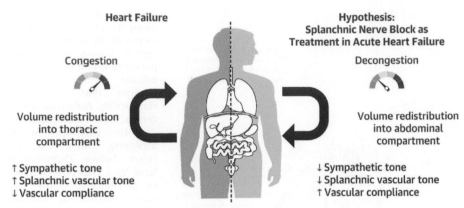

Fig. 4. The splanchnic vascular compartment is the largest reservoir for intravascular blood volume and is major regulator of volume redistribution in heart failure. Activation of the splanchnic nerves results in vasoconstriction of the splanchnic vasculatures, reduction in splanchnic capacitance, and central recruitment of blood volume. (*From* Fudim M, Jones WS, Boortz-Marx RL, Ganesh A, Green CL, Hernandez AF, Patel MR. Splanchnic Nerve Block for Acute Heart Failure. Circulation. 2018 Aug 28;138(9):95153.)

pressures and an increase in cardiac index.[39] These hemodynamic changes were subsequently replicated in patients with chronic HFrEF.[40] Following these encouraging results in HFrEF, splanchnic nerve blockade via surgical ablation of the right greater splanchnic nerve was evaluated in patients with HFpEF in a prospective, single-arm study that included 10 patients with HFpEF with NYHA class III with PCWP greater than or equal to 15 mm Hg at rest or greater than or equal to 25 mm Hg with exercise. Ablation of the right greater splanchnic nerve in these patients resulted in reduction in exercise PCWP at 3 months and improvement in NYHA functional class and quality of life as assessed by MLWHFQ at 12 months.[33] Rebalance-HF (Endovascular Ablation of the Right Greater Splanchnic Nerve in Subjects Having HFpEF; NCT04592445) is an ongoing sham-controlled trial that aims to assess the efficacy and safety of catheter-based unilateral ablation of the right greater splanchnic nerve in patients with HFpEF.

Respiratory Modulation: Phrenic Nerve Stimulation for Central Sleep Apnea

Central sleep apnea (CSA) is common in patients with HF, with 20% prevalence among patients with HFpEF.[41] CSA is characterized by intermittent withdrawal of central respiratory drive that leads to temporary cessation of respiratory muscle activity.[41] In patients with HF, CSA manifests in a Cheyne-Stokes respiration pattern and alternating phases of apnea and hyperpnea.[41] CSA is associated with neurohumoral and hemodynamic changes that contribute to HF progression via inflammation, oxidative stress, and endothelial injury.[42–44]

Continuous positive airway pressure failed to show meaningful benefits in patients with concurrent HF and CSA[45]; therefore, phrenic nerve stimulation via the implantable remedē system has been developed as an alternative approach to induce diaphragmatic contraction, thus restoring normal breathing pattern and stabilizing the Pao_2 and $Paco_2$ balance during sleep.[46] The pilot and pivotal trials of phrenic nerve stimulation, which involved patients with moderate to severe CSA, showed that phrenic nerve stimulation significantly reduces apnea-hypopnea index and improves oxygenation, sleep quality, and quality of life with consistent results in patients with concurrent HF (regardless of LVEF).[47,48] Phrenic nerve stimulation also demonstrated a good safety profile with 92% freedom from adverse events at 1 year.[48] Based on these results, phrenic nerve stimulation via the remedē system was approved by the US FDA for patients with moderate to severe CSA in 2017.[6]

SUMMARY

HFpEF is a complex and heterogeneous syndrome with limited effective pharmacologic therapies. Device therapy has emerged as a promising approach in patients with HFpEF and has targeted structural and neurohormonal abnormalities that have not been amenable to pharmacologic approaches. Current approaches include left-to-right atrial shunts (IASD, V-Wave shunt device, Occlutech atrial flow regulator), CCM using the OPTIMIZER system, autonomic modulation (BAT, and splanchnic nerve modulation), and respiratory modulation (ie, phrenic nerve stimulation in patients with CSA) with several devices that were initially investigated in patients with HFrEF currently being evaluated in patients with HFpEF given mechanistical plausibility.

CLINICS CARE POINTS

- Current evidence does not support the use of left-to-right shunt in HFpEF; however, there is a signal of possible beneficial effects in those with a peak exercise PVR of less than 1.74 Wood units that warrants further investigation

- CCM therapy should be considered in patients with QRS duration of less than 130 ms, LVEF 25% to 45%, NYHA functional class III, and no concurrent longstanding or permanent atrial fibrillation; its efficacy and safety in HFpEF is currently being evaluated

- BAT should be considered in patients with LVEF less than or equal to 35%, NYHA functional class III, and NT-proBNP less than 1600 pg/mL who are not candidates for cardiac resynchronization therapy; its efficacy and safety in HFpEF is currently being evaluated

- Phrenic nerve stimulation should be considered in patients with moderate to severe CSA (regardless of LVEF)

- Investigational studies of splanchnic nerve modulation are ongoing

DISCLOSURE

Dr M. Fudim was supported by the National Heart, Lung, and Blood Institute (NHLBI) (K23HL151744), the American Heart Association (20IPA35310955), Mario Family Award, Duke Chair's Award, Translating Duke Health Award, Bayer, Bodyport, BTG Specialty Pharmaceuticals, and Verily. He receives consulting fees from Abbott, Alleviant, Audicor, AxonTherapies, Bayer, Bodyguide, Bodyport, Boston Scientific, CVRx, Daxor, Deerfield Catalyst, Edwards LifeSciences, Feldschuh Foundation, Fire1, Gradient, Intershunt, NXT Biomedical, Pharmacosmos, PreHealth, Shifamed, Splendo, Vironix, Viscardia, and Zoll. All other authors declare no disclosures.

FINANCIAL SUPPORT

None

REFERENCES

1. Shah SJ, Katz DH, Deo RC. Phenotypic spectrum of heart failure with preserved ejection fraction. Heart Fail Clin 2014;10(3):407–18.

2. Pfeffer MA, Shah AM, Borlaug BA. Heart failure with preserved ejection fraction in perspective. Circ Res 2019;124(11):1598–617.

3. Fudim M, Sobotka PA, Dunlap ME. Extracardiac abnormalities of preload reserve. Circ Heart Fail 2021; 14(1):e007308.

4. Salah HM, Pandey A, Soloveva A, et al. Relationship of nonalcoholic fatty liver disease and heart failure with preserved ejection fraction. JACC: Basic Translational Sci 2021;6(11):918–32.

5. Anker SD, Butler J, Filippatos G, et al. Empagliflozin in heart failure with a preserved ejection fraction. N Engl J Med 2021;385(16):1451–61.

6. Fudim M, Abraham WT, Bardeleben RSv, et al. Device therapy in chronic heart failure. J Am Coll Cardiol 2021;78(9):931–56.

7. Reddy YNV, Olson TP, Obokata M, et al. Hemodynamic correlates and diagnostic role of cardiopulmonary exercise testing in heart failure with preserved ejection fraction. JACC: Heart Fail 2018; 6(8):665–75.

8. Borlaug BA, Nishimura RA, Sorajja P, et al. Exercise hemodynamics enhance diagnosis of early heart failure with preserved ejection fraction. Circ Heart Fail 2010;3(5):588–95.

9. Miyagi C, Miyamoto T, Karimov JH, et al. Device-based treatment options for heart failure with preserved ejection fraction. Heart Fail Rev 2021;26(4): 749–62.

10. Hasenfuß G, Hayward C, Burkhoff D, et al. A transcatheter intracardiac shunt device for heart failure with preserved ejection fraction (REDUCE LAP-HF): a multicentre, open-label, single-arm, phase 1 trial. Lancet 2016;387(10025): 1298–304.

11. Feldman T, Mauri L, Kahwash R, et al. Transcatheter interatrial shunt device for the treatment of heart failure with preserved ejection fraction (reduce lap-hf i [reduce elevated left atrial pressure in patients with heart failure]). Circulation 2018; 137(4):364–75.

12. Shah SJ, Borlaug BA, Chung ES, et al. Atrial shunt device for heart failure with preserved and mildly reduced ejection fraction (REDUCE LAP-HF II): a randomised, multicentre, blinded, sham-controlled trial. Lancet 2022. https://doi.org/10.1016/S0140-6736(22)00016-2.

13. Del Trigo M, Bergeron S, Bernier M, et al. Unidirectional left-to-right interatrial shunting for treatment of patients with heart failure with reduced ejection fraction: a safety and proof-of-principle cohort study. Lancet 2016;387(10025):1290–7.

14. Rodés-Cabau J, Bernier M, Amat-Santos IJ, et al. Interatrial shunting for heart failure: early and late results from the first-in-human experience with the V-wave system. JACC: Cardiovasc Interventions 2018;11(22):2300–10.

15. Gupta A, Bailey SR. Update on devices for diastolic dysfunction: options for a no option condition? Curr Cardiol Rep 2018;20(10):85.

16. Rajeshkumar R, Pavithran S, Sivakumar K, et al. Atrial septostomy with a predefined diameter using a novel occlutech atrial flow regulator improves symptoms and cardiac index in patients with severe pulmonary arterial hypertension. Catheter Cardiovasc Interv 2017;90(7):1145–53.

17. Paitazoglou C, Bergmann MW, Özdemir R, et al. One-year results of the first-in-man study investigating the Atrial Flow Regulator for left atrial shunting in symptomatic heart failure patients: the PRELIEVE study. Eur J Heart Fail 2021;23(5): 800–10.

18. Yano M, Ikeda Y, Matsuzaki M. Altered intracellular Ca2+ handling in heart failure. J Clin Invest 2005; 115(3):556–64.

19. Abraham WT, Kuck K-H, Goldsmith RL, et al. A randomized controlled trial to evaluate the safety and efficacy of cardiac contractility modulation. JACC: Heart Fail 2018;6(10):874–83.

20. Abi-Samra F, Gutterman D. Cardiac contractility modulation: a novel approach for the treatment of heart failure. Heart Fail Rev 2016;21(6):645–60.

21. Giallauria F, Cuomo G, Parlato A, et al. A comprehensive individual patient data meta-analysis of the effects of cardiac contractility modulation on functional capacity and heart failure-related quality of life. ESC Heart Fail 2020;7(5):2922–32.

22. Anker SD, Borggrefe M, Neuser H, et al. Cardiac contractility modulation improves long-term survival and hospitalizations in heart failure with reduced ejection fraction. Eur J Heart Fail 2019;21(9): 1103–13.

23. Ferguson DW, Abboud FM, Mark AL. Selective impairment of baroreflex-mediated vasoconstrictor responses in patients with ventricular dysfunction. Circulation 1984;69(3):451–60.

24. Badrov MB, Mak S, Floras JS. Cardiovascular autonomic disturbances in heart failure with preserved ejection fraction. Can J Cardiol 2021; 37(4):609–20.

25. Burgoyne S, Georgakopoulos D, Belenkie I, et al. Systemic vascular effects of acute electrical baroreflex stimulation. Am J Physiology-Heart Circulatory Physiol 2014;307(2):H236–41.

26. Abraham WT, Zile MR, Weaver FA, et al. Baroreflex activation therapy for the treatment of heart failure with a reduced ejection fraction. JACC: Heart Fail 2015;3(6):487–96.

27. Zile MR, Lindenfeld J, Weaver FA, et al. Baroreflex activation therapy in patients with heart failure with reduced ejection fraction. J Am Coll Cardiol 2020; 76(1):1–13.

28. Georgakopoulos D, Little WC, Abraham WT, et al. Chronic baroreflex activation: a potential therapeutic approach to heart failure with preserved ejection fraction. J Card Fail 2011;17(2):167–78.

29. Wallbach M, Koziolek MJ, Wachter R. Barorezeptoraktivierungstherapie. Internist (Berl) 2018;59(10): 1011–20.

30. Zile MR, Bennett TD, Sutton MSJ, et al. Transition from chronic compensated to acute decompensated heart failure. Circulation 2008;118(14): 1433–41.

31. Chaudhry SI, Wang Y, Concato J, et al. Patterns of weight change preceding hospitalization for heart failure. Circulation 2007;116(14):1549–54.

32. Fudim M, Hernandez AF, Felker GM. Role of volume redistribution in the congestion of heart failure. J Am Heart Assoc 2017;6(8):e006817.

33. Málek F, Gajewski P, Zymliński R, et al. Surgical ablation of the right greater splanchnic nerve for the treatment of heart failure with preserved ejection fraction: first-in-human clinical trial. Eur J Heart Fail 2021;23(7):1134–43.

34. Barnes RJ, Bower EA, Rink TJ. Haemodynamic responses to stimulation of the splanchnic and cardiac sympathetic nerves in the anaesthetized cat. J Physiol 1986;378:417–36.

35. Bapna A, Adin C, Engelman ZJ, et al. Increasing blood pressure by greater splanchnic nerve stimulation: a feasibility study. J Cardiovasc Translational Res 2020;13(4):509–18.

36. Fudim M, Yalamuri S, Herbert JT, et al. Raising the pressure: hemodynamic effects of splanchnic nerve stimulation. J Appl Physiol 2017;123(1): 126–7.

37. Gelman S, Warner David S, Warner Mark A. Venous function and central venous pressure: a physiologic story. Anesthesiology 2008;108(4):735–48.

38. Fudim M, Neuzil P, Malek F, et al. Greater splanchnic nerve stimulation in heart failure with preserved ejection fraction. J Am Coll Cardiol 2021;77(15):1952–3.

39. Fudim M, Jones WS, Boortz-Marx RL, et al. Splanchnic nerve block for acute heart failure. Circulation 2018;138(9):951–3.

40. Fudim M, Boortz-Marx RL, Ganesh A, et al. Splanchnic nerve block for chronic heart failure. JACC: Heart Fail 2020;8(9):742–52.

41. Costanzo MR, Khayat R, Ponikowski P, et al. Mechanisms and clinical consequences of untreated central sleep apnea in heart failure. J Am Coll Cardiol 2015;65(1):72–84.

42. Lavie L, Lavie P. Molecular mechanisms of cardiovascular disease in OSAHS: the oxidative stress link. Eur Respir J 2009;33(6):1467–84.

43. SCHULZ R, MAHMOUDI S, HATTAR K, et al. Enhanced release of superoxide from polymorphonuclear neutrophils in obstructive sleep apnea. Am J Respir Crit Care Med 2000;162(2):566–70.

44. Seddon M, Looi YH, Shah AM. Oxidative stress and redox signalling in cardiac hypertrophy and heart failure. Heart 2007;93(8):903–7.

45. Bradley TD, Logan AG, Kimoff RJ, et al. Continuous positive airway pressure for central sleep apnea and heart failure. N Engl J Med 2005;353(19):2025–33.

46. Costanzo MR, Augostini R, Goldberg LR, et al. Design of the remedē system pivotal trial: a prospective, randomized study in the use of respiratory rhythm management to treat central sleep apnea. J Card Fail 2015;21(11):892–902.

47. Fudim M, Spector AR, Costanzo MR, et al. Phrenic nerve stimulation for the treatment of central sleep apnea: a pooled cohort analysis. J Clin Sleep Med 2019;15(12):1747–55.

48. Costanzo MR, Ponikowski P, Coats A, et al. Phrenic nerve stimulation to treat patients with central sleep apnoea and heart failure. Eur J Heart Fail 2018; 20(12):1746–54.

Geriatric Domains in Patients with Heart Failure with Preserved Ejection Fraction

Parag Goyal, MD, MSc[a],*, Omar Zainul BS, MD[b], Dylan Marshall, MD[a],
Dalane W. Kitzman, MD[c]

KEYWORDS

- HFpEF • Multimorbidity • Polypharmacy • Cognitive impairment • Depression • Frailty • Falls
- Social isolation

KEY POINTS

- To care for HFpEF, it is necessary to evaluate and consider multiple domains of health including medical, mind and brain, physical function, and social environment.
- Multimorbidity, polypharmacy, cognitive impairment, depression, frailty, falls, and social isolation are common geriatric syndromes that have important clinical implications on adults with HFpEF.
- There are multiple strategies to screen for geriatric syndromes that can be administered quickly in routine clinical practice by medical team members with minimal training.
- Evidence-based interventions to modify and/or mitigate the consequences of geriatric syndromes are available, and should be incorporated into routine management of adults with HFpEF.

INTRODUCTION

As the population ages, the prevalence of heart failure with preserved ejection fraction (HFpEF) continues to increase. As of 2022, HFpEF is the predominant subtype of heart failure (HF) and affects more than 3 million people in the United States[1] . The mean age of patients with HFpEF is 76 years,[2] and the prevalence increases exponentially with advancing age[3]; this is in large part because its pathophysiology is closely intertwined with aging processes.[4] Comorbid conditions that increase in prevalence with age such as diabetes and lung disease, changes in cardiovascular and noncardiovascular organ structure, and aging-related processes such as systemic inflammation and sarcopenia all contribute to the pathophysiology of HFpEF.[5,6] Accordingly, HFpEF has been described as the quintessential geriatric syndrome[7]; this supports the concept that geriatric domains are important to integrate into the care of adults with HFpEF.

A multidomain approach was recently outlined by the American College of Cardiology Geriatric Cardiology Section Leadership Council as a holistic framework to guide clinicians in regarding best care for older adults with HF (**Fig. 1**).[8] This framework outlines 4 key domains of health that are often impaired among older adults with HF—medical, mind and brain, physical function, and social environment. This review outlines the prevalence of deficits across these domains among adults with HFpEF, highlights etiologic contributions, enumerates implications for patient care, and proposes potential strategies and interventions (**Table 1** and **Table 2**) that can optimize care and/or alter the health trajectory of this vulnerable population.

[a] Department of Medicine, Weill Cornell Medicine, 1300 York Avenue, New York, NY 10023, USA; [b] Weill Cornell Medical College, 1300 York Avenue, New York, NY 10023, USA; [c] Department of Internal Medicine, Sections on Cardiovascular Disease and Geriatrics, Wake Forest School of Medicine, 1 Medical Center Boulevard, Winston-Salem, NC 27157-1045, USA
* Corresponding author. Division of Cardiology, Division of General Internal Medicine, Department of Medicine, Weill Cornell Medicine, 420 East 70th Street, LH-365, New York, NY 10063.
E-mail address: pag9051@med.cornell.edu

Cardiol Clin 40 (2022) 517–532
https://doi.org/10.1016/j.ccl.2022.06.006
0733-8651/22/© 2022 Elsevier Inc. All rights reserved.

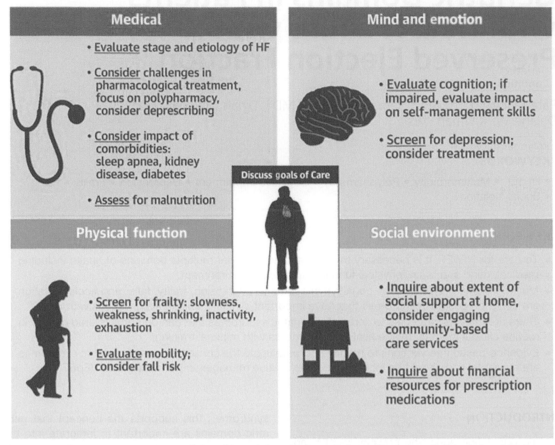

Fig. 1. Domain management approach for older adults with heart failure. (*From* Gorodeski EZ, Goyal P, Hummel SL, et al. Domain management approach to heart failure in the geriatric patient: present and future. J Am Coll Cardiol 2018;71(17):1921–36.)

Medical Domain: Multimorbidity

Prevalence and implications

Multimorbidity refers to the condition of having multiple chronic conditions[9] and is nearly universal in HFpEF.[10] One recent study estimated that the average hospitalized patient with HFpEF had 5 other medical conditions.[11] Common conditions include hypertension (prevalence as high as 87%), coronary artery disease (prevalence as high as 70%), and atrial fibrillation (AF) (prevalence ~ 44%), and several noncardiovascular conditions including lung disease (prevalence ~31% to 41%), chronic kidney disease (prevalence ~15% to 53%), diabetes (prevalence ~33% to 45%), and anemia (prevalence ~22% to 53%).[2,11–13] Variations in prevalence depend on patient population (ambulatory vs hospitalized) and method for ascertainment (case report form vs chart abstraction vs claims data). The high prevalence of multimorbidity and specific cardiovascular and noncardiovascular conditions is not surprising because several of

these conditions are directly linked to the pathophysiology of HFpEF. For example, AF and HFpEF likely have a bidirectional relationship, whereby AF begets HF and HF begets AF[14,15]; diabetes and lung disease are closely linked with the pathophysiology of HFpEF through promotion of inflammation and microvascular dysfunction.[4]

Multimorbidity has a major impact on overall prognosis. With the onset of each condition, life expectancy declines. Indeed, patients with HFpEF experience noncardiac mortality much more commonly (62%) compared with those with HF with reduced ejection fraction (35%)[16]; this underscores the importance of understanding and considering the concept of competing risk when making treatment decisions for patients with HFpEF. Patients with limited life expectancy from other comorbid conditions may not have the opportunity to derive as much lifetime benefit from a cardiovascular procedure or pharmacotherapy.[17]

Table 1
Validated screening tools for geriatric conditions in heart failure with preserved ejection fraction

Geriatric Condition	Screening Tool	Screening Thresholds	Duration of Administration	Special Training or Personnel Necessary	Diagnostic Performance
Multimorbidity	History taking and EMR Review	—	—	Clinician	—
Polypharmacy	History taking and EMR Review	—	—	Clinician	—
Cognitive Impairment	Mini-Cog[48]	Score < 3	3 min	None	Sensitivity: 79%[49] Specificity: 89%[49]
	MoCA[50]	Score < 26	10 min	Online training	Sensitivity: 81%[51] Specificity: 92%[51]
Depression	PHQ-9[69]	Score ≥ 4	3 min	None	Sensitivity: 70%[69] Specificity: 92%[69]
Frailty	Frail scale[82,138]	Score > 2	1–2 min	None	Sensitivity: 88%[92] Specificity: 85%[92]
	TUG	Time > 10 s	15 s–2 min	None	Sensitivity: 72%[92] Specificity: 82%[92]
	SPPB[139]	Score ≤ 8	5–10 min	None	Sensitivity: 82%–100%[96] Specificity: 36%–41%[96]
	HIIFRM[116]	Score ≥ 5	5–10 min	None	Sensitivity: 75%[116] Specificity: 74%[116]
Falls	12-Item FRQ[140]	Score ≥ 4	3–5 min	None	Sensitivity: 65%[117] Specificity: 65%[117]
	LSNS-6[133,141]	Score < 12	5 min	None	Not known
Social Isolation	UCLA 3-item loneliness scale[134]	Score ≥ 6	2 min	None	Not known

Abbreviations: EMR, electronic medical record; FRQ, Fall Risk Questionnaire; HIIFRM, Hendrich II Fall Risk Model; LSNS-6, Lubben Social Network Scale 6; MoCA, Montreal Cognitive Assessment; PHQ, Patient Health Questionnaire; SPPB, Short Physical Performance Battery; TUG, timed-up-and-go; UCLA, The University of California, Los Angeles.

Screening and Interventions

Screening for multimorbidity begins with a history and/or review of the electronic medical record. Considering diagnostic testing for common comorbid conditions may also be important. For example, patients who present with shortness of breath may merit formal spirometry to rule out concurrent lung disease. Routine screening for obstructive sleep apnea may also be important given its high prevalence in HFpEF,[18] and the fact that its diagnosis is often delayed leading to undertreatment for many years.[19]

Interventions for multimorbidity include optimizing treatment of each condition, which may require multiple clinicians and/or specialists, highlighting the importance of interdisciplinary communication. Pharmacologic agents that can concurrently treat multiple conditions is also an emerging and appealing strategy, well illustrated by sodium-glucose cotransport-2 inhibitors, which can concurrently treat HFpEF, diabetes, and chronic kidney disease.[20] Finally, exercise has pleiotropic effects, which can positively impact multiple conditions and improve overall health.[6]

Medical Domain: Polypharmacy

Prevalence and implications

Polypharmacy has been variably defined in the literature, with some using a threshold count of 5 medications and others using a threshold of 10 to describe a more extreme version called "hyperpolypharmacy."[21] Polypharmacy based on a threshold of 5 is nearly universal in HFpEF, and more than 50% of patients with HFpEF have hyperpolypharmacy.[11] Polypharmacy is prevalent in large part because multimorbidity is nearly

Table 2
Interventions for geriatric conditions in heart failure with preserved ejection fraction

Geriatric Condition	Interventions
Multimorbidity	Optimize treatment of comorbidities Use of pharmacologic agents to treat multiple conditions (ie, sodium-glucose cotransport-2 inhibitors)[20] Exercise[6]
Polypharmacy	Deprescribe agents with limited benefit (ie, beta-blockers)[34,35] Deprescribe medications without clear, expired, or resolved indication Deprescribe medications with drug-drug, drug-disease, or drug-person interactions
Cognitive impairment	Treat underlying conditions (ie, heart failure, atrial fibrillation, obstructive sleep apnea)[52–54] Accommodate for deficiencies in self-care (ie, simplifying medication regimens, engaging social support)[55] Referral to memory specialist, neuropsychological testing and brain imaging for definitive diagnosis
Depression	Optimize HFpEF therapy including use of spironolactone[66] Cognitive behavioral therapy[71] Exercise (ie, Tai Chi and resistance band)[72,73]
Frailty	Exercise and physical rehabilitation[76,102]
Falls	Multicomponent exercise programs (balance, strength, flexibility, and endurance training)[119] Physical rehabilitation[102] Home hazard modification (ie, removing or changing loose floor mats, painting the edges of steps, reducing glare, installing grab bars and stair rails, removing clutter, and improving lighting)[122]
Social isolation and loneliness	Use of Internet and cellular technologies[136] Community arts programs[123] Use of social care provision (ie, volunteer visitations to community-dwelling elderly)[137]

universal. As a consequence, much of polypharmacy may actually represent guideline-concordant therapy. In addition to diuretics and antihypertensive agents, patients frequently take medication for coronary artery disease and AF, as well as medication for diabetes, lung disease, and osteoarthritis.[11] Importantly, medication regimens for older adults with HFpEF often include medications that may be harmful. For example, in a single-center study of ambulatory patients with HFpEF, prevalence of HF-exacerbating medications was 52%, prevalence of Beers criteria medications (agents deemed to cause more harm than benefit in most clinical situations involving older adults) was 73%,[22] and prevalence of medications that could potentially worsen geriatric conditions was 100%.[23]

There are several important implications of polypharmacy. Across a variety of conditions, polypharmacy is associated with a broad range of adverse outcomes including falls,[24] disability,[25] and hospitalization.[26,27] Much of this is a direct result of adverse drug events, which can result from drug-drug interactions, drug-disease interactions, or drug-person interactions. Polypharmacy is also associated with treatment burden, defined as the workload imposed by health care on patients,[28] and reduced medication adherence.[29]

Screening and Interventions

Screening for polypharmacy is simple and involves a standard intake of medications and/or a review of the electronic medical record. Screening tools using implicit criteria to identify potentially harmful agents such as the Medication Appropriateness Index and the STOPP/START (Screening Tool of Older Persons' Potentially Inappropriate Prescriptions/Screening Tool to Alert Doctors to the Right

Treatment)[30,31] can provide additional guidance for medication review and potential identification of agents whose risk for harm could outweigh the potential for benefit.

Deprescribing has emerged as an important intervention for managing polypharmacy and mitigating its potential risks. Deprescribing is defined as the "systematic process of discontinuing drugs when existing/potential harms outweigh existing/potential benefits in the context of an individual's care goals, level of functioning, life expectancy, values, and preferences," and is part of a comprehensive medication optimization process for ensuring safe and effective prescribing practice.[32] Although there is a paucity of data on its benefits among patients with HFpEF, there is intuitive rationale that eliminating medications whose risks outweigh potential benefits is likely to improve outcomes in older adults with HFpEF. As a first step, it may be reasonable to deprescribe medications without a clear indication, expired indication, or resolved indication. Deprescribing medications with drug-drug interactions (aspirin and warfarin), drug-disease interactions (HF-exacerbating medications), and/or drug-person interactions (Beers criteria medications; or digoxin) may be reasonable as well, although this may require a multidisciplinary discussion involving the patient's other physicians. Finally, it may be reasonable to consider deprescribing commonly used agents with limited benefit—for example, beta-blockers are commonly used in HFpEF (86% prevalence in a recent randomized controlled trial),[33] but they have limited data supporting benefits specifically for HFpEF,[34,35] and some emerging data indicating potential for harm.[36]

Mind and Brain Domain: Cognitive Impairment

Prevalence and implications

The reported prevalence of cognitive impairment among patients with HF ranges from 22% to 78%.[37,38] These differences reflect variations in the populations studied and diagnostic tools used across studies. Adults with HFpEF[2] have several major risk factors for cognitive impairment including advanced age, hypertension, diabetes, and obesity.[39] HF itself is also thought to be a major etiologic contributor to cognitive impairment through multiple postulated mechanisms. First, reduced cardiac output can contribute to impaired cerebral blood flow,[40] especially in the setting of the increased arterial stiffness and reduced vasodilatory reserve found in HFpEF.[41] Second, deep brain structures at watershed areas are particularly vulnerable to hypoperfusion and subsequent

ischemic injury and resulting cognitive impairment.[42] Third, neurohormonal and inflammatory mechanisms common to HFpEF such as elevated levels of cortisol, interleukin-6 (IL-6), tumor necrosis factor-alpha, and total plasma homocysteine can cause a cardiocerebral syndrome through atrophy and decreased neurogenesis.[42,43]

Cognitive impairment among adults with HF has been linked to increased disability, and elevated risk of clinical events including emergency room visits, hospitalization and rehospitalization, and mortality.[44] For example, a multicenter study of 1583 hospitalized patients with HF found that cognitive impairment was associated with a 6-fold increased odds for disability, defined as the inability to perform at least 1 activity of daily living.[45] Among 246 ambulatory adults with HF (inclusive of HFpEF and heart failure with reduced ejection fraction [HFrEF]), a Montreal Cognitive Assessment (MoCA) score of less than 26 of 30 was associated with a 70% increased hazard of experiencing an emergency room visit, hospitalization, or death within 180 days.[46] It is posited that self-care is an important mediator of these associations, because intact cognition is necessary for patients to engage in self-care behaviors like symptom monitoring and medication adherence.[47]

Screening and Interventions

Given its implications on prognosis and management, screening of cognitive impairment may be important to integrate into routine workflow when caring for patients with HFpEF. The Mini-Cog is a validated[44,48,49] ultrashort cognitive "vital sign" that was developed as a screening tool for dementia with excellent sensitivity and specificity,[48] takes 3 minutes on average to administer, and can be conducted by any member of the health care team. The MoCA is another validated tool[50,51] with strong psychometric properties that incorporates multiple domains (including executive functioning, word recall, counting, naming, fluency), and therefore takes a bit longer to administer (10 minutes). The MoCA can be conducted by any member of the health care team, although brief training and certification are required. Although there is no consensus regarding the best screening tool for cognitive impairment, consideration for the routine use of the Mini-Cog or MoCA based on time availability and personnel is reasonable.

Interventions for cognitive impairment are multiple. First, it is important to treat underlying contributors—this includes treating HF[52]; other cardiac and vascular conditions like AF,[53] which are highly prevalent in HFpEF[53]; and other noncardiovascular conditions such as obstructive sleep apnea.[54] It is also important to accommodate for deficiencies in self-care that result from cognitive impairment. This may require modifications to medication regimens and/or engagement of the patient's social support structure because patients with cognitive impairment are more likely to make medication errors.[55] Finally, referral to a memory specialist (eg, neurologist and/or geriatrician) as well as neuropsychological testing and brain imaging for more definitive diagnoses may be reasonable.

Mind and Brain Domain: Depression

Prevalence and implications

Depression is common among patients with HFpEF, with 30% prevalence in a recent meta-analysis of more than 80,000 patients with HF across ambulatory and hospitalized settings.[56] Although this study did not differentiate between HFpEF and HFrEF, smaller studies specifically among patients with HFpEF have shown similar prevalence.[38,57–59] The hippocampus, which is the center for emotion, memory, and the autonomic nervous system,[60] is vulnerable to cerebral hypoxia and may be affected by low cardiac output and poor cerebral blood flow similar to the mechanism by which HF can cause cognitive impairment. Indeed, brain imaging studies to assess cerebral blood flow have demonstrated that patients with HF with poor flow to the hippocampus have a higher rate of depression.[61] Depression is also closely associated with reduced cognitive function,[62] and may be driven by a similar process of elevated levels of inflammatory (IL-6)[63] and neurohormonal biomarkers (eg, cortisol)[64] commonly seen in HFpEF.[42]

Depression is relevant in HFpEF because it has been associated with a greater than 2-fold risk for hospitalizations and mortality.[65] In a study specific to HFpEF, a secondary analysis from the Treatment of Preserved Cardiac Function Heart Failure with an Aldosterone Antagonist (TOPCAT) study showed that higher baseline 9-item Patient Health Questionnaire (PHQ-9) scores were associated with 9% increased hazard for all-cause mortality and worsening depressive symptoms at 12 months were associated with cardiovascular death and all-cause mortality.[66] Similar to cognitive impairment, it is thought that the increased risk from depression can partially be explained by impaired self-care. Indeed, a study of 400 hospitalized patients with HF (including HFpEF and HFrEF) showed that depression based on PHQ-9 was independently associated with poor self-care maintenance, management, and confidence.[67] It is noteworthy that even in the absence of a formal depression diagnosis based on *Diagnostic and Statistical Manual of Mental Disorders, Fifth Edition* (*DSM-V*) criteria, subthreshold levels of depressive symptoms are associated with poor self-care.[67]

Screening and Interventions

The American Heart Association recommends 2-step depression screening of all patients with heart disease using the 2-item PHQ-2, followed by the PHQ-9 for positive-screen patients. The PHQ-2 assesses the frequency of depressed mood and anhedonia in the prior 2 weeks.[68] If a patient answers affirmatively to either question, then 7 additional questions can be administered for a complete PHQ-9. The PHQ-9 includes questions that align with the 9 criteria for DSM-based diagnosis of depression, and has good sensitivity and specificity.[69] The PHQ-2 takes about 1 minute to administer, and the complete PHQ-9 takes about 3 minutes. PHQ-9 can be administered by any member of the medical team via interview format,[69] or through a self-reported questionnaire that the patient can complete before the visit or while in the waiting room.

Interventions including management of underlying HF, cognitive behavioral therapy (CBT), and exercise have shown promise for depression specifically in HFpEF. In a secondary analysis from the TOPCAT trial, spironolactone was associated with a modest but statistically significant reduction in depressive symptoms, suggesting potential benefit from selected pharmacotherapy.[66] CBT refers to a family of interventions that combine cognitive, behavioral, and emotion-focused techniques to change false and distressing beliefs.[70] A single-center randomized clinical trial of 158 patients inclusive of both ambulatory patients with HFrEF and HFpEF found that CBT led to improvements in quality of life, depressive symptoms, anxiety, and fatigue. Notably, the study was not sufficiently powered to evaluate cardiovascular events.[71] Exercise is also emerging as an important intervention to improve depression. For example, a multicenter randomized clinical trial of 64 ambulatory patients with HFpEF found that 3 months of exercise improved PHQ-9 by 2 points.[72] A single-center randomized clinical trial of 70 HFpEF and HFrEF outpatients similarly found that Tai Chi and resistance band exercise each demonstrated significant improvements in depression at 16 weeks.[73] Studies of traditional pharmacologic therapies such as selective serotonin reuptake inhibitors have failed to improve clinical outcomes in HFrEF,[74,75] and have yet to be studied in HFpEF.

Functional Domain: Frailty

Prevalence and implications

Frailty is a condition of "increased vulnerability to stressors due to decreased physiologic reserves."[76] There are 2 fundamental approaches to characterizing frailty: the Fried physical frailty phenotype[77] and the cumulative deficit definition of frailty.[78,79] The Fried physical frailty phenotype incorporates quantifiable physical attributes and abilities based on 5 criteria: unintentional weight loss, self-reported exhaustion, slow walking speed, weakness, and low physical activity. Physical frailty is present when 3 of these 5 criteria are met. Alternatively, the Rockwood cumulative deficit definition of frailty integrates multiple domains of health and is characterized by "a heterogeneous combination of decreased mobility, weakness, reduced muscle mass, poor nutritional status and diminished cognitive function."[80] This definition is operationalized by multi-item weighted calculations like the frailty index.[81] Given the multiple definitions and hundreds of tools by which to identify frailty,[82] the prevalence of frailty ranges from 50% to 94% among adults with HFpEF.[83,84] This prevalence is because the pathophysiology of frailty and HFpEF are intertwined.[85] Similar to HFpEF, frailty is driven by a chronic inflammatory process associated with oxidative stress and mitochondrial dysfunction, and this in turn causes metabolic dysfunction, cell senescence, and ultimately cell necrosis. As a result, adipocytes proliferate and lipids accumulate, which impairs skeletal muscle function.[86] The result is exercise intolerance and limited functional reserve.[6]

Frailty is associated with loss of independence, hospitalization, and mortality. Although not well studied in the HF population, frailty is a well-known risk factor for nursing home placement, conferring an up to 6-fold risk compared with nonfrail adults.[87] Frailty is also associated with hospitalization, with a 50% increased risk observed in the TOPCAT trial based on the cumulative deficit definition.[88] Moreover, in a study of hospitalized Medicare beneficiaries, frailty emerged as the most important predictor of 1-year readmission among nearly 50 variables studied.[89] There have also been multiple studies showing that frailty is also associated with mortality among patients with HFpEF,[84,89,90] conferring a 2-fold increased risk for death.[84,91]

Screening and Interventions

Validated screening tools for Fried's physical frailty that effectively predict worse outcomes include the FRAIL scale, timed-up-and-go (TUG) test, and the Short Physical Performance Battery (SPPB).[92–94] The FRAIL scale screens for 5 frailty-based deficits including fatigue, resistance (ability to climb a single flight of stairs), ambulation (ability to walk 1 block), illnesses (more than 5), and loss of weight (more than 5%); frailty is defined as more than 2 deficits.[82] The TUG test is a physical test in which a patient stands from a seated position, walks 10 ft, turns around and returns to sit in the original chair—a patient is considered frail if the test lasts longer than 10 seconds.[95] Finally, the SPPB is a 3-item measure commonly used in clinical trials that assigns values to patients based on performance of gait speed, timed chair stands, and standing balance[80]; a score less than or equal to 8 indicates frailty with high sensitivity (82-100%).[96] Importantly, these tools only take a few minutes to complete and do not require formal training.[97,98] Tools that screen for the cumulative deficit definition of frailty also exist, and the most effective of these tools are embedded into the electronic medical records given its nature as a multidomain and multi-item index.[99] The use of an electronic frailty index is growing and has been recommended by the British Geriatrics Society and National Health Service guidelines for frailty management.[100]

Frailty is believed to be a modifiable condition.[76] Exercise-based interventions have demonstrated the greatest potential to improve outcomes among frail adults with HFpEF, with some indication that it even reverses some aspects of frailty.[76] Through its effects on myocardial, vascular, and skeletal muscle function,[56] exercise can mitigate pathophysiologic features and consequences of frailty.[101] The recently published Rehabilitation Therapy in Older Acute Heart Failure Patients (REHAB-HF) trial demonstrated 3-month improvements in frailty (as well as physical functioning and quality of life) with progressive exercise-based rehabilitation[102] as measured by the SPPB among older adults hospitalized for HF. Notably, this effect was most robust among patients with HFpEF,[103] and a larger pivotal trial specifically for HFpEF is being planned.

Functional Domain: Falls

Prevalence and implications

The prevalence of falls among ambulatory older adults with HF may be as high as 43% over a 2-year period,[104,105] which is higher than that of the general older adult population (30%).[106] Although limited data specific to HFpEF exist, this is consistent with data from the REHAB-HF trial, which showed that the 3-month prevalence of falls among patients with HF preceding a hospitalization was 15%, and as high as 53% over the following 6 months.[103] The link between HFpEF and risk for falls is mediated by many factors. Several age-related changes to cardiovascular structure and function have been implicated in predisposing older adults with HF to falls, including attenuated barore-ceptor and autonomic reflexes, decreased adren-ergic responsiveness, and impaired maintenance of intravascular volume related to decreased salt/water handling.[107] This situation can be exacer-bated by several medications commonly prescribed to older adults with HFpEF including antihyperten-sives, diuretics, beta-blockers, antiarrhythmics, antidiabetic agents, and Beers criteria medica-tions.[23,108] Finally, this risk is further increased by multimorbidity, polypharmacy, frailty, and cognitive impairment,[109,110] which are also highly prevalent in older adults with HFpEF.[58]

Falls are a common cause of health care utiliza-tion among older adults and are associated with substantial morbidity and mortality.[104,105] Approxi-mately 35% of adults who fall suffer physical harm.[111] Hip fracture is a major consequence of falls and results in a 25% reduction in life expectancy and institutionalization rates of 8% to 34% for patients from the community.[112] These injuries can have long-lasting effects: for example, 40% to 60% of pa-tients following a hip fracture are never able to return to the same functional capacity as before the injury.[113] Falls also contribute to patient fear and anxiety regarding future falls, which impair quality of life and lead to declines in mobility (70%), self-care (41%), and activities of daily living (64%).[114]

Screening and Interventions

The American Geriatrics Society recommends annual screening for falls in patients aged 65 years and older,[115] which applies to most adults with HFpEF.[7] Screening tools for falls include the vali-dated Hendrich II Fall Risk Model (HIIFRM), which takes 5 to 10 minutes to complete, can be admin-istered by any member of the health care team, and evaluates 8 variables including measures of mental status, depression, altered elimination, dizziness/vertigo, 2 categories of medications (an-tiepileptics and benzodiazepines), gender, and functional status.[116] The tool is scored by adding up the risk factors: greater than or equal to 5 indi-cates a high fall risk.[116] The validated 12-item Fall Risk Questionnaire (FRQ) created by the US Cen-ters for Disease Control and Prevention may also be a reasonable screening tool, can be adminis-tered by any member of the health care team, and takes only 3 to 5 minutes to administer. This instrument is composed of 12 yes/no questions related to risk factors for falls.[117] This tool is also scored by adding up risk factors, and greater than or equal to 4 indicates moderate to high risk for falls.[117] Although screening instruments likely have superior diagnostic performance, asking pa-tients about their history of falls may be a reason-able screen because fall history is the strongest predictor of future falls.[118]

Given the substantial morbidity and mortality of falls, preventing falls should be a priority for clini-cians caring for adults with HFpEF. Multicompo-nent exercise programs, physical rehabilitation, and home hazard modifications can mitigate fall risk.[102,119] Multicomponent exercise programs should include a combination of the following components: balance, strength, flexibility, and endurance training—when at least 2 are incorpo-rated, fall risk decreases by 17%.[120,121] Home hazard modifications can decrease the fall rate by 44%; this involves removing or changing loose floor mats, painting the edges of steps, reducing glare, installing grab bars and stair rails, removing clutter, and improving lighting.[122]

Social Domain: Social Isolation and Loneliness

Prevalence and implications

Social isolation is an objective lack of meaningful and sustained communication.[123] This isolation occurs when a person's social network size is reduced, resulting in a paucity of social contacts and interactions.[124] Social isolation can result in loneliness, which is the feeling of being alone, separated, or apart from others, and may be considered as the psychological embodiment of social isolation.[125] The prevalence of social isola-tion is estimated to be about 25% among ambu-latory patients with HF,[126] and 49% among hospitalized patients with HF.[127] Although these studies did not specifically differentiate between HFpEF or HFrEF, these are reasonable estimates for both subtypes of HF. Older adults with HFpEF are at especially high risk for social isolation for several reasons. Social isolation becomes increasingly common with age due to a shrinking social network that can result from dispersion of family and/or the death of spouses and friends over time—indeed, patients with HFpEF frequently live alone(25%).[58,128] Even when social contacts are present, HF symptoms can lead to a decline in capacity to engage in social interac-tions due to high symptom burden and well-described physical limitations, further contrib-uting to social isolation among older adults with HFpEF.[129] The high prevalence of depressive symptoms among older adults with HFpEF may additionally undermine motivation to engage in social interactions, and subsequently lead to further social isolation.[130]

Social isolation is associated with worse health-related quality of life, and increased morbidity and mortality.[124,125] These findings have been described among ambulatory and hospitalized patients with HF.[131,132] For example, in a study of 312 patients with HF (inclusive of HFpEF and HFrEF) over a period of 2 years, perceived social isolation was associated with an almost 4-fold times increased risk of death, 57% increased risk of emergency department visits, and 68% increased risk of hospitalization.[126]

Screening and Interventions

Social isolation can be assessed through the Lubben Social Network Scale (LSNS-6), which consists of 6 questions focused on perceived social support from family and friends. The LSNS-6 is a validated tool,[133] can be administered by any member of the health care team, and takes about 5 minutes to complete. The total score ranges from 0 to 30, with scores less than 12 indicating the presence of social isolation.[133] To understand the psychological embodiment of social isolation, it may be reasonable to also screen older adults with HFpEF for loneliness—this can be done via the validated The University of California, Los Angeles 3-item loneliness score and can again be administered by a nonclinical team member in just 2 minutes.[134] This survey consists of 3 questions that assesses 3 dimensions of loneliness (relational connectedness, social connectedness, and self-perceived isolation) and is scored on a scale from 3 to 9 with scores greater than or equal to 6 indicating loneliness.[134]

Identification of social isolation is important because interventions are possible. Internet access and cellular technologies have the power to overcome the social and spatial barriers of social interaction by facilitating interactions among older adults via convenient and affordable platforms like mobile devices.[135] A recent systematic review found that Internet access and cellular technologies alleviated social isolation through 4 main mechanisms: connection to the outside world, increasing social support, engaging in activities of interest, and boosting self-confidence.[136] Community arts programs are also promising, with data demonstrating that they significantly reduce the perception of social isolation and feeling of loneliness by helping older adults expand their community connections, establish supportive relationships with others participants, and develop meaningful roles through art.[123] There are also effective one-on-one interventions that use social care provisions; for example, one study used nursing students to aid socialization through visitations in community-dwelling older adults and found that those receiving the intervention were 12 times less likely to report feeling socially isolated.[137] Although there is no clear consensus as to which intervention is best,[123] tailoring interventions to suit the needs of each individual is likely to provide the greatest benefit.

SUMMARY

Multimorbidity, polypharmacy, cognitive impairment, depressive symptoms, frailty, falls, and social isolation are highly prevalent in HFpEF due to common risk factors and the direct contributions of HF. These conditions each have important implications for quality of life, clinical events important to older adults including hospitalization, and mortality. A summary of this is illustrated in **Fig. 2**. There are multiple strategies to screen for these conditions, and many can be administered quickly in routine clinical practice by medical team members with minimal training. Finally, evidence-based interventions to modify the consequences of these conditions are available. Taken together, this narrative review underscores the importance of screening for multiple geriatric conditions, integrating these conditions into decision making, and addressing these conditions when caring for older adults with HFpEF. Future work should focus on developing approaches to integrate assessments and interventions of these conditions into the routine provision of care to this vulnerable population.

DISCLOSURES

Dr Goyal has received personal fees for medico-legal consulting related to heart failure, and has received honoraria from Akcea Inc and Bionest Inc. Dr Kitzman has received honoraria as a consultant outside the present study for Bayer, Merck, Pfizer, Corvia Medical, Boehringer Ingelheim, Ketyo, Rivus, NovoNordisk, AstraZeneca, and Novartis; grant funding from Novartis, Bayer, Pfizer, NovoNordisk, and AstraZeneca; and has stock ownership in Gilead Sciences.

SOURCES OF FUNDING

Dr Goyal is supported by American Heart Association grant 20CDA35310455, National Institute on Aging (NIA) grant K76AG064428, and Loan Repayment Program award L30AG060521. Dr Kitzman is supported by NIA grants R01AG045551, R01AG1

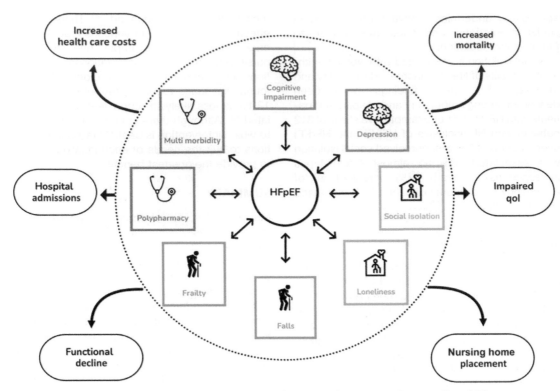

Fig. 2. Intertwined relationship of HFpEF, geriatric conditions, and outcomes. QoL, quality of life.

8915, P30AG021332, and U24AG059624, and by NHLBI grant U01HL160272. Dr Kitzman is also supported in part by the Kermit Glenn Phillips II Chair in Cardiovascular Medicine at Wake Forest School of Medicine.

CLINICS CARE POINTS

Multimorbidity

- To screen for multimorbidity, conduct a thorough history and consider screening for common comorbid conditions.

- When present, optimization of treatment for each condition and maintaining effective communication with other treating clinicians is beneficial.

Polypharmacy

- To screen for polypharmacy, a standard intake of medications and/or review of the electronic medical record, with potential integration of tools that screen for potential harmful agents like the STOPP/START tool may be beneficial.

- When present, consider deprescribing medications whose risks outweigh benefits

Cognitive impairment

- To screen for cognitive impairment, consider administering the Mini-Cog, which takes only 3 minutes to conduct.

- When present, treat underlying contributing factors, accommodate for deficiencies in self-care, and consider referring to a memory specialist and/or additional testing.

Depression

- To screen for depression, consider administering the PHQ-2, and proceeding with the PHQ-9 if the PHQ-2 is positive.

- When present, consider exercise and/or referring for cognitive behavioral therapy.

Frailty

- To screen for frailty, there are myriad instruments that can be used including the TUG and SPPB.

- When present, consider exercise-based interventions.

Falls

- To screen for falls risk, consider asking patients about a history of falls and/or administer the HIIFRM or FRQ.

- When present, consider multicomponent exercise programs, physical rehabilitation, and/or home hazard modifications.

Social

- isolation To screen for social isolation and/or loneliness, consider the LSNS-6 and/or the UCLA 3-item loneliness scale.
- When present, consider increasing social interactions through technology, community programs, and/or one-on-one socialization interventions.

ACKNOWLEDGMENTS

None

REFERENCES

1. Tsao CW, Aday AW, Almarzooq ZI, et al. Heart disease and stroke statistics-2022 update: a report from the American heart association. Circulation 2022;145(8):e153–639 (In eng).

2. Goyal P, Almarzooq ZI, Horn EM, et al. Characteristics of hospitalizations for heart failure with preserved ejection fraction. Am J Med 2016;129(6): 635 e15–26.

3. Kitzman DW, Gardin JM, Gottdiener JS, et al. Importance of heart failure with preserved systolic function in patients > or = 65 years of age. CHS Research Group. Cardiovascular Health Study. Am J Cardiol 2001;87(4):413–9 (In eng).

4. Paulus WJ, Tschöpe C. A novel paradigm for heart failure with preserved ejection fraction: comorbidities drive myocardial dysfunction and remodeling through coronary microvascular endothelial inflammation. J Am Coll Cardiol 2013;62(4):263–71 (In eng).

5. Mathew S, Maurer SLH, Parag G. Heart failure. In: Halter JB, Ouslander JG, Studenski S, et al, editors. Hazzard's Geriatric Medicine and Gerontology, 7e. New York, NY: McGraw-Hill Education; 2017.

6. Pandey A, Shah SJ, Butler J, et al. Exercise intolerance in older adults with heart failure with preserved ejection fraction: JACC state-of-the-art review. J Am Coll Cardiol 2021;78(11):1166–87. https://doi.org/10.1016/j.jacc.2021.07.014 (In eng).

7. Upadhya B, Taffet GE, Cheng CP, et al. Heart failure with preserved ejection fraction in the elderly: scope of the problem. J Mol Cell Cardiol 2015;83: 73–87.

8. Gorodeski EZ, Goyal P, Hummel SL, et al. Domain management approach to heart failure in the geriatric patient: present and future. J Am Coll Cardiol 2018;71(17):1921–36. https://doi.org/10.1016/j.jacc.2018.02.059.

9. Forman DE, Maurer MS, Boyd C, et al. Multimorbidity in older adults with cardiovascular disease. J Am Coll Cardiol 2018;71(19):2149–61.

10. Redfield MM. Heart failure with preserved ejection fraction. N Engl J Med 2017;376(9):897 (In eng).

11. Unlu O, Levitan EB, Reshetnyak E, et al. Polypharmacy in older adults hospitalized for heart failure. Circ Heart Fail 2020;13(11):e006977.

12. Mentz RJ, Kelly JP, von Lueder TG, et al. Noncardiac comorbidities in heart failure with reduced versus preserved ejection fraction. J Am Coll Cardiol 2014;64(21):2281–93.

13. Khan MS, Samman Tahhan A, Vaduganathan M, et al. Trends in prevalence of comorbidities in heart failure clinical trials. Eur J Heart Fail 2020;22(6): 1032–42 (In eng).

14. Santhanakrishnan R, Wang N, Larson MG, et al. Atrial fibrillation begets heart failure and vice versa: temporal associations and differences in preserved versus reduced ejection fraction. Circulation 2016;133(5):484–92. https://doi.org/10.1161/CIRCULATIONAHA.115.018614.

15. Carlisle MA, Fudim M, DeVore AD, et al. Heart failure and atrial fibrillation, like fire and fury. JACC Heart Fail 2019;7(6):447–56. https://doi.org/10.1016/j.jchf.2019.03.005.

16. Vergaro G, Ghionzoli N, Innocenti L, et al. Noncardiac versus cardiac mortality in heart failure with preserved, midrange, and reduced ejection fraction. J Am Heart Assoc 2019;8(20):e013441. https://doi.org/10.1161/jaha.119.013441 (In eng).

17. Goyal P, Sauer AJ, Rich MW. All-cause mortality as an end point for heart failure with preserved ejection fraction: underperformance or overambitious? J Card Fail 2022;28(5):863–5 (In eng).

18. Baniak LM, Chasens ER. Sleep disordered breathing in older adults with heart failure with preserved ejection fraction. Geriatr Nurs 2018;39(1):77–83 (In eng).

19. Suen C, Wong J, Ryan CM, et al. Prevalence of undiagnosed obstructive sleep apnea among patients hospitalized for cardiovascular disease and associated in-hospital outcomes: a scoping review. J Clin Med 2020;9(4). https://doi.org/10.3390/jcm9040989 (In eng).

20. Goyal P, Kneifati-Hayek J, Archambault A, et al. Reply: toward improved understanding of potential harm in heart failure. JACC Heart Fail 2020;8(3): 247–8. https://doi.org/10.1016/j.jchf.2019.12.003 (In eng).

21. Kennel PJ, Kneifati-Hayek J, Bryan J, et al. Prevalence and determinants of hyperpolypharmacy in adults with heart failure: an observational study from the national health and nutrition examination survey (NHANES). BMC Cardiovasc Disord 2019; 19(1):76. https://doi.org/10.1186/s12872-019-1058-7 (In eng).

22. American geriatrics society 2019 updated AGS Beers Criteria® for potentially inappropriate medication use in older adults. J Am Geriatr Soc 2019; 67(4):674–94. https://doi.org/10.1111/jgs.15767 (In eng).

23. Brinker LM, Konerman MC, Navid P, et al. Complex and potentially harmful medication patterns in heart failure with preserved ejection fraction. Am J Med 2021;134(3):374–82. https://doi.org/10.1016/j.amjmed.2020.07.023 (In eng).

24. Freeland KN, Thompson AN, Zhao Y, et al. Medication use and associated risk of falling in a geriatric outpatient population. Ann Pharmacother 2012; 46(9):1188–92. https://doi.org/10.1345/aph.1Q689 (In eng).

25. Jyrkkä J, Enlund H, Lavikainen P, et al. Association of polypharmacy with nutritional status, functional ability and cognitive capacity over a three-year period in an elderly population. Pharmacoepidemiol Drug Saf 2011;20(5):514–22 (In eng).

26. Marcum ZA, Amuan ME, Hanlon JT, et al. Prevalence of unplanned hospitalizations caused by adverse drug reactions in older veterans. J Am Geriatr Soc 2012;60(1):34–41 (In eng).

27. Picker D, Heard K, Bailey TC, et al. The number of discharge medications predicts thirty-day hospital readmission: a cohort study. BMC Health Serv Res 2015;15:282. https://doi.org/10.1186/s12913-015-0950-9 (In eng).

28. Boyd CM, Darer J, Boult C, et al. Clinical practice guidelines and quality of care for older patients with multiple comorbid diseases: implications for pay for performance. JAMA 2005;294(6):716–24. https://doi.org/10.1001/jama.294.6.716.

29. Goyal P, Mangal S, Krishnaswami A, et al. Polypharmacy in heart failure: progress but also problem. Am J Med 2021;134(9):1071–3 (In eng).

30. Samsa GP, Hanlon JT, Schmader KE, et al. A summated score for the medication appropriateness index: development and assessment of clinimetric properties including content validity. J Clin Epidemiol 1994;47(8):891–6 (In eng).

31. O'Mahony D, O'Sullivan D, Byrne S, et al. STOPP/START criteria for potentially inappropriate prescribing in older people: version 2. Age Ageing 2015;44(2):213–8. https://doi.org/10.1093/ageing/afu145 (In eng).

32. Krishnaswami A, Steinman MA, Goyal P, et al. Deprescribing in older adults with cardiovascular disease. J Am Coll Cardiol 2019;73(20):2584–95 (In eng).

33. Anker SD, Butler J, Filippatos G, et al. Empagliflozin in heart failure with a preserved ejection fraction. N Engl J Med 2021;385(16):1451–61. https://doi.org/10.1056/NEJMoa2107038.

34. Yamamoto K, Origasa H, Hori M, et al. Effects of carvedilol on heart failure with preserved ejection fraction: the Japanese Diastolic Heart Failure Study (J-DHF). Eur J Heart Fail 2013;15(1):110–8. https://doi.org/10.1093/eurjhf/hfs141.

35. Cleland JGF, Bunting KV, Flather MD, et al. Beta-blockers for heart failure with reduced, mid-range, and preserved ejection fraction: an individual patient-level analysis of double-blind randomized trials. Eur Heart J 2018;39(1):26–35. https://doi.org/10.1093/eurheartj/ehx564.

36. Palau P, Seller J, Dominguez E, et al. Effect of beta-blocker withdrawal on functional capacity in heart failure and preserved ejection fraction. J Am Coll Cardiol 2021;78(21):2042–56. https://doi.org/10.1016/j.jacc.2021.08.073.

37. Cannon JA, Moffitt P, Perez-Moreno AC, et al. Cognitive impairment and heart failure: systematic review and meta-analysis. J Card Fail 2017;23(6):464–75. https://doi.org/10.1016/j.cardfail.2017.04.007 (In eng).

38. Pastva AM, Hugenschmidt CE, Kitzman DW, et al. Cognition, physical function, and quality of life in older patients with acute decompensated heart failure. J Card Fail 2021;27(3):286–94. https://doi.org/10.1016/j.cardfail.2020.09.007 (In eng).

39. Luck T, Luppa M, Briel S, et al. Mild cognitive impairment: incidence and risk factors: results of the leipzig longitudinal study of the aged. J Am Geriatr Soc 2010;58(10):1903–10 (In eng).

40. Jefferson AL, Himali JJ, Beiser AS, et al. Cardiac index is associated with brain aging: the Framingham Heart Study. Circulation 2010;122(7):690–7 (In eng).

41. Weber T, Wassertheurer S, O'Rourke MF, et al. Pulsatile hemodynamics in patients with exertional dyspnea: potentially of value in the diagnostic evaluation of suspected heart failure with preserved ejection fraction. J Am Coll Cardiol 2013;61(18):1874–83. https://doi.org/10.1016/j.jacc.2013.02.013 (In eng).

42. Havakuk O, King KS, Grazette L, et al. Heart failure-induced brain injury. J Am Coll Cardiol 2017;69(12):1609–16 (In eng).

43. Chetty S, Friedman AR, Taravosh-Lahn K, et al. Stress and glucocorticoids promote oligodendrogenesis in the adult hippocampus. Mol Psychiatry 2014;19(12):1275–83 (In eng).

44. Yzeiraj E, Tam DM, Gorodeski EZ. Management of cognitive impairment in heart failure. Curr Treat Options Cardiovasc Med 2016;18(1):4 (In eng).

45. Zuccalà G, Onder G, Pedone C, et al. Cognitive dysfunction as a major determinant of disability in patients with heart failure: results from a multicentre survey. On behalf of the GIFA (SIGG-ONLUS) Investigators. J Neurol Neurosurg Psychiatry 2001;70(1):109–12 (In eng).

46. Gelow JM, Mudd JO, Chien CV, et al. Usefulness of cognitive dysfunction in heart failure to predict cardiovascular risk at 180 days. Am J Cardiol 2015;115(6):778–82 (In eng).

47. Currie K, Rideout A, Lindsay G, et al. The association between mild cognitive impairment and self-care in adults with chronic heart failure: a systematic review and narrative synthesis. J Cardiovasc Nurs 2015;30(5):382–93 (In eng).

48. Patel A, Parikh R, Howell EH, et al. Mini-cog performance: novel marker of post discharge risk among patients hospitalized for heart failure. Circ Heart Fail 2015;8(1):8–16 (In eng).

49. Borson S, Scanlan JM, Chen P, et al. The Mini-Cog as a screen for dementia: validation in a population-based sample. J Am Geriatr Soc 2003;51(10):1451–4 (In eng).

50. Harkness K, Demers C, Heckman GA, et al. Screening for cognitive deficits using the Montreal cognitive assessment tool in outpatients ≥65 years of age with heart failure. Am J Cardiol 2011;107(8):1203–7 (In eng).

51. Alagiakrishnan K, Mah D, Dyck JR, et al. Comparison of two commonly used clinical cognitive screening tests to diagnose mild cognitive impairment in heart failure with the golden standard European Consortium Criteria. Int J Cardiol 2017;228:558–62 (In eng).

52. Kindermann I, Fischer D, Karbach J, et al. Cognitive function in patients with decompensated heart failure: the Cognitive Impairment in Heart Failure (CogImpair-HF) study. Eur J Heart Fail 2012;14(4):404–13 (In eng).

53. Leto L, Feola M. Cognitive impairment in heart failure patients: role of atrial fibrillation. J Geriatr Cardiol 2015;12(6):690 (In eng).

54. Canessa N, Castronovo V, Cappa SF, et al. Obstructive sleep apnea: brain structural changes and neurocognitive function before and after treatment. Am J Respir Crit Care Med 2011;183(10):1419–26 (In eng).

55. Douglas A, Letts L, Richardson J. A systematic review of accidental injury from fire, wandering and medication self-administration errors for older adults with and without dementia. Arch Gerontol Geriatr 2011;52(1) (In eng). e1–10.

56. Sokoreli I, de Vries JJG, Pauws SC, et al. Depression and anxiety as predictors of mortality among heart failure patients: systematic review and meta-analysis. Heart Fail Rev 2016;21(1):49–63. https://doi.org/10.1007/s10741-015-9517-4 (In eng).

57. Liu J, Guo Z, Fan M, et al. Major depression and clinical outcomes in patients with heart failure with preserved ejection fraction. Eur J Clin Invest 2021;51(3):e13401 (In eng).

58. Navid P, Nguyen L, Jaber D, et al. Attitudes toward deprescribing among adults with heart failure with preserved ejection fraction. J Am Geriatr Soc 2021;69(7):1948–55. https://doi.org/10.1111/jgs.17204 (In eng).

59. Warraich HJ, Kitzman DW, Whellan DJ, et al. Physical function, frailty, cognition, depression, and quality of life in hospitalized adults ≥60 Years with acute decompensated heart failure with preserved versus reduced ejection fraction. Circ Heart Fail 2018;11(11):e005254. https://doi.org/10.1161/circheartfailure.118.005254 (In eng).

60. Alves TC, Busatto GF. Regional cerebral blood flow reductions, heart failure and Alzheimer's disease. Neurol Res 2006;28(6):579–87. https://doi.org/10.1179/016164106x130416 (In eng).

61. Suzuki H, Matsumoto Y, Ota H, et al. Hippocampal blood flow abnormality associated with depressive symptoms and cognitive impairment in patients with chronic heart failure. Circ J 2016;80(8):1773–80. https://doi.org/10.1253/circj.CJ-16-0367 (In eng).

62. Saczynski JS, Beiser A, Seshadri S, et al. Depressive symptoms and risk of dementia: the framingham heart study. Neurology 2010;75(1):35–41. https://doi.org/10.1212/WNL.0b013e3181e62138 (In eng).

63. Schiepers OJ, Wichers MC, Maes M. Cytokines and major depression. Prog Neuropsychopharmacol Biol Psychiatry 2005;29(2):201–17. https://doi.org/10.1016/j.pnpbp.2004.11.003 (In eng).

64. Bhagwagar Z, Hafizi S, Cowen PJ. Increased salivary cortisol after waking in depression. Psychopharmacology (Berl) 2005;182(1):54–7. https://doi.org/10.1007/s00213-005-0062-z (In eng).

65. Rutledge T, Reis VA, Linke SE, et al. Depression in heart failure a meta-analytic review of prevalence, intervention effects, and associations with clinical outcomes. J Am Coll Cardiol 2006;48(8):1527–37. https://doi.org/10.1016/j.jacc.2006.06.055 (In eng).

66. Chandra A, Alcala MAD, Claggett B, et al. Associations between depressive symptoms and HFpEF-related outcomes. JACC Heart Fail 2020;8(12):1009–20. https://doi.org/10.1016/j.jchf.2020.06.010 (In eng).

67. Freedland KE, Skala JA, Steinmeyer BC, et al. Effects of depression on heart failure self-care. J Card Fail 2021;27(5):522–32. https://doi.org/10.1016/j.cardfail.2020.12.015 (In eng).

68. Kroenke K, Spitzer RL, Williams JB. The Patient Health Questionnaire-2: validity of a two-item depression screener. Med Care 2003;41(11):1284–92. https://doi.org/10.1097/01.Mlr.0000093487.78664.3c (In eng).

69. Hammash MH, Hall LA, Lennie TA, et al. Psychometrics of the PHQ-9 as a measure of depressive symptoms in patients with heart failure. Eur J Cardiovasc Nurs 2013;12(5):446–53. https://doi.org/10.1177/1474515112468068 (In eng).

70. David D, Cristea I, Hofmann SG. Why cognitive behavioral therapy is the current gold standard of psychotherapy. Front Psychiatry 2018;9:4. https://doi.org/10.3389/fpsyt.2018.00004 (In eng).

71. Freedland KE, Carney RM, Rich MW, et al. Cognitive behavior therapy for depression and self-care in heart failure patients: a randomized clinical trial. JAMA Intern Med 2015;175(11):1773–82. https://doi.org/10.1001/jamainternmed.2015.5220 (In eng).

72. Nolte K, Herrmann-Lingen C, Wachter R, et al. Effects of exercise training on different quality of life dimensions in heart failure with preserved ejection fraction: the Ex-DHF-P trial. Eur J Prev Cardiol 2015;22(5):582–93. https://doi.org/10.1177/2047487314526071 (In eng).

73. Redwine LS, Wilson K, Pung MA, et al. A randomized study examining the effects of mild-to-moderate group exercises on cardiovascular, physical, and psychological well-being in patients with heart failure. J Cardiopulm Rehabil Prev 2019;39(6):403–8. https://doi.org/10.1097/hcr.0000000000000430 (In eng).

74. O'Connor CM, Jiang W, Kuchibhatla M, et al. Safety and efficacy of sertraline for depression in patients with heart failure: results of the SADHART-CHF (Sertraline against Depression and Heart Disease in Chronic Heart Failure) trial. J Am Coll Cardiol 2010;56(9):692–9. https://doi.org/10.1016/j.jacc.2010.03.068 (In eng).

75. Angermann CE, Gelbrich G, Störk S, et al. Effect of escitalopram on all-cause mortality and hospitalization in patients with heart failure and depression: the MOOD-HF randomized clinical trial. JAMA 2016;315(24):2683–93. https://doi.org/10.1001/jama.2016.7635 (In eng).

76. Ijaz N, Buta B, Xue QL, et al. Interventions for frailty among older adults with cardiovascular disease: JACC state-of-the-art review. J Am Coll Cardiol 2022;79(5):482–503. https://doi.org/10.1016/j.jacc.2021.11.029 (In eng).

77. Fried LP, Tangen CM, Walston J, et al. Frailty in older adults: evidence for a phenotype. J Gerontol A Biol Sci Med Sci 2001;56(3):M146–56. https://doi.org/10.1093/gerona/56.3.m146 (In eng).

78. Rockwood K, Fox RA, Stolee P, et al. Frailty in elderly people: an evolving concept. CMAJ 1994;150(4):489–95 (In eng).

79. Mitnitski AB, Mogilner AJ, Rockwood K. Accumulation of deficits as a proxy measure of aging. ScientificWorldJournal 2001;1:323–36. https://doi.org/10.1100/tsw.2001.58 (In eng).

80. Martín-Sánchez FJ, Christ M, Miró Ò, et al. Practical approach on frail older patients attended for acute heart failure. Int J Cardiol 2016;222:62–71 (In eng).

81. Searle SD, Mitnitski A, Gahbauer EA, et al. A standard procedure for creating a frailty index. BMC Geriatr 2008;8:24 (In eng).

82. Walston J, Buta B, Xue QL. Frailty screening and interventions: considerations for clinical practice. Clin Geriatr Med 2018;34(1):25–38 (In eng).

83. Pandey A, Kitzman D, Whellan DJ, et al. Frailty among older decompensated heart failure patients: prevalence, association with patient-centered outcomes, and efficient detection methods. JACC Heart Fail 2019;7(12):1079–88 (In eng).

84. Sanders NA, Supiano MA, Lewis EF, et al. The frailty syndrome and outcomes in the TOPCAT trial. Eur J Heart Fail 2018;20(11):1570–7 (In eng).

85. Pandey A, Kitzman D, Reeves G. Frailty is intertwined with heart failure: mechanisms, prevalence, prognosis, assessment, and management. JACC Heart Fail 2019;7(12):1001–11 (In eng).

86. Bellumkonda L, Tyrrell D, Hummel SL, et al. Pathophysiology of heart failure and frailty: a common inflammatory origin? Aging Cell 2017;16(3):444–50 (In eng).

87. Kojima G. Frailty as a predictor of nursing home placement among community-dwelling older adults: a systematic review and meta-analysis. J Geriatr Phys Ther 2018;41(1):42–8 (In eng).

88. McNallan SM, Singh M, Chamberlain AM, et al. Frailty and healthcare utilization among patients with heart failure in the community. JACC Heart Fail 2013;1(2):135–41 (In eng).

89. Goyal P, Yum B, Navid P, et al. Frailty and post-hospitalization outcomes in patients with heart failure with preserved ejection fraction. Am J Cardiol 2021;148:84–93 (In eng).

90. Hegde SM, Claggett B, Shah AM, et al. Physical activity and prognosis in the TOPCAT Trial (treatment of preserved cardiac function heart failure with an aldosterone antagonist). Circulation 2017;136(11):982–92 (In eng).

91. McNallan SM, Chamberlain AM, Gerber Y, et al. Measuring frailty in heart failure: a community perspective. Am Heart J 2013;166(4):768–74 (In eng).

92. Sukkriang N, Punsawad C. Comparison of geriatric assessment tools for frailty among community elderly. Heliyon 2020;6(9):e04797 (In eng).

93. Afilalo J, Alexander KP, Mack MJ, et al. Frailty assessment in the cardiovascular care of older adults. J Am Coll Cardiol 2014;63(8):747–62 (In eng).

94. Hornsby WE, Sareini MA, Golbus JR, et al. Lower extremity function is independently associated with hospitalization burden in heart failure with preserved ejection fraction. J Card Fail 2019;25(1):2–9 (In eng).

95. Turner G, Clegg A. Best practice guidelines for the management of frailty: a British geriatrics society, age UK and royal College of general practitioners report. Age Ageing 2014;43(6):744–7 (In eng).

96. Phu S, Kirk B, Bani Hassan E, et al. The diagnostic value of the Short physical performance Battery for sarcopenia. BMC Geriatr 2020;20(1):242. https://doi.org/10.1186/s12877-020-01642-4 (In eng).

97. Sze S, Pellicori P, Zhang J, et al. Identification of frailty in chronic heart failure. JACC Heart Fail 2019;7(4):291–302. https://doi.org/10.1016/j.jchf.2018.11.017 (In eng).

98. Bellettiere J, Lamonte MJ, Unkart J, et al. Short physical performance Battery and incident cardiovascular events among older women. J Am Heart Assoc 2020;9(14):e016845 (In eng).

99. Sepehri K, Braley MS, Chinda B, et al. A computerized frailty assessment tool at points-of-care: development of a standalone electronic comprehensive geriatric assessment/frailty index (eFI-CGA). Front Public Health 2020;8. https://doi.org/10.3389/fpubh.2020.00089 (Technology and Code) (In English).

100. Clegg A, Bates C, Young J, et al. Development and validation of an electronic frailty index using routine primary care electronic health record data. Age Ageing 2016;45(3):353–60 (In eng).

101. Theou O, Stathokostas L, Roland KP, et al. The effectiveness of exercise interventions for the management of frailty: a systematic review. J Aging Res 2011;2011:569194 (In eng).

102. Kitzman DW, Whellan DJ, Duncan P, et al. Physical rehabilitation for older patients hospitalized for heart failure. N Engl J Med 2021;385(3):203–16. https://doi.org/10.1056/NEJMoa2026141 (In eng).

103. Mentz RJ, Whellan DJ, Reeves GR, et al. Rehabilitation intervention in older patients with acute heart failure with preserved versus reduced ejection fraction. JACC Heart Fail 2021;9(10):747–57. https://doi.org/10.1016/j.jchf.2021.05.007 (In eng).

104. Lee PG, Cigolle C, Blaum C. The co-occurrence of chronic diseases and geriatric syndromes: the health and retirement study. J Am Geriatr Soc 2009;57(3):511–6 (In eng).

105. Tinetti ME, Williams CS. Falls, injuries due to falls, and the risk of admission to a nursing home. N Engl J Med 1997;337(18):1279–84 (In eng).

106. Tromp AM, Pluijm SM, Smit JH, et al. Fall-risk screening test: a prospective study on predictors for falls in community-dwelling elderly. J Clin Epidemiol 2001;54(8):837–44 (In eng).

107. Forman DE, Lipsitz LA. Syncope in the elderly. Cardiol Clin 1997;15(2):295–311 (In eng).

108. Jaber D, Vargas F, Nguyen L, et al. Prescriptions for potentially inappropriate medications from the Beers criteria among older adults hospitalized for heart failure. J Card Fail 2021;S1071-9164(21):00479–86 (In eng).

109. Sibley KM, Voth J, Munce SE, et al. Chronic disease and falls in community-dwelling Canadians over 65 years old: a population-based study exploring associations with number and pattern of chronic conditions. BMC Geriatr 2014;14:22 (In eng).

110. Tchalla AE, Dufour AB, Travison TG, et al. Patterns, predictors, and outcomes of falls trajectories in older adults: the MOBILIZE Boston Study with 5 years of follow-up. PLoS One 2014;9(9):e106363 (In eng).

111. Healey F, Scobie S, Oliver D, et al. Falls in English and Welsh hospitals: a national observational study based on retrospective analysis of 12 months of patient safety incident reports. Qual Saf Health Care 2008;17(6):424–30 (In eng).

112. Braithwaite RS, Col NF, Wong JB. Estimating hip fracture morbidity, mortality and costs. J Am Geriatr Soc 2003;51(3):364–70 (In eng).

113. Dyer SM, Crotty M, Fairhall N, et al. A critical review of the long-term disability outcomes following hip fracture. BMC Geriatr 2016;16(1):158 (In eng).

114. Hartholt KA, van Beeck EF, Polinder S, et al. Societal consequences of falls in the older population: injuries, healthcare costs, and long-term reduced quality of life. J Trauma 2011;71(3):748–53 (In eng).

115. Moncada LVV, Mire LG. Preventing falls in older persons. Am Fam Physician 2017;96(4):240–7. https://www.ncbi.nlm.nih.gov/pubmed/28925664.

116. Hendrich AL, Bufalino A, Groves C. Validation of the Hendrich II Fall Risk Model: the imperative to reduce modifiable risk factors. Appl Nurs Res 2020;53:151243 (In eng).

117. Lohman MC, Crow RS, DiMilia PR, et al. Operationalisation and validation of the Stopping Elderly Accidents, Deaths, and Injuries (STEADI) fall risk algorithm in a nationally representative sample. J Epidemiol Community Health 2017;71(12):1191–7 (In eng).

118. Berry SD, Miller RR. Falls: epidemiology, pathophysiology, and relationship to fracture. Curr Osteoporos Rep 2008;6(4):149–54 (In eng).

119. Karlsson MK, Vonschewelov T, Karlsson C, et al. Prevention of falls in the elderly: a review. Scand J Public Health 2013;41(5):442–54 (In eng).

120. Li F, Harmer P, Fisher KJ, et al. Tai Chi and fall reductions in older adults: a randomized controlled trial. J Gerontol A Biol Sci Med Sci 2005;60(2):187–94 (In eng).

121. Province MA, Hadley EC, Hornbrook MC, et al. The effects of exercise on falls in elderly patients. A preplanned meta-analysis of the FICSIT Trials. Frailty and Injuries: cooperative Studies of Intervention Techniques. Jama 1995;273(17):1341–7 (In eng).

122. Gillespie LD, Robertson MC, Gillespie WJ, et al. Interventions for preventing falls in older people living in the community. Cochrane Database Syst Rev 2012;2012(9):Cd007146 (In eng).

123. Poscia A, Stojanovic J, La Milia DI, et al. Interventions targeting loneliness and social isolation among the older people: an update systematic review. Exp Gerontol 2018;102:133–44. https://doi.org/10.1016/j.exger.2017.11.017 (In eng).

124. Steptoe A, Shankar A, Demakakos P, et al. Social isolation, loneliness, and all-cause mortality in older

men and women. Proc Natl Acad Sci U S A 2013; 110(15):5797–801 (In eng).

125. Molloy GJ, McGee HM, O'Neill D, et al. Loneliness and emergency and planned hospitalizations in a community sample of older adults. J Am Geriatr Soc 2010;58(8):1538–41 (In eng).

126. Manemann SM, Chamberlain AM, Roger VL, et al. Perceived social isolation and outcomes in patients with heart failure. J Am Heart Assoc 2018;7(11) (In eng).

127. Saito H, Kagiyama N, Nagano N, et al. Social isolation is associated with 90-day rehospitalization due to heart failure. Eur J Cardiovasc Nurs 2019;18(1): 16–20 (In eng).

128. Zhu W, Wu Y, Zhou Y, et al. Living alone and clinical outcomes in patients with heart failure with preserved ejection fraction. Psychosom Med 2021; 83(5):470–6 (In eng).

129. Cortis JD, Williams A. Palliative and supportive needs of older adults with heart failure. Int Nurs Rev 2007;54(3):263–70 (In eng).

130. Friedmann E, Thomas SA, Liu F, et al. Relationship of depression, anxiety, and social isolation to chronic heart failure outpatient mortality. Am Heart J 2006;152(5):940.e1–8 (In eng).

131. Årestedt K, Saveman BI, Johansson P, et al. Social support and its association with health-related quality of life among older patients with chronic heart failure. Eur J Cardiovasc Nurs 2013;12(1): 69–77 (In eng).

132. Krumholz HM, Butler J, Miller J, et al. Prognostic importance of emotional support for elderly patients hospitalized with heart failure. Circulation 1998;97(10):958–64. Available at: https://www. ncbi.nlm.nih.gov/pubmed/9529263.

133. Lubben J, Blozik E, Gillmann G, et al. Performance of an abbreviated version of the Lubben Social Network Scale among three European community-dwelling older adult populations. Gerontologist 2006;46(4):503–13. https://doi.org/ 10.1093/geront/46.4.503 (In eng).

134. Russell DW. UCLA Loneliness Scale (Version 3): reliability, validity, and factor structure. J Pers Assess 1996;66(1):20–40. https://doi.org/10.1207/ s15327752jpa6601_2 (In eng).

135. Krishnaswami A, Beavers C, Dorsch MP, et al. Gerotechnology for older adults with cardiovascular diseases: JACC state-of-the-art review. J Am Coll Cardiol 2020;76(22):2650–70 (In eng).

136. Chen YR, Schulz PJ. The effect of information communication technology interventions on reducing social isolation in the elderly: a systematic review. J Med Internet Res 2016;18(1):e18 (In eng).

137. Nicholson NR Jr, Shellman J. Decreasing social isolation in older adults: effects of an empowerment intervention offered through the CARELINK program. Res Gerontol Nurs 2013;6(2):89–97 (In eng).

138. Abellan van Kan G, Rolland Y, Bergman H, et al. The I.A.N.A Task Force on frailty assessment of older people in clinical practice. J Nutr Health Aging 2008;12(1):29–37 (In eng).

139. Gómez JF, Curcio CL, Alvarado B, et al. Validity and reliability of the Short physical performance Battery (SPPB): a pilot study on mobility in the Colombian andes. Colomb Med (Cali) 2013;44(3): 165–71 (In eng).

140. Stevens JA, Phelan EA. Development of STEADI: a fall prevention resource for health care providers. Health Promot Pract 2013;14(5):706–14 (In eng).

141. Chang Q, Sha F, Chan CH, et al. Validation of an abbreviated version of the Lubben Social Network Scale ("LSNS-6") and its associations with suicidality among older adults in China. PLoS One 2018; 13(8):e0201612 (In eng).

Pulmonary Hypertension in Heart Failure with Preserved Ejection Fraction

Victor M. Moles, MD[a],*, Gillian Grafton, DO[b]

KEYWORDS

- Heart failure with preserved ejection fraction ● Pulmonary arterial hypertension
- pulmonary hypertension

KEY POINTS

- Pulmonary hypertension can be frquently associated with HFpEF and is associated with worsened symptoms and mortality.
- Although right heart catheterization is the gold standard for diagnosing pulmonary hypertension, the echocardiogram raimains the screening test of choice and provides insightful information about hemodynamics.
- Currently, therer are no pulmonary hypertension sppecific medications approved for PH-HFpEF and treatment remains focused to optimizing co-morbidities.

INTRODUCTION

Heart failure with preserved ejection fraction (HFpEF) is a common entity that predominately affects older adults. Epidemiologic trends show that the incidence of HFpEF has not declined as profoundly as heart failure with reduced ejection fraction (HFrEF), and overall mortality remains unchanged.[1] Pulmonary hypertension (PH) is a heterogeneous condition defined hemodynamically as an elevation of pulmonary artery (PA) pressures and is commonly associated with HFpEF. Clinically, PH can be classified into 5 distinct categories based on the etiology, underlying pathophysiology, and potential treatment options.[2] Of these categories, PH due to left heart disease (PH-LHD) is frequently seen in clinical practice and is most commonly a consequence of the underlying left heart condition and probably related to its severity and duration.[3,4] The association of PH and HFpEF (PH-HFpEF) can be found in a majority of patients with HFpEF and is associated with worse symptoms and increased mortality.[5]

Despite the advancements in the treatment of other forms of PH, such as pulmonary arterial hypertension (PAH), pulmonary hypertension due to interstitial lung disease (PH-ILD) and chronic thromboembolic pulmonary hypertension (CTEPH), effective treatment of PH-LHD has not been found yet.[6–9]

HOW SHOULD PULMONARY HYPERTENSION-HEART FAILURE WITH PRESERVED EJECTION FRACTION BE DEFINED?

PH was traditionally defined as a mean PA pressure $\geq$ 25 mm Hg based on a resting right heart catheterization (RHC). This threshold has been considered arbitrary and inconsistent with recent hemodynamic data of healthy individuals showing an average mean PA pressure of 14 ± 3.3 mm Hg, a value that was minimally influenced by age. This had led to a recent change in the cutoff for elevated pulmonary pressures as a mean PA pressure > 20 mm Hg during the most recent World Symposium in Pulmonary Hypertension.[10] Despite

[a] Division of Cardiovascular Medicine, Department of Internal Medicine, University of Michigan, 1500 East Medical Center Drive, Cardiovascular Center, Floor 2, Ann Arbor, MI 48103, USA; [b] Division of Cardiovascular Medicine, Department of Internal Medicine, Henry Ford Hospital, 2799 West Grand Boulevard, K14, Detroit, MI MI 48202, USA
* Corresponding author.
E-mail address: vmoles@med.umich.edu

Cardiol Clin 40 (2022) 533–540
https://doi.org/10.1016/j.ccl.2022.06.007
0733-8651/22/© 2022 Elsevier Inc. All rights reserved.

the recognition of this lower diagnostic threshold, PH-LHD continues to be defined as a mean PA $\geq$ 25 mm Hg and a pulmonary capillary wedge pressure (PCWP) > 15 mm Hg.[7] The definition of PH-LHD relies heavily on the accurate measurement of PCWP and special attention should be placed on measurements at end of expiration. In sinus rhythm, this corresponds to the mean of the A-wave.[7]

PH-LHD can be a result of several factors, including the passive transmission of elevated left-sided filling pressures, pulmonary vasculopathy, increased pulmonary blood flow, or a combination of these elements. Understanding the underlying pathophysiology may help in guiding medical management and selecting future therapeutic options. PH-LHD can be further divided into 2 categories based on PCWP and pulmonary vascular resistance (PVR): (1) isolated postcapillary pulmonary hypertension (IpcPH) when PCWP > 15 mm Hg and PVR < 3 WU; and (2) combined pre and postcapillary pulmonary hypertension (CpcPH) when PCWP > 15 and PVR $\geq$ 3 Wood units. Although previously the diastolic pressure gradient (DPG = PA diastolic–PCWP) was introduced to distinguish between IpcPH and CpcPH, this definition was found restrictive and exposed to interpretation, leading to PVR being subsequently reintroduced as part of the definition.[7] The importance of differentiating CpcPH from IpcPH is highlighted by a meta-analysis of 10 retrospective analyses showing that PVR was a strong predictor of survival.[11] Similarly, a recent large retrospective analysis also showed that PVR was a predictor of mortality and hospitalizations in HFpEF.[12]

As routine invasive RHC is often not performed as part of the diagnosis of HFpEF, the initial assessment of PH may rely heavily on an echocardiogram. Many studies which studied PH-HFpEF did so by using the echocardiogram to define PH. The probability of PH can be estimated based on the peak tricuspid regurgitation velocity and the presence of other supporting PH signs -RV/LV ratio >1.0, flattening of interventricular septum, right ventricular outflow tract notching or short acceleration time, elevated right atrial pressures based on IVC measurements- (**Table 1**), although most of these signs reflect an elevated PVR which not may necessarily be abnormal in PH-HFpEF.[13]

IS PULMONARY HYPERTENSION-HEART FAILURE WITH PRESERVED EJECTION FRACTION COMMON?

Lam and colleagues[5] reported an incidence of the PH of 83% based on echocardiographic data with a median right ventricular systolic pressure (RVSP) of 48 mm Hg in patients with HFpEF in Olmsted County. Also, the TOPCAT study showed that 36% of patients with had estimated systolic PA pressure of at least 35 mm Hg plus right trial pressure measured by echocardiogram.[14]

Strange and colleagues[3] performed a large observational population cohort study in Australia which showed that 9.1% of echocardiograms performed showed evidence of PH (estimated RVSP > 40 mm Hg). Based on clinical and echocardiographic data, patients were classified into in one of the 5 distinctive groups based on the updated classification at the time from the Third World Symposium on Pulmonary Hypertension.[15] PH-LHD was the most common type of PH diagnosed accounting for 68% of cases and an estimated incidence of 250 cases per 100,000. The presence of PH was significantly associated with poor survival. The mean survival rate for patients with PH-LHD was 4.3 $\pm$ 0.3 years. Interestingly, the survival for patients with PAH was better than those with PH-LHD, presumably because medical therapy was available.

WHAT ARE THE CLINICAL IMPLICATIONS OF PULMONARY HYPERTENSION IN HEART FAILURE WITH PRESERVED EJECTION FRACTION?

The deleterious association of PH-LHD and survival were also assessed by Lam and colleagues[5] who used a random sample of patients with available echocardiographic data from Olmsted County, Minnesota. The increase in RVSP was coupled with increases in pulse pressure and echocardiography-derived PCWP, suggesting that age-associated blood vessel stiffness and diastolic dysfunction contribute to changes in pulmonary artery pressure. After adjusting for estimated PCWP, RVSP was higher in HFpEF compared to hypertensive individuals without heart failure. This suggests that beyond the postcapillary contribution of pulmonary venous congestion, a precapillary component may contribute to greater PH in HFpEF. The presence of PH defined by an RVSP above 35 mm Hg was strongly associated with mortality. Moreover, mortality was higher in those with an RVSP above the median of 48 mm Hg.

The presence of PH-HFpEF and RV dysfunction is associated with increased mortality.[16,17] Mohammed and colleagues[18] demonstrated in a community-based study that any degree of RV dysfunction was found in about 21–35% of patients -semi qualitatively or tricuspid annular plane systolic excursion (TAPSE) derived, respectively,

Table 1
Echocardiography probability of PH

Peak TR Velocity (m/sec)	Other Echocardiogram Findings Suggestive of PH	Echocardiographic Probability of PH
≤ 2.8 or unable to measure	Absent	Low
≤ 2.8 or unable to measure	Present	Intermediate
2.9–3.4	Absent	Intermediate
2.9–3.4	Present	High
>3.4	Not required	High

Supporting echocardiographic findings of PH: right ventricular to left ventricular basal diameter ratio> 1, flattening of the interventricular septum (eccentricity index > 1.1 in systole and/or diastole), right ventricular outflow tract Doppler acceleration time < 105 msec and/or midsystolic notching, early pulmonary regurgitation velocity > 2,2 m/sec, pulmonary artery diameter > 25 mm, inferior vena cava diameter > 21 mm with decreased respiratory variation (<50% with sniff or < 20% quiet inspiration, right atrial area at end of systole > 18 cm^2.

with HFpEF. Both RV dysfunction and elevated RVSP were associated with worse cardiovascular mortality and more frequent heart failure hospitalizations. Melenovsky and colleagues[19] described that 33% of patients with HFpEF had RV dysfunction -as defined by fractional area change < 35%- in a single-center study of patients who underwent RHC. Those with RV dysfunction had higher right heart filling pressures and more severe pulmonary vascular disease (higher PA pressures and PVR). Patients with HFpEF with RV dysfunction had higher mortality when compared to patients without RV dysfunction (median 2-year survival 56% vs 93%), and RV dysfunction was the strongest predictor for mortality (HR 2.4 CI 1.6–2.6).

HOW CAN PULMONARY ARTERIAL HYPERTENSION AND PULMONARY HYPERTENSION-HEART FAILURE WITH PRESERVED EJECTION FRACTION BE DIFFERENTIATED?

PH is usually suspected after an echocardiogram is performed in the setting of dyspnea on exertion and shows an elevated estimated RVSP. Although RHC is the definitive test of choice to define PH, echocardiography remains the screening test of preference for the initial evaluation and management of this condition. When findings such as decreased left ventricular systolic function or severe aortic or mitral valve pathology are present, the diagnosis of PH-LHD may be evident. On the other side, an elevated RVSP in the setting of preserved left ventricular ejection fraction may represent a diagnostic dilemma between PAH and PH-HFpEF. The echocardiogram is essential in generating an initial suspicion of the cause of PH and to predict hemodynamics (**Table 2**).[20]

The accuracy of echocardiography to diagnose PH was assessed in the Registry to Evaluate Early and Long-term PAH Disease Management (REVEAL), a large United States-based PH registry.[21] In patients who had both an echocardiogram and RHC performed on the same day, echocardiography underestimated RVSP in 29% of the cases, it overestimated RVSP in 31% of the cases and RVSP was within 10 mm Hg of RHC in 40% of the cases. This correlation did not change significantly whether the tests occurred on the same day or within 12 months. This study highlights the importance of invasive hemodynamic assessment when suspecting significant PH.

An assessment of the morphology of the RV can help predict hemodynamics and the cause of PH.[22] Raza and colleagues showed that an end-systolic RV base/apex ratio < 1.5 strongly correlates with an elevated PVR. In contrast, the RV base was twofold wider—end-systolic RV base/apex ratio > 2—than the apex in patients with PH-LHC. Of note, patients with CpcPH showed a low end-systolic RV base/apex ratio < 1.5, resembling those with PH due to pulmonary vascular disease. These findings are likely explained by the impact elevated RV afterload on the RV compared to elevated pressures due to passive left-sided pressure transmission.

Arkles and colleagues[23] demonstrated that a simple visual inspection of the right ventricular outflow tract (RVOT) Doppler provides a powerful insight into the hemodynamics in a diverse PH cohort. The presence of a midsystolic notch in the RVOT Doppler was highly sensitive and specific for the triad of markedly elevated PVR, decreased pulmonary vascular compliance, and RV dysfunction seen in patients with PH due to pulmonary vascular disease. On the other

Table 2
Echocardiographic findings that help differentiate precapillary PH vs postcapillary PH in patients with normal left ventricular systolic function

Precapillary PH (PAH)	Echocardiogram Parameter	Postcapillary PH (PH-HFpEF)
Usually normal or small	Left atrial size	Usually dilated
Bows right to left	Interatrial septum	Bows left to right
< 1.5	Right ventricle morphology (end-systolic RV base/apex ratio)	> 2
Present	RVOT Doppler midsystolic notch and/or short RVOT acceleration time < 80 ms.	Absent
Higher score	Prediction rule: LA diameter: < 3.2 cm = +1 LA diameter: > 4.2 cm = −1 RVOT notching and/or AT < 80 ms = +1 Lateral mitral E/e': > 10 = −1	Lower score
< 1	Mitral E/A ratio	> 1

Abbreviations: LA, left atrium; PAH, pulmonary arterial hypertension; PH, pulmonary hypertension; PH-HFpEF: pulmonary hypertension due to heart failure with preserved ejection fraction; RV, right ventricle; RVOT, right ventricular outflow tract.

hand, PH in the absence of RVOT notching typically occurred in the setting of left heart congestion.

A simple prediction rule including left atrial diameter (+1 point for diameter < 3.2 cm and −1 point for diameter > 4.2 cm), RVOT Doppler notching assessment (+1 if present) or RVOT acceleration time (1+ if < 80 msec) and lateral mitral E/e' (−1 if > 10) accurately defines PH hemodynamics.[24] In this study of patients with normal left ventricular ejection fraction referred for the evaluation of PH, PVR increased stepwise with higher scores (score range −2 to +2). Negative scores argue strongly against PH due to a pulmonary vasculopathy. In addition, a negative score in conjunction with normal RVOT acceleration time and preserved RV function essentially excluded elevated PVR.

ARE THERE TREATMENT OPTIONS FOR PATIENTS WITH PULMONARY HYPERTENSION-HEART FAILURE WITH PRESERVED EJECTION FRACTION?

While pulmonary vasodilators are the standard of care in the treatment of PAH, results have not been consistently replicated in patients with PH-LHD; although these medications are sometimes tried in a patient with PH-HFpEF because of the significant symptoms and poor prognosis that is associated with this patient population. There have been trials using phosphodiesterase 5 inhibitors (PD5i),

soluble guanylate cyclase (sGC) stimulator, endothelin receptor antagonists (ERA), and prostacyclin with mixed results.

Experimental models and human studies have shown that nitric oxide-dependent pulmonary vasodilation is impaired in heart failure and contributes to endothelial dysfunction.[25] These observations led to the investigation of PD5i and sGC as potential treatment options for PH-LHD.

Guazzi and colleagues studied sildenafil 50 mg three times a day for up to 12 months in a double-blind, randomized, placebo-controlled trial. Forty-four patients with HFpEF with echocardiographic evidence of PH (estimated RVSP ≥ 40 mm Hg) were enrolled, and sildenafil showed improvement in mean PA pressures, PVR, and RV function.[26] On the other hand, the RELAX study, which included patients with HFpEF with ejection fraction (EF) > 50%, failed to show a significant effect of sildenafil 60 mg three times a day in the primary endpoint of change in peak oxygen consumption at 24 weeks of therapy.[27] Secondary endpoints of 6-minute walk distance and a clinical rank score -composite of death, hospitalization and change in heart failure questionnaire- were also negative. Of note, RELAX did not require the presence of PH as part of the inclusion criteria. Hoendermis and colleagues studied the use of sildenafil 60 mg three times a day for 12 weeks in 52 patients with PH-HFpEF in a single-center, randomized, double-blind, placebo-controlled trial. There was no change in the primary endpoint of mean pulmonary artery pressure at 12 weeks.[28] Interestingly, neither of these studies required an elevated PVR as part of the inclusion criteria and most patients had an IpcPH hemodynamic profile.

DILATE-1 evaluated the hemodynamic effect of a single dose of riociguat in patients with PH-HFpEF (EF > 50%, mean PA ≥ 25 mm Hg, and PCWP 15 mm Hg). There was no change in the primary endpoint of mean PA pressure compared to placebo. However, riociguat significantly increased stroke volume and decreased systolic blood pressure and RV end-diastolic area without changing PCWP, transpulmonary gradient, and PVR. As a follow-up, the phase IIb DYNAMIC study was designed to evaluate the efficacy, safety, and kinetics of riociguat in PH-HFpEF over 26 weeks with a primary endpoint of change in cardiac output. The results are not yet available. Pieske and colleagues[29] evaluated vericiguat in patients with EF ≥ 45% in the SOCRATES PRE-SERVED trial. The primary outcomes of this study were changed from baseline to week 12 in NT-proBNP and left atrial volume, which showed no improvement.

In patients with heart failure, plasma levels of endothelin-1 are elevated and associated with increased pulmonary pressure and higher risk for mortality.[30,31] Based on this observation, ERA have been evaluated as potential treatment options for heart failure.

The MELODY-1 study enrolled 63 patients with CpcPH confirmed by RHC and an EF >30%. In this phase II trial, patients were randomized to macitentan 10 mg daily or matching placebo for 12 weeks stratified by EF (<50% vs ≥ 50%). The median PVR was 5.8 WU, PCWP 20 mm Hg, and mean PA pressure 47 mm Hg; and 25% had EF <50%. At 12 weeks, the macitentan group showed no significant change in PVR, mean right atrial pressure, PCWP, and cardiac index. Notably, macitentan-treated patients were qualitatively more likely to experience fluid retention (10% treatment difference).[32] Bosentan, another ERA, was also previously evaluated in patients with HFrEF in the REACH-1 and ENABLE studies. Both of these trials were neutral for their primary outcome and were associated with worsening heart failure early in the treatment course.[33,34]

Levosimendan, an intravenous calcium sensitizer and inodilator, was evaluated in patients with PH-HFpEF, with mean PA ≥ 35 mm Hg, PCWP ≥ 20 mm Hg and EF ≥ 40%.[35] Six weeks of once-weekly infusions did not reduce the primary endpoint of peak exercise PCWP, but patients were noted to have a decrease in resting PCWP as well as improvement in 6-minute walk distance compared to placebo.

Currently, the CADENCE study (clinicaltrials.gov) is evaluating the effect of sotatercept—a first-in-class ligand trap for TGF-β superfamily ligands-in patients with PH-HFpEF and CpcPH. The rationale for performing this study comes from the PULSAR trial, which studied sotatercept in patients with PAH and showed a significant decrease in the primary endpoint of PVR, as well as improvements in prespecified secondary outcomes of 6-minute walk distance, NT-proBNP, and World Health Organization functional class.[36]

As seen, pulmonary vasodilators have shown mixed results in the treatment of PH-LHD with most results showing negative results and even signals of harm. Many of these trials studied pulmonary vasodilators in HFrEF. Of those who studied these medications in PH-HFpEF, the definition of PH was not uniform and not always based on invasive hemodynamics. Moreover, a distinction between IpcPH and CpcPH was not mandatory in most studies.

There has been significant interest in further understanding the cardiac and vascular changes leading to PH-HFpEF to help guide potential future therapies outside of traditional pulmonary vasodilators.[7] Vascular remodeling, metabolic syndrome oxidative stress, and fibrosis are all targets for future therapies. The vascular changes that occur in PH-HFpEF are different than what is seen in a patient with idiopathic PAH as well as patients with PH-HFrEF, and therefore respond differently to currently available therapeutic options. As well as arterial remodeling, there is significant venous remodeling and luminal narrowing that is similar to changes observed in pulmonary veno-occlusive disease.[37] The increased left atrial pressures and the associated back pressure leads causes barotrauma to the lung capillary and small arteries. These changes lead to a breakdown of the endothelial layer and increased permeability, resulting in gas exchange inefficiency, disrupted fluid filtration and reabsorption, and increased risk of pulmonary edema.[38] Patients with PH-HFpEF compared with PH-HFrEF have been found to have increased stiffness in the pulmonary circulation and vascular changes when compared to patients with the same pulmonary capillary wedge pressure leading to reduced pulmonary artery compliance (PAC = stroke volume/pulmonary artery pulse pressure).[39] Along with elevated pulmonary vascular changes and the uncoupling, further assessment of the RV shows diffuse fibrosis out of proportion to the degree of pulmonary hypertension in patients with PH-HFpEF.[40]

Table 3
Results of completed clinical trials PH-HFpEF

First Author/Study	Study Drug/Dose	Population (n)	Duration	Primary Outcome	Result
Guazzi et al,[26] 2011	Sildenafil 50 mg TID	HFpEF n = 44	12 months	PVR, RV performance, CPET	Improvement
Hoendermis et al,[28] 2015	Sildenafil 60 mg TID	HFpEF n = 52	12 weeks	mPAP vs placebo	No change
MELODY-1 [32]	Macitentan 10 mg daily	HF (EF> 30%) 75% HFpEF n = 48	12 weeks	Safety and tolerability	+10% fluid retention in active group
Burkhoff et al,[35] 2021	Levosimendan Weekly infusion (0.075–0.1 ug/kg/min for 24 hr)	HFpEF n = 37	6 weeks	Peak exercise PCWP	No change

Abbreviations: CPET, cardiopulmonary exercise testing; EF, ejection fraction; HF, heart failure; HFpEF, Heart failure with preserved ejection fraction; mPAP: mean pulmonary arterial pressure; PCWP: pulmonary capillary wedge pressure; PVR, pulmonary vascular resistance; RV: right ventricular.

The variability of cardiac and vascular changes for each individual patient has made it more difficult to assess the efficacy of therapy. The importance of separating patients into specific phenotypes (i.e. IphPH, CpcPH, exercise PH, and so forth) has been an important step to further understanding the pathophysiology of the cardiac and vascular changes, defining prognosis, and serving as a basis for clinical trial design.[7]

To date, there are currently no FDA-approved therapies for PH-HFpEF. Diagnosis and management of the underlying comorbidities—sleep apnea, hypoxia, arrhythmias, hypertension, coronary artery, obesity disease, and diabetes mellitus others—remains a focus of treatment of patients with PH-HFpEF.

SUMMARY

PH is frequently seen in patients with HFpEF and is associated with significantly greater symptom burden and increased mortality. The echocardiogram remains the initial screening test for PH in HFpEF and can generate an initial impression of the type of PH present and RV function. The RHC is the test of choice to define PH-HFpEF, and also importantly, understand the underlying hemodynamic profile (IpcPH vs CpcPH). The use of pulmonary vasodilators in PH-HFpEF has been evaluated in multiple clinical trials with mixed results. There are currently no FDA-approved therapies for PH-HFpEF . There is a significant interest in finding an effective therapeutic option for this population and clinical trials are currently

underway using novel mechanistic approaches in well-defined phenotypes. Improving the understanding of the different phenotypes and mechanisms of injury in each subset of patients with PH-HFpEF will be a critical step to improving the treatment in the future (**Table 3**).

CLINICS CARE POINT

- There are currently no FDA approved medical therapy for PH associated with HFpEF (PH-HFpEF).
- Differentiating between pulmonary arterial hypertension (PAH) and PH-HFpEF can be difficult and requires a high degree of suspicion. Referral to a tertiary center may be needed.

DISCLOSURE

The authors have nothing to disclose.

REFERENCES

1. Gerber Y, Weston SA, Redfield MM, et al. A contemporary appraisal of the heart failure epidemic in Olmsted County, Minnesota, 2000 to 2010. JAMA Intern Med 2015;175(6):996–1004.
2. Simonneau G, Montani D, Celermajer DS, et al. Haemodynamic definitions and updated clinical

classification of pulmonary hypertension. Eur Respir J 2019;53(1):1801913.

3. Strange G, Playford D, Stewart S, et al. Pulmonary hypertension: prevalence and mortality in the Armadale echocardiography cohort. Heart 2012;98(24):1805–11.

4. Vachiery JL, Adir Y, Barbera JA, et al. Pulmonary hypertension due to left heart diseases. J Am Coll Cardiol 2013;62(25 Suppl):D100–8.

5. Lam CS, Roger VL, Rodeheffer RJ, et al. Pulmonary hypertension in heart failure with preserved ejection fraction: a community-based study. J Am Coll Cardiol 2009;53(13):1119–26.

6. Galie N, Channick RN, Frantz RP, et al. Risk stratification and medical therapy of pulmonary arterial hypertension. Eur Respir J 2019;53(1):1801889.

7. Vachiery JL, Tedford RJ, Rosenkranz S, et al. Pulmonary hypertension due to left heart disease. Eur Respir J 2019;53(1):1801897.

8. Kim NH, Delcroix M, Jais X, et al. Chronic thromboembolic pulmonary hypertension. Eur Respir J 2019;53(1):1–10.

9. Waxman A, Restrepo-Jaramillo R, Thenappan T, et al. Inhaled treprostinil in pulmonary hypertension due to interstitial lung disease. N Engl J Med 2021;384(4):325–34.

10. Kovacs G, Berghold A, Scheidl S, et al. Pulmonary arterial pressure during rest and exercise in healthy subjects: a systematic review. Eur Respir J 2009;34(4):888–94.

11. Caravita S, Dewachter C, Soranna D, et al. Haemodynamics to predict outcome in pulmonary hypertension due to left heart disease: a meta-analysis. Eur Respir J 2018;51(4):1702427.

12. Vanderpool RR, Saul M, Nouraie M, et al. Association between hemodynamic markers of pulmonary hypertension and outcomes in heart failure with preserved ejection fraction. JAMA Cardiol 2018;3(4):298–306.

13. Galie N, Humbert M, Vachiery JL, et al. 2015 ESC/ERS guidelines for the diagnosis and treatment of pulmonary hypertension: the joint task force for the diagnosis and treatment of pulmonary hypertension of the European society of cardiology (ESC) and the European respiratory society (ERS): endorsed by: association for European paediatric and congenital cardiology (AEPC), international society for heart and lung transplantation (ISHLT). Eur Respir J 2015;46(4):903–75.

14. Shah AM, Claggett B, Sweitzer NK, et al. Cardiac structure and function and prognosis in heart failure with preserved ejection fraction: findings from the echocardiographic study of the Treatment of Preserved Cardiac Function Heart Failure with an Aldosterone Antagonist (TOPCAT) Trial. Circ Heart Fail 2014;7(5):740–51.

15. Simonneau G, Galie N, Rubin LJ, et al. Clinical classification of pulmonary hypertension. J Am Coll Cardiol 2004;43(12 Suppl S):5S–12S.

16. Lam CS, Borlaug BA, Kane GC, et al. Age-associated increases in pulmonary artery systolic pressure in the general population. Circulation 2009;119(20):2663–70.

17. Kjaergaard J, Akkan D, Iversen KK, et al. Prognostic importance of pulmonary hypertension in patients with heart failure. Am J Cardiol 2007;99(8):1146–50.

18. Mohammed SF, Hussain I, AbouEzzeddine OF, et al. Right ventricular function in heart failure with preserved ejection fraction: a community-based study. Circulation 2014;130(25):2310–20.

19. Melenovsky V, Hwang SJ, Lin G, et al. Right heart dysfunction in heart failure with preserved ejection fraction. Eur Heart J 2014;35(48):3452–62.

20. McLaughlin VV, Shah SJ, Souza R, et al. Management of pulmonary arterial hypertension. J Am Coll Cardiol 2015;65(18):1976–97.

21. Farber HW, Foreman AJ, Miller DP, et al. REVEAL Registry: correlation of right heart catheterization and echocardiography in patients with pulmonary arterial hypertension. Congest Heart Fail 2011;17(2):56–64.

22. Raza F, Dillane C, Mirza A, et al. Differences in right ventricular morphology, not function, indicate the nature of increased afterload in pulmonary hypertensive subjects with normal left ventricular function. Echocardiography 2017;34(11):1584–92.

23. Arkles JS, Opotowsky AR, Ojeda J, et al. Shape of the right ventricular Doppler envelope predicts hemodynamics and right heart function in pulmonary hypertension. Am J Respir Crit Care Med 2011;183(2):268–76.

24. Opotowsky AR, Ojeda J, Rogers F, et al. A simple echocardiographic prediction rule for hemodynamics in pulmonary hypertension. Circ Cardiovasc Imaging 2012;5(6):765–75.

25. Moraes DL, Colucci WS, Givertz MM. Secondary pulmonary hypertension in chronic heart failure: the role of the endothelium in pathophysiology and management. Circulation 2000;102(14):1718–23.

26. Guazzi M, Vicenzi M, Arena R, et al. Pulmonary hypertension in heart failure with preserved ejection fraction: a target of phosphodiesterase-5 inhibition in a 1-year study. Circulation 2011;124(2):164–74.

27. Redfield MM, Chen HH, Borlaug BA, et al. Effect of phosphodiesterase-5 inhibition on exercise capacity and clinical status in heart failure with preserved ejection fraction: a randomized clinical trial. JAMA 2013;309(12):1268–77.

28. Hoendermis ES, Liu LC, Hummel YM, et al. Effects of sildenafil on invasive haemodynamics and exercise capacity in heart failure patients with preserved ejection fraction and pulmonary hypertension: a

randomized controlled trial. Eur Heart J 2015;36(38): 2565–73.

29. Pieske B, Maggioni AP, Lam CSP, et al. Vericiguat in patients with worsening chronic heart failure and preserved ejection fraction: results of the SOluble guanylate Cyclase stimulatoR in heArT failurE patientS with PRESERVED EF (SOCRATES-PRESERVED) study. Eur Heart J 2017;38(15):1119–27.

30. Cody RJ, Haas GJ, Binkley PF, et al. Plasma endothelin correlates with the extent of pulmonary hypertension in patients with chronic congestive heart failure. Circulation 1992;85(2):504–9.

31. Pousset F, Isnard R, Lechat P, et al. Prognostic value of plasma endothelin-1 in patients with chronic heart failure. Eur Heart J 1997;18(2):254–8.

32. Vachiery JL, Delcroix M, Al-Hiti H, et al. Macitentan in pulmonary hypertension due to left ventricular dysfunction. Eur Respir J 2018;51(2).

33. Kalra PR, Moon JC, Coats AJ. Do results of the ENABLE (Endothelin Antagonist Bosentan for Lowering Cardiac Events in Heart Failure) study spell the end for non-selective endothelin antagonism in heart failure? Int J Cardiol 2002;85(2–3): 195–7.

34. Packer M, McMurray J, Massie BM, et al. Clinical effects of endothelin receptor antagonism with bosentan in patients with severe chronic heart failure: results of a pilot study. J Card Fail 2005;11(1):12–20.

35. Burkhoff D, Borlaug BA, Shah SJ, et al. Levosimendan improves hemodynamics and exercise tolerance in PH-HFpEF: results of the randomized placebo-controlled HELP trial. JACC Heart Fail 2021;9(5):360–70.

36. Humbert M, McLaughlin V, Gibbs JSR, et al. Sotatercept for the treatment of pulmonary arterial hypertension. N Engl J Med 2021;384(13):1204–15.

37. Fayyaz AU, Edwards WD, Maleszewski JJ, et al. Global pulmonary vascular remodeling in pulmonary hypertension associated with heart failure and preserved or reduced ejection fraction. Circulation 2018;137(17):1796–810.

38. Nguyen QT, Nsaibia MJ, Sirois MG, et al. PBI-4050 reduces pulmonary hypertension, lung fibrosis, and right ventricular dysfunction in heart failure. Cardiovasc Res 2020;116(1):171–82.

39. Adir Y, Guazzi M, Offer A, et al. Pulmonary hemodynamics in heart failure patients with reduced or preserved ejection fraction and pulmonary hypertension: similarities and disparities. Am Heart J 2017;192:120–7.

40. Patel RB, Li E, Benefield BC, et al. Diffuse right ventricular fibrosis in heart failure with preserved ejection fraction and pulmonary hypertension. ESC Heart Fail 2020;7(1):253–63.

Transthyretin Cardiac Amyloidosis
An Evolution in Diagnosis and Management of an "Old" Disease

Dia A. Smiley, DO*, Carlos M. Rodriguez, MD, Mathew S. Maurer, MD

KEYWORDS

- Amyloidosis • Cardiac amyloidosis • Amyloid cardiomyopathy • Transthyretin
- Transthyretin cardiomyopathy • Cardiac scintigraphy • Heart failure with preserved ejection fraction

KEY POINTS

- HFpEF is a heterogeneous clinical syndrome with multiple underlying causes, possibly explaining why many of the therapies used to treat HFrEF have not shown a mortality benefit in patients with HFpEF.
- ATTR cardiac amyloidosis (ATTR-CA) is a progressive, infiltrative, and restrictive cardiomyopathy that is often an overlooked and an underdiagnosed cause of HFpEF.
- CA is increasingly recognized due to better diagnostic imaging and enhanced clinical awareness, as well as the recent introduction of novel therapies that meaningfully reduce morbidity and mortality from this condition.
- Because of the unique physiologic and hemodynamic features of CA, patients poorly tolerate traditional heart failure medications and experience worse outcomes compared with other causes of HFpEF.
- Early diagnosis and treatment in TTR-CA are imperative, as novel treatments have been shown to slow the progression of cardiomyopathy and neurologic impairment.

Abbreviations	
HFpEF	Heart failure with preserved ejection fraction
ATTR-CA	ATTR cardiac amyloidosis
ATTR	myloid transthyretin
AL	amyloidosisimmunoglobulin light chain
HFrEF	heart failure with reduced ejection fraction

INTRODUCTION

Heart failure with preserved ejection fraction (HFpEF) currently accounts for more than half of all heart failure and is associated with significant morbidity and mortality, with an event rate post-heart failure hospitalization that is similar to heart

Funding: This work was supported by K24AG036778 from the National Institute on Aging, and by fellowship support from the Amyloidosis Foundation.
Cardiac Amyloidosis Program, Columbia University Irving Medical Center, New York Presbyterian Hospital, New York, NY 10032, USA
* Corresponding author. Clinical Cardiovascular Research Laboratory for the Elderly, 21 Audubon Avenue, New York, NY 10032.
E-mail address: ds4031@cumc.columbia.edu

Cardiol Clin 40 (2022) 541–558
https://doi.org/10.1016/j.ccl.2022.06.008

Table 1
Epidemiology, pathophysiology, and clinical differences between ATTRwt and ATTRv

Characteristics	ATTRwt	ATTRv
Precursor protein	Normal TTR	Variant TTR
Age at diagnosis	60–100	18–80
Epidemiology	80%–90% men	male predominance, autosomal dominant genetic inheritance pattern
Cardiac involvement	May be responsible for as many as 15% of HFpEF cases in patients >75 years old. Predominant cardiac phenotype with restrictive cardiomyopathy, atrial and ventricular arrhythmias.	Variable depending on the mutation. Val122Ile predominately cardiac, Thr60Ala mixed, and Val30Met predominately neuropathic
Extracardiac involvement	Carpal tunnel syndrome, lumbar spine stenosis, gastrointestinal tract	Nerves, kidney, gastrointestinal tract, ocular
Pathophysiology	Transthyretin has a heavy beta-pleated sheet structure and has propensity to dissociate into monomers that can misfold, aggregate, and deposit as amyloid fibrils individuals age	Amino acid substitutions result in tetramer instability and the development of monomers prone to aggregation and deposition as amyloid fibrils in affected organs.

failure with reduced ejection fraction (HFrEF).[1] HFpEF is a heterogeneous clinical syndrome with multiple underlying causes, possibly explaining why many of the therapies used to treat HFrEF have not shown a mortality benefit in patients with HFpEF.[2] ATTR cardiac amyloidosis (ATTR-CA) is a progressive, infiltrative, and restrictive cardiomyopathy that is often an overlooked and an underdiagnosed cause of HFpEF.[3] ATTR-CA is present in 13% to 17% of hospitalized HFpEF patients with an increased wall thickness on echocardiography,[3,4] and cardiac ATTR deposits have been found in up to 25% of individuals greater than 85 years of age at autopsy.[5,6]

There are more than 30 different precursor proteins implicated in various amyloidosis diseases, arising as localized with different organ involvement or systemic, hereditary, or nonhereditary, and with differing prognoses.[7,8] Five of these proteins are known to infiltrate the heart and cause CA: amyloid transthyretin (ATTR), immunoglobulin light chain (AL amyloidosis), immunoglobulin heavy chain, serum amyloid A, and apolipoprotein AI. The 2 types that account for more than 95% of all CA are AL amyloidosis and ATTR. Differentiating these causes is difficult given their similar phenotype, but essential as they differ in their natural history, genetics, and treatment. In this review, we will focus on the most common form of CA,

namely ATTR-CA. ATTR-CA can be due to variants in the TTR gene (hereditary, mutant variant, familial, ATTRv) which are inherited in an autosomal dominant fashion, and wild-type (senile, nonhereditary, ATTRwt)[6,9] (**Table 1**).

CA is increasingly recognized due to better diagnostic imaging and enhanced clinical awareness, as well as the recent introduction of novel therapies that meaningfully reduce morbidity and mortality from this condition. What cardiologists learned about CA more than a decade ago has changed tremendously. There have been several seminal events in the evaluation and management of ATTR-CA including the advent of nuclear scintigraphy to establish the diagnosis without the need for biopsy and the development of novel therapeutics, such as TTR stabilizers and silencers. A disease we had no intrinsic treatment for, now has life-extending potential, with other promising therapies in the pipeline.

HISTORY OF CARDIAC AMYLOIDOSIS

As can be seen in **Fig. 1**, this "old" disease has been described for decades in the medical literature with a rapid increasing number of important diagnostic and therapeutic developments. The term "amyloid" is derived from the Latin word "amylym" which means starch and was coined

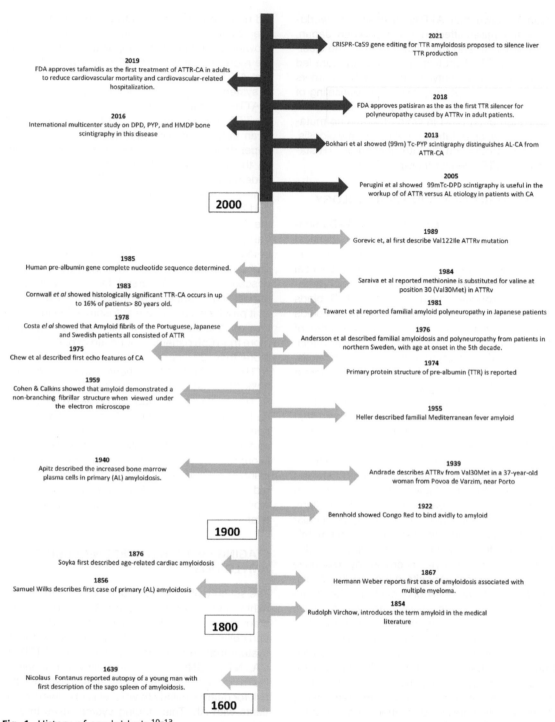

Fig. 1. History of amyloidosis.[10–13]

by the German botanist Matthias Schleiden (1804–1881). German pathologist Rudolph Virchow first introduced the term "amyloid" in the medical literature in 1854, to denote a macroscopic tissue abnormality that exhibited a positive iodine staining reaction, describing the "starch-like," properties of the amyloid fibrils. The first report of age-related deposition of amyloid in the heart and use of the term senile amyloid is attributed to Soyka in 1876.[10] Since Corino Andrade brought attention to the transthyretin type of peripheral neuropathy in Portugal in the 1930s, it soon became known that ATTRv disease was worldwide with families affected also in Sweden, Japan, South America, and the United States. The elucidation of the TTR protein and gene structure led to methods for identifying mutant gene carriers and allowed prompt diagnosis and counseling of family members. Further, progress included the recognition of ATTRwt in which there is no mutation, liver transplantation for ATTRv amyloidosis, and later introduction the introduction of TTR stabilizer and TTR silencer therapies.[11,12]

PATHOPHYSIOLOGY AND EPIDEMIOLOGY

TTR, also known as prealbumin, is a 56-kDa non-glycosylated protein composed of 4 identical 127-amino acid monomers circulating in the serum. Noncovalent bonds hold these 4 identical monomers together, and a single gene on chromosome 18 produces each monomer. TTR binds approximately 10% of T_4 and 10% of T_3 and binds retinol-binding protein as the sole transporter of vitamin A or retinol. TTR is mostly of liver origin, but it is also synthesized in pancreatic islet cells, the retina, and epithelial cells of the choroid plexus.[14] Aging and amylogenic mutations destabilize the native quaternary structures of TTR; thereby inducing conformational changes that lead to the dissociation of the tetramers into partially unfolded subunits, which can subsequently self-assemble into amyloid fibrils that deposit in tissues, including the heart. Misfolded TTR proteins form insoluble fibers, and in the heart occupy interstitial spaces in the myocardium, making it stiff and rigid and reducing ventricular capacitance, leading to diastolic and ultimately systolic dysfunction. Amyloid deposits can also directly cause myocyte necrosis by oxidative stress, and amyloid deposits in the conduction tissue can affect electrical conduction. Further, amyloid deposition in the valves can lead to valve thickening, and amyloid protein can deposit in the media and adventitia of coronary arteries and veins, as well as in the pericardium, which sometimes causes pericardial effusions.[15] ATTR infiltration of the atria causes significantly increased atrial stiffness, loss of normal architecture, remodeling of the vessels, capillary disruption, and upregulation of the collagen at the level of the subendocardium.[16] TTR deposition also causes myocardial fibrosis, exacerbating impairments in left ventricular filling and systolic function.[17]

Most cases of ATTR-CA are due to ATTRwt disease. The TTR gene in ATTRwt has a normal sequence and the development of disease is associated with aging, usually developing in the seventh and eighth decades of life.[6] Accordingly, the old nomenclature referred to this condition as senile systemic amyloidosis. Since the fastest growing segment of the population is those who are more than the age of 80 years, we anticipate that ATTRwt will become the most common form of systemic amyloidosis over the next few years.

ATTRv is caused by more than 130 variants in the TTR gene on chromosome 18, and is inherited in an autosomal dominant fashion, with an age-dependent penetrance that is highly dependent on the variant and whether individuals are from endemic or nonendemic areas[18] (**Table 2**). In the United States, the most common variants are Val122Ile, in which isoleucine replaces valine at the 122nd position of the protein.[4,9,19–21,24] The Val122Ile variant is observed almost exclusively in individuals of West African descent, while the Thr60Ala variant is common in individuals of Irish descent.[20,21,24,25] A careful family history is of utmost importance in hereditary forms of ATTR, as it provides clues to the autosomal dominant nature of inheritance. In our clinical experience of more than 650 patients diagnosed at our institution more than 20 years, ~50% (350 patients) had ATTRwt, ~21% (144 patients) had ATTRv, and 29% (200 patients) had AL-CA. Out of the 144 ATTRv patients, 91 had Val122Ile mutation, 23 had the Thr60Ala mutation, 4 had Val30Met mutation, and the rest (n = 26) had other less common mutations. Most of the patients diagnosed with CA in our registry are men. ATTRwt presents predominantly in Caucasian men more than 70 years old.[9,19] However, ATTRwt is more common in women than previously believed, and develops at a later age.[4,17]

STAGING OF TRANSTHYRETIN-CARDIAC AMYLOIDOSIS

The severity of ATTR-CA varies widely among patients, and currently, there are 3biomarker-based staging systems that have been proposed. Grogan and colleagues demonstrated in the Mayo staging system that, in a cohort of patients with ATTRwt-CA, NT-proBNP and high-sensitivity troponin T (hsTnT) plasma values were able to stratify the risk for death similarly to what was observed in patients with AL. This staging system uses thresholds of troponin T (0.05 ng/mL) and N-terminal pro-B-type natriuretic peptide (3000 pg/mL). The respective 4-year overall survival estimates were 57% for stage I (both values below cutoff), 42% for stage II (1 above), and 18% for stage III (both above), respectively. Stage III patients were at an increased risk of mortality after adjustment for age and sex compared with stage I patients (hazard ratio: 3.6; $P < .001$).[26] On the other hand,

Table 2
Most common ATTR variant mutations causing ATTRv-CA[4,9,13,14,18–23]

Variant	Mutation in the TTR Gene mRNA Sequence Variance/Codon Change/Location	Age at Onset	Organs Involved	Ethnic Origin/ Geographic Focus	Historical/Clinical Facts
Val122Ile (V122I; p.V142I)	Substitution of isoleucine for valine at position 122. c.424 G > A/GTC > ATC/ Exon 4	>60 year old Clinical penetrance varies, resulting in substantial heart disease in some carriers and few symptoms in others	Heart, PNS, soft tissues	Africa, Caribbean, United States	Most common variant worldwide Originated in West Africa Carried by 3.9% of African Americans Found in 10% of African Americans older than age 65 with severe CHF.
Val30Met (V30 M; p. Val50Met)	Substitution of methionine for valine at position 30 c.148 G > A/ GTG > ATG/Exon 2	Late 20s–early 40 s in the endemic area with a high penetrance rate >50 y of age in nonendemic areas with low penetrance	heart, PNS, ANS, leptomeninges, GI, Eyes	Portugal, Japan, Sweden, Cyprus, and Majorca	First TTR variant discovered First described in Portugal in the 1950s and later in Japan and Sweden Most widespread variant worldwide Most common cause of FAP
Thr60Ala (T60 A; p. Thr80Ala)	Substitution of alanine for threonine at position 60 c.238 A > G/ ACT > GCT/Exon 3	>45 y of age	Heart, PNS, ANS, GI, CTS	United Kingdom, Ireland Australian, German, Irish, British, US	First described in an Irish family in 1986, and a cluster of cases was identified in the County Donegal region of North-West Ireland. Affects up to 1% of the population of Northwestern Ireland. Second most frequent form of ATTR in the US

(continued on next page)

Table 2
(continued)

Variant	Mutation in the TTR Gene mRNA Sequence Variance/Codon Change/Location	Age at Onset	Organs Involved	Ethnic Origin/ Geographic Focus	Historical/Clinical Facts
Ile68Leu (I68 L; p. Ile88Leu)	Substitution of leucine for isoleucine at position 68 c.262 A > T/C/ATA > C/ TTA/Exon 3	>65 y of age	Heart, PNS	Central-northern Italy, Germany, United States	>15% of Italian patients with ATTRv referred to specialized amyloidosis centers have a late-onset cardiac phenotype, which is almost indistinguishable from ATTRwt
Leu111Met (L111 M; p. Leu131Met)	Substitution of methionine for leucine at position 111 c.391 C > A/ CTG > ATG/Exon 4	>40 y of age, with high penetrance	Heart, PNS, CTS	Denmark	Identified only in Danish families
Ser50Ile (S50I; p. Ser70Ile)	Substitution of isoleucine for serine at position 50 c.209 G > T/AGT > ATT/ Exon 3	>40 y of age	Heart, ANS, PNS	Spain, Japan	Less common cause of FAP
Asp18Glu (A18 G; p. Asp38Glu)	Substitution of glutamine for aspartate at position 18 c.114 T > A or G/ GAT > GAA/G/Exon 2	Very few patients reported, diagnosed in middle age (>45 y of age)	Heart, PNS, Eyes, Kidneys	Few patients reported from South America, American of Italian descent, Canadian of British descent	Only reported in the literature 4 times

Abbreviations: AS, autonomic nervous system; CTS, carpal tunnel syndrome; FAP, familial amyloid polyneuropathy; GI, gastrointestinal; PNS, peripheral nervous system.

Table 3
ATTR-CA staging systems[26–28]

	Mayo Staging
Stage I	Troponin T ≤0.05 ng/mL *and* NT-proBNP ≤3000 pg/mL (Both Normal)
Stage II	Troponin T ≥0.05 ng/mL *or* NT-proBNP ≥3000 pg/mL (one abnormal)
Stage III	Troponin T ≥0.05 ng/mL *or* NT-proBNP ≥3000 pg/mL (Both abnormal)
	UK Staging (Gilmore)
Stage I	NT-proBNP ≤3000 ng/L *and* eGFR ≥45 mL/min (Both Normal)
Stage II	NT-proBNP ≥3000 ng/L *or* eGFR ≤45 mL/min (One abnormal)
Stage III	NT-proBNP ≥3000 ng/L *and* eGFR <45 mL/min (Both abnormal)
	Columbia Staging
Stage I	1–3 points
Stage II	4–6 points
Stage III	7–9 points

Mayo score + diuretic dose + NYHA functional class
Or
UK score + diuretic dose + NYHA functional class
Daily diuretic dosing is categorized into furosemide equivalents assigned to a point system:
0 points for 0 mg/kg
1 point for > 0–0.5 mg/kg
2 points for >0.5–1 mg/kg
3 points for >1 mg/kg
NHYA class assigned to a point system:
1 point NYHA functional class I
2 points NYHA functional class II
3 points NYHA functional class III
4 points NYHA functional class IV

Gillmore *and colleagues* defined the stages further in the UK staging system by combining NT-proBNP and estimated glomerular filtration rate (eGFR) in both ATTRwt-CA and ATTRv-CA. Stage I is defined as NT-proBNP ≤3000 ng/L and eGFR ≥45 mL/min, Stage III was defined as NT-proBNP greater than 3000 ng/L and eGFR less than 45 mL/min, and the remainder were Stage II.[27] Most recently, Cheng and colleagues showed that adding diuretic dose and NYHA functional class to either the Mayo or UK risk scores for ATTR-CM, provides incremental predictive and discriminative utility[28] (**Table 3**).

SYMPTOMS AND CLINICAL FINDINGS

The diagnosis of ATTR-CA is frequently delayed, in part because patients present with varied symptoms, which are nonspecific. A high index of suspicion is the most important factor in identifying ATTR-CA as a cause of heart failure. The predominant symptoms of patients presenting with ATTR-CA are edema, shortness of breath, dyspnea on exertion, paroxysmal nocturnal dyspnea (PND), and orthopnea. Jugular venous pressure frequently reveals an inspiratory rise (Kussmaul sign), which is also present in patients with constrictive pericarditis. Further, unlike patients with severe heart failure caused by most other etiologies, third and fourth heart sounds are uncommon in CA. The absence of a fourth heart sound is attributable to the infiltration of the atria causing atrial mechanical dysfunction. Other symptoms that should raise suspicion of ATTR-CA are hypotension, dizziness, autonomic dysfunction, syncope, and peripheral neuropathy. There is also "normalization" of previous hypertension, as the blood pressure in patients with ATTR-CA is frequently low, due to a combination of reduced cardiac output and low peripheral vascular tone. ATTR-CA is a multi-systemic infiltrative disease associated with noncardiac soft

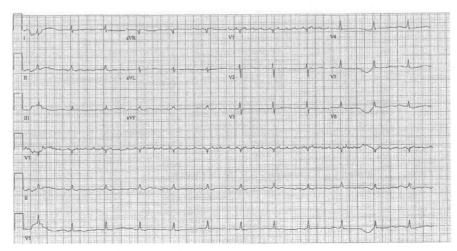

An ECG of a patient with TTR-CA, showing atrial flutter and low voltage.

Fig. 2. Electrrodiagram of a patient with TTR-CA. An ECG of a patient with TTR-CA, showing atrial flutter and low voltage.

tissue deposition, and patients often have carpal tunnel syndrome, lumbar spinal stenosis, biceps tendon rupture, and hip, knee, and shoulder replacements. Additionally, the presence of autonomic and/or sensory polyneuropathy is an important clue to the diagnosis. It is important to note that these systemic noncardiac manifestations of TTR deposition may precede the cardiac diagnosis of ATTR-CA by several years.[24,29–31]

Further, ATTR-CA is present in one out of 7 patients with degenerative aortic stenosis who need a valve replacement, and occult ATTR-CA has been found in 16% of patients' post-TAVR.[32,33] Aortic stenosis (AS) is associated with left ventricular hypertrophy and dysfunction, similar to that observed in ATTR-CA. Hence, AS and TTR-CA frequently coexist in older adults and share several clinical and echocardiographic features, which complicates the diagnosis and management of both conditions. Further, as both ATTR and AS share signs and symptoms, mainly those of heart failure, dizziness, and syncope, the indication for aortic valve replacement is often difficult to determine, especially as most patients with ATTR-CA have a low flow, low gradient phenotype. The accumulation of amyloid fibrils within the myocardium of patients with ATTR results in wall thickening and stiffening, which lead to restrictive cardiomyopathy with both LV and right ventricular dysfunction. Left ventricular ejection fraction (LVEF) is often preserved in patients with ATTR-CA, but low cardiac output and thus a low transvalvular flow state are frequent and may complicate the evaluation of AS severity. Low flow-low gradient pattern of severe AS (ie, AVA ≤1.0 cm2,

mean gradient <40 mm Hg, and stroke volume index <35 mL/m2) has been observed in 30% to 80% of patients with dual pathology of AS and CA, compared with less than 30% in patients with AS without CA.[34–37]

CLINICAL FINDINGS (BIOMARKERS, ECHO, MAGNETIC RESONANCE IMAGING , SCINTIGRAPHY, BIOPSY, AND GENETIC TESTING)

Serum cardiac biomarkers can be useful in detecting cardiac involvement in systemic amyloidosis or in evaluating the severity of the disease. B-type natriuretic peptide (BNP) and NT-proBNP are raised in all cases of heart failure and are often disproportionately high in CA. Additionally, patients will frequently have chronic troponin elevations without a definite anginal syndrome.[25,38,39] All patients with the suspicion of CA should get an electrocardiogram (ECG) (**Fig. 2**), and the hallmark ECG finding in ATTR-CA is low voltage QRS complexes due to amyloid infiltration. However, low voltage on EKG is only present in 20% to 30% in ATTR-CA and is a relatively late phase phenomenon. Thus, it is specific but not sensitive for identifying CA.[9,40] More importantly, discordance between EKG voltage and left ventricular wall thickness occurs due to myocardial infiltration by amyloidosis and is often mistakenly referred to as "left ventricular hypertrophy," but is not really LVH, as the there is no hypertrophy of the myocytes, but rather infiltration of the extracellular spaces by amyloid. ECG voltages tend to decrease as ATTR-CA progresses. More

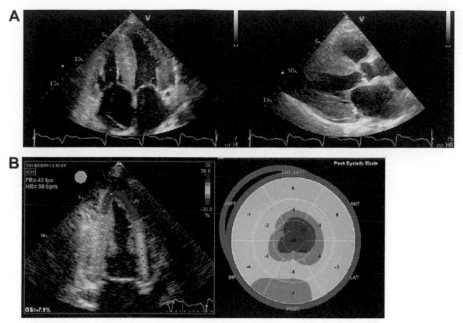

Fig. 3. Echocardiography of a patient with TTR-CA. (*A*) Four chamber and long access views of a patient with TTR-CA. Note the thickening of both LV and RV, as well as biatrial enlargement. (*B*) Longitudinal strain in the above patient with TTR. Note decreased strain, with almost preserved strain at the apex.

commonly, in approximately 50% to 70% of patients with ATTR-CA, pseudoinfarct patterns are present.[4,40] Further, conduction disorders occur frequently, and the occurrence of atrioventricular block in patients with increased wall thickness should raise suspicion for CA.[41]

Echocardiographic evaluation is a cornerstone of the noninvasive evaluation of ATTR-CA. Echocardiographic findings of infiltrative disease include LV wall thickening, small LV cavity size, biatrial enlargement, thickening of RV-free wall, thickened valves, and granular sparkling appearance (speckling) of the myocardial wall (**Fig. 3**). Amyloid deposits produce, in older nonharmonic 2D echo imaging, a pathognomonic hyperreflective appearance, defined as "granular sparkling," of the thickened ventricular myocardium. More recent harmonic 2D echo imaging often gives a speckled appearance to the myocardium, which is suggestive of CA. In the advanced stages of CA and, sometimes, in the early stage, even papillary muscles are thickened.[42] Amyloid infiltration also leads to valvular thickening and valvular regurgitation, although usually not significant.[42,43] Diastolic LV dysfunction is invariably present, with findings dependent on the stage of disease, and a restrictive LV pathology is found in advanced disease.[44] Pericardial effusions and systolic heart failure develop in the later stages of ATTR-CA. Longitudinal strain measurement by tissue Doppler and echocardiographic speckle

tracking have emerged as useful measurements for the identification of ATTR-CA, as they could help differentiate CA from other causes of left ventricular hypertrophy (LVH). Two-dimensional (2D) strain mapping shows relative preservation of apical function, which can be an early clue to amyloidosis because it gives rise to a "bulls-eye" pattern when the segmental strain is plotted, which is rare in other cardiomyopathies.[41,42]

Cardiovascular magnetic resonance (CMR) has unique advantages over echo in identifying cardiac infiltration in ATTR-CA, as it provides insights into tissue characterization. Although any pattern of late gadolinium enhancement (LGE) can be seen, a diffuse subendocardial pattern of LGE is highly suggestive of CA (specificity 95%), although diffuse transmural LGE is more common. Furthermore, diffuse transmural LGE is more common in ATTR than in AL, whilst a diffuse subendocardial pattern is more common in AL amyloidosis.[44,45] While useful for differentiating amyloidosis from nonamyloid diseases, neither echocardiography nor CMR can reliably differentiate ATTR-CM from AL amyloidosis.

Cardiac scintigraphy with 99mTc-pyrophosphate scintigraphy (99mTc-PYP) has revolutionized the diagnosis of ATTR-CA in the last decade. 99mTc-PYP scans are highly sensitive and specific for diagnosing cardiac ATTR amyloidosis and may reliably distinguish other causes of cardiomyopathy that mimic amyloidosis such as hypertrophic

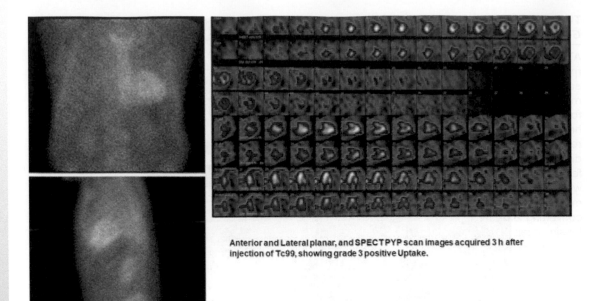

Anterior and Lateral planar, and SPECT PYP scan images acquired 3 h after injection of Tc99, showing grade 3 positive Uptake.

Fig. 4. Tc99 PYP scan image showing grade 3 positive Uptake in a Patient with TTR-CA. Anterior and Lateral planar, and SPECTPYP scan images were acquired 3 hours after the injection of Tc99, showing grade 3 positive uptake.

cardiomyopathy.[46] The sensitivity of grade 2 or 3 cardiac uptake on a radionuclide scan for cardiac ATTR amyloid deposits is 90% with a specificity of 97%.[6] ^{99m}Tc-PYP scintigraphy may identify cardiac ATTR amyloid deposits early in the course of the disease, sometimes before the development of abnormalities on echocardiography or CMR (**Fig. 4**).[45,47]

All patients with the suspicion or new diagnosis of CA need to be assessed for plasma cell dyscrasias, which is achieved with the use of serum-free light chain (FLC) measurements and serum and urine immunofixation electrophoresis (IFE). A ratio of kappa/lambda free light chains measured less than 0.26 or greater than 1.65 is abnormal and is present in more than 90% of untreated AL cases. However, the presence of a monoclonal protein does not ensure that AL is the cause of amyloidosis as up to 40% of patients with ATTR can have a monoclonal gammopathy of unknown significance (MGUS). In this setting ^{99m}Tc-PYP, scintigraphy alone cannot ensure a diagnosis with 100% specificity, and an endomyocardial biopsy sometimes is necessary to definitively diagnose ATTR. If no monoclonal protein is detected, then a diagnosis of AL CA is excluded, and ^{99m}Tc-PYP scintigraphy alone without an endomyocardial biopsy can be used to diagnose ATTR-CA.[6,39]

Endomyocardial biopsy and histologic analysis are the gold standard for identifying and typing ATTR-CA. The sensitivity and specificity are up to 100% if cardiac biopsies are obtained from 4 or more intracardiac sites. Endomyocardial biopsy is associated with a low risk of complications, including myocardial perforation and tamponade when performed by experienced operators. Unfortunately, is it not routinely performed in all centers and thus the diagnosis can be delayed. The sensitivity of extracardiac tissue biopsy varies significantly and is usually not recommended.[48–50] Biopsy of subcutaneous fat, salivary gland, or rectum has a low sensitivity (50% to 80% of patients with AL amyloidosis) and a much lower yield in patients with ATTR. Thus, a negative fat pad biopsy is insufficient to exclude CA.[49,50] Amyloid deposits are detected with the Congo red stain in association with polarized light microscopy, which shows a typical red–green birefringence when analyzed under polarized light microscopy.[51] In experienced laboratories, immunochemistry and tandem mass spectroscopy can be used to identify the type and nature of misfolded precursor protein.

In patients with confirmed ATTR-CA, TTR gene sequencing is necessary even if they do not have a family history of amyloidosis or evidence of polyneuropathy because the penetrance of ATTRv varies among the variants and in families. If ATTRv is detected, genetic counseling for relatives of the affected patient is indicated.[52]

THERAPY
General management and supportive therapy

ATTR-CA management requires supportive treatment to address heart failure symptoms. Patient education and multidisciplinary care are paramount. Heart failure therapy in ATTR-CA is focused on volume management, using basic heart failure recommendations of sodium and fluid restriction, daily weights, and the titration of loop diuretics and an aldosterone antagonist. A key difference in the heart failure management of patients with ATTR-CA is that conventional heart failure medications such as beta-blockers, angiotensin-converting enzyme inhibitors (ACEi), and angiotensin receptor blockers (ARB) are often poorly tolerated especially in high doses. They can further reduce cardiac output and contribute to systemic hypotension, thereby worsening symptoms. Physiologically, this occurs because patients with ATTR-CA have low stroke volumes and as the disease progresses, increasing heart rate is the main way to increase cardiac output. Nondihydropyridine calcium channel blockers should also be avoided because they often produce a significant negative inotropic effect by avidly binding to amyloid fibrils and causing shock and high degree heart block.[53,54] Although there is a general recommendation to avoid digoxin as first-line therapy in CA, it can still be administered cautiously, at lower doses with close monitoring of drug levels, renal function, and electrolytes; in patients with CA and atrial fibrillation with uncontrolled ventricular rate or low output heart failure when no other reasonable options exist.[55,56] Orthostatic hypotension is common and can be treated with midodrine and compression stockings; and avoiding vasodilators including ACEi/ARB, nitrates and hydralazine.[24,57] In the TOPCAT (Treatment of Preserved Cardiac Function Heart Failure with an Aldosterone Antagonist) study, a subset of patients enriched with structural and functional echocardiographic features of CA had the worst prognosis in the study but benefited from spironolactone therapy.[58] Future studies of mineralocorticoid receptor antagonists (MRA) in patients with CA are warranted. There are no studies currently supporting the use of the other pillars of heart failure therapy: angiotensin receptor neprilysin inhibitors (ARNI) and sodium-glucose cotransporter-2 (SGLT2) inhibitors in heart failure caused by ATTR-CA. These agents represent an area of active investigation.

Atrial arrhythmias are common among patients with CA. Atrial fibrillation is the most common arrhythmia in patients with CA and is present in as many as 70%.[17,59] Management of arrhythmic issues in patients with CA is largely based on expert consensus. Due to the significant restrictive cardiomyopathy in CA, loss of the atrial contribution to ventricular filling is poorly tolerated and associated with clinical deterioration and recurrent hospitalizations.[60] However, studies have not shown an effect on survival in CA. Whether to pursue a rate or rhythm control strategy is unknown, and medications traditionally used to slow the heart rate may be harmful in patients with CA due to dysautonomia, impairment of cardiac output in the setting of restrictive physiology, and concomitant reduced stroke volumes. Conversion to sinus rhythm may be preferred, particularly in symptomatic individuals. The rate of atrial fibrillation recurrence is high, and which antiarrhythmic to use and the role of catheter ablation remain unknown.[60–66] Anticoagulation is recommended in all patients with atrial fibrillation and CA, irrespective of their CHADS-VASC score, as CA is associated with high rates of atrial thrombus.[60,61] Further, anticoagulation may be considered even in patients with sinus rhythm and enlarged atria with low atrial strain due to a high risk of left atrial thrombus.[62–66]

Due to the progressive amyloid deposition throughout the heart, sinus node dysfunction and conduction disease often worsen over time. Bradyarrhythmias have been linked to sudden death in patients with CA, and therefore for patients with symptomatic bradycardia from conduction system abnormalities, pacemaker implantation is recommended as per traditional guidelines.

Lead placement should be carefully considered and many favor placement of a biventricular pacer, given the potential for further LV decrement in stroke volume from RV pacing and resulting ventricular dyssynchrony. Currently, there are no studies that can provide definitive guidance on which type of pacing should be routinely recommended in patients with CA but small series suggest a benefit of biventricular pacing.[3,62–64,67] Further, recommendations regarding implantable cardioverter-defibrillators (ICD) remain unclear.[68,69] Studies to date have been retrospective and observational, with small heterogeneous cohorts, with most of the patients having AL-CA. Results have shown a high prevalence of nonsustained ventricular arrhythmia, but variable rates of appropriate ICD therapies and no impact on survival.[68–70] There is a critical need for research in this field, as defining the natural history and significance of the electrical problems associated with CA will enable us to better understand which patients would benefit from antiarrhythmic therapy, and pacemakers or ICDs.

Table 4
Current and emerging therapies for the treatment of TTR-CA[71–78]

Mode of Action	Therapy	Indication	Phase of Study	Primary Endpoints	Dose	Side Effects	Concomitant Medications/ Monitoring	Cost
Approved Therapies								
Stabilizer	Tafamidis meglumine60 (Vyndaqel) Tafamidis free salt (Vyndamax)	ATTRv and ATTRwt-CA (NYHA class I–III)	Approved	All-cause mortality lower with tafamidis (29.5% vs 42.9%) Frequency of CV-related hospitalizations lower with tafamidis (RRR, 0.68)	80 mg PO qd 61 mg PO qd	No safety signals of potential clinical concern	None	~$235 000
	Diflunisal	ATTRv and ATTRwt-CA	Approved	Difference in polyneuropathy progression was slowed by diflunisal as measured by NIS+7	250 mg PO BID	Bleeding Hypertension Fluid retention Renal dysfunction	Proton pump inhibitor Monitor CBC and BMP q 3–6 mo	$420
Silencer	Inotersen (Tegsedi)	ATTRv with or without cardiomyopathy	NEURO-TTR phase 3 trial-FDA approved for the treatment of stage 1 or 2 polyneuropathy due to ATTRv Given side effects and toxicity profile, it is no longer being developed for use in ATTR-CA	Difference in the modified NIS+7 and QOL as measured by Norfolk QOL-DN questionnaire in those given Inotersen compared with placebo	300 mg SC q1 week	Glomerulonephritis Thrombocytopenia Vitamin A deficiency	Vitamin A supplementation CBC, BMP, and UA every 2 wk	~$450 000
	Patisiran (Onpattro)	ATTRv polyneuropathy with or without cardiomyopathy	Approved APOLLO	Change from baseline in mNIS+7 at 18 mo was less with patisiran compared with placebo.	0.3 mg/kg IV infusion q3 weeks	Infusion reactions Vitamin A deficiency	Steroid IV, APAP, H1 and H2 blocker IV, Vitamin A Supplementation	~450,000
Emerging Therapies								
Stabilizer	AG-10 (Acoramidis)	ATTRv and ATTRwt-CA (NYHA class I–III)	Phase 3 ATTRIBUTE-CM NCT03860935	Part A: Change in 6MWT at 12 mo Part B: All-cause mortality and CV-related hospitalizations at 30 mo	800 mg PO BID	Unknown	None	Unknown
Silencer	Patisiran (Onpattro)	ATTRv or ATTRwt cardiac amyloidosis	Phase 3 APOLLO-B NCT03997383	Change from baseline at month 12 in 6-MWT	0.3 mg/kg IV infusion q3 weeks	Infusion reactions Vitamin A deficiency	Steroid IV, APAP, H1 and H2 blocker IV,	~450,000

Drug	Population	Phase/Trial	Primary Outcome	Dose			Status
Vutrisiran	ATTRv and ATTRwt-CA (NYHA class I–III)	Phase 3HELIOS-B NCT04153149	Composite outcome of all-cause mortality and recurrent CV hospitalizations at 30–36 mo	25 mg SC q3 months	Unknown Vitamin A deficiency	Vitamin A Supplementation Vitamin A supplementation	Unknown
Eplontersen	ATTRv and ATTRwt-CA (NYHA class I–III)	Phase 3Cardio-TTRansform NCT04136171	Composite of CV mortality and frequency of CV clinical events at 140 wk	45 mg SC q4 weeks	Unknown Vitamin A deficiency	Vitamin A supplement, Platelets every week BMP, LFTs, and UPCR every 2 wk	Unknown
CRISPR (NTLA-2001)	ATTRv	Phase 1 Open-label and Single-Dose Expansion Study	Adverse events, pharmacokinetics, pharmacodynamics Change from baseline in serum TTR, prealbumin, antidrug antibody, and anti-Cas9 antibody levels	IV single dose	Unknown	H2 blockers and steroids used in phase I trial	Unknown

ASO indicates antisense oligonucleotide.

Abbreviations: 6-MWD/6-MWT, 6-min walk distance or time; ATTRv, variant transthyretin amyloid; ATTRwt, wild-type ATTR; CRISPR, clustered regularly interspaced short palindromic repeats; CV, cardiovascular; NIS+7, Neuropathy Impairment Score plus 7 nerve tests; NSAID, nonsteroidal antiinflammatory; NYHA, New York Heart Association heart failure class; QOL-DN, Quality of Life–Diabetic Neuropathy questionnaire; RISC, RNA-induced silencing complex; TUDCA, tauroursodeoxycholic acid.

Novel disease-specific therapeutic options

Early diagnosis and treatment in TTR-CA are imperative, as novel treatments have been shown to slow the progression of cardiomyopathy and neurologic impairment, but do not address existing amyloid deposits. Thus, the institution of therapy before significant cardiac dysfunction is key to best leveraging emerging therapies. Several novel therapeutic strategies are currently available for patients or are actively being investigated in human clinical trials (**Table 4**). TTR tetramer stabilizers and TTR silencers are the main available agents currently. Tafamidis is the first novel treatment to reduce morbidity and mortality in TTR-CA. Tafamidis is an orally available TTR stabilizer that binds with high affinity and selectivity to the thyroxine site of TTR, slowing the dissociation of TTR tetramers into monomers and preventing aggregation in amyloid fibrils. In the ATTR-ACT trial, 441 patients with ATTR-CA, NYHA class I–III HF were randomized to receive tafamidis 80 mg, 20 mg, or placebo daily for 30 months. Tafamidis was associated with lower all-cause mortality versus placebo (29.5% vs 42.9%, absolute reduction of 13.4%) and a 32% lower risk of cardiovascular hospitalizations.[79] Early benefit of treatment of patients with ATTR-CA with tafamidis has been shown in the long-term extension (LTE) data after the ATTR-ACT trial, whereby patients who initiated tafamidis after ATTR-ACT had poorer outcomes than those on continuous tafamidis treatment.[79,80] Another stabilizer, AG10 (Acoramidis) has been shown to be a potent and selective stabilizer of TTR, exceeding the efficacy of tafamidis in stabilizing ATTRwt and ATTRv in serum. In the phase 2 AG10 to 201 study, there was near complete stabilization (>90%) of TTR at peak and trough serum levels and is being currently investigated in a phase 3 trial, the Eidos AG10 study (ATTRIBUTE-CM).[71] Part A results from ATTRibute-CM failed to show improvements in functional status as measured by six-minute walk distance (6MWD) relative to placebo at 12 months, but acoramidis demonstrated improvement in NT-ProBNP and serum TTR measurements, as well as improvements in quality of life by the Kansas City Cardiomyopathy Questionnaire Overall Summary (KCCQ-OS). Part B results focused on clinical endpoints are anxiously awaited. Diflunisal is a nonsteroidal antiinflammatory (NSAID) agent which binds to the T4 binding sites on ATTR, though with lower affinity than tafamidis and with less potency for tetramer stabilization. Given that diflunisal is an NSAID, its potential for adverse effects such as renal dysfunction, gastrointestinal bleeding, hypertension, and fluid retention, makes it less appealing to use in patients with heart failure ATTR-CA. It may be considered for off-label use in selected patients with ATTR-CM, but more extensive studies of diflunisal in ATTR-CA are necessary.[72]

There are currently 4 TTR silencers that are available to patients or are undergoing phase III trials (see **Table 4**). Inotersen is a 2'-O-methoxyethyl-modified antisense oligonucleotide inhibitor of TTR production in the liver and is currently FDA approved in the United States for the treatment of stage 1 or 2 polyneuropathy due to ATTRv, but not for ATTR-CA.[73] Patisiran is another first-generation TTR silencer, which is a small interfering RNA (siRNA) that blocks the expression of both ATTRv and ATTRwt and is approved for the treatment of adults with ATTRv-related polyneuropathy.[74] The APOLLO-B trial (A Study to Evaluate Patisiran in Participants with Transthyretin Amyloidosis with Cardiomyopathy) is currently underway, and is a phase III study of patisiran in 300 patients with ATTR-CA. Vutrisiran is siRNA that is conjugated to an N-acetyl galactosamine (GalNAc), specifically targeting hepatocytes. HELIOS-A (A Study of Vutrisiran in Patients with Hereditary Transthyretin Amyloidosis) was a phase III study that enrolled 164 patients with ATTRv and polyneuropathy with or without cardiac involvement (excluding NYHA class III–IV heart failure). Vutrisiran met the primary endpoint of a change in modified neurologic impairment score+7 from baseline at month 9. HELIOS-B is a phase III study of ≈600 patients with ATTR-CA, randomized 1:1 to receive 25 mg of vutrisiran every 3 months or placebo, and is currently underway. Eplontersen (is a ligand (GalNAc linked to the 5' end) conjugated ASO (ligand conjugated antisense oligonucleotide) for which the ASO portion shares the same base sequence as inotersen. It is currently undergoing a phase III trial, Cardio-TTRansform, which plans to enroll 900 patients with ATTR-CA, randomized 1:1 to receive 45 mg of Eplontersen or placebo subcutaneously once every 4 weeks.[15]

Lastly, Clustered Regularly Interspaced Short Palindromic Repeats (CRISPR) and CRISPR-associated protein 9 (Cas9) is a genome-editing approach that is currently in phase I human trials, being leveraged to knock down the production of hepatic TTR. Formulations in phase 1 human trials include NTLA-2001 which is composed of human single-guide RNA and an mRNA sequence encoding Cas9 protein encapsulated in an LNP (lipid nanoparticle), that facilitates delivery to hepatocytes. The phase I study showed durable knockout of TTR after a single dose on day 28, with a mean reduction from baseline in serum

TTR protein concentration of 52% in the group receiving the lower dose of NTLA-2001 per kilogram, and 87% in the group that received the higher dose of NTLA-2001 per kilogram. Serial assessments of safety during the first 28 days after infusion in patients revealed few adverse events, and those that did occur were mild in grade.[75]

SUMMARY AND CONCLUSION

ATTR-CA is a progressive, infiltrative, and restrictive cardiomyopathy, which remains an under-appreciated and under-diagnosed cause of HFpEF. The importance of enhanced suspicion and early diagnosis cannot be overemphasized, as emerging therapies are more effective early in the course of the disease. Further, because of the unique physiologic and hemodynamic features of CA, patients poorly tolerate traditional heart failure medications and experience worse outcomes compared with other causes of HFpEF. ATTR CA is increasingly recognized due to enhanced clinical awareness, advances in diagnostic imaging that allow noninvasive diagnosis, as well as the recent introduction of novel disease-modifying treatments.

CLINICS CARE POINTS

- The importance of enhanced suspicion and early diagnosis cannot be overemphasized for cardiac amyloidosis, as emerging therapies are more effective early in the course of the disease.
- Always suspect cardiac amyloidosis in a patient with LVH on echo, normal-low voltage on EKG, and normal to low blood pressure or normalization of hypertension.

DISCLOSURE

Dr M.S. Maurer has grant support from NIH R01HL139671, R21AG058348, and K24AG036778. Consulting income from Eidos, Prothena, Ionis, and Alnylam and Intellia. Institutional support in the form of clinical trial funding from Pfizer, Ionis, Eidos, and Alnylam.

REFERENCES

1. Butler J, Fonarow GC, Zile MR, et al. Developing therapies for heart failure with preserved ejection fraction: current state and future directions. JACC Heart Fail 2014;2(2):97–112.
2. Oghina S, Bougouin W, Bézard M, et al. The impact of patients with cardiac amyloidosis in HFpEF trials. JACC Heart Fail 2021;9(3):169–78.
3. Mohammed SF, Mirzoyev SA, Edwards WD, et al. Left ventricular amyloid deposition in patients with heart failure and preserved ejection fraction. JACC Heart Fail 2014;2(2):113–22.
4. González-López E, Gagliardi C, Dominguez F, et al. Clinical characteristics of wild-type transthyretin cardiac amyloidosis: disproving myths. Eur Heart J 2017;38(24):1895–904.
5. Tanskanen M, Peuralinna T, Polvikoski T, et al. Senile systemic amyloidosis affects 25% of the very aged and associates with genetic variation inalpha2-macroglobulinandtau: a population-based autopsy study. Ann Med. 2008;40(3):232-239.
6. Gillmore JD, Maurer MS, Falk RH, et al. Nonbiopsy diagnosis of cardiac transthyretin amyloidosis. Circulation 2016;133(24):2404–12.
7. Sipe JD, Benson MD, Buxbaum JN, et al. Nomenclature 2014: amyloid fibril proteins and clinical classification of the amyloidosis. Amyloid 2014;21(4):221–4.
8. Merlini G, Bellotti V. Molecular mechanisms of amyloidosis. N Engl J Med 2003;349(6):583–96.
9. Rapezzi C, Merlini G, Quarta CC, et al. Systemic cardiac amyloidoses: disease profiles and clinical courses of the 3 main types. Circulation 2009;120(13):1203–12.
10. Kyle RA. Amyloidosis: a convoluted story: historical review. Br J Haematol 2001;114(3):529–38.
11. Benson MD. Transthyretin amyloidosis: a little history of hereditary amyloidosis. Amyloid 2017;24(sup1):76–7.
12. Cohen A, Kyle RA. History of amyloidosis. J Intern Med 1992;232(6):509–10.
13. Gorevic PD, Prelli FC, Wright J, et al. Systemic senile amyloidosis. Identification of a new prealbumin (transthyretin) variant in cardiac tissue: immunologic and biochemical similarity to one form of familial amyloidotic polyneuropathy. J Clin Invest 1989;83(3):836–43.
14. Connors LH, Lim A, Prokaeva T, et al. Tabulation of human transthyretin (TTR) variants. Amyloid 2003;10(3):160–84.
15. Falk RH, Gertz MA, Benson MD, et al. Rationale and Design of a Phase 3 study to evaluate the efficacy and safety of ION-682884 in patients with transthyretin-mediated amyloid cardiomyopathy (ATTR-CM). Blood 2019;134(Supplement_1):5764.
16. Bandera F, Martone R, Chacko L, et al. Clinical importance of left atrial infiltration in cardiac transthyretin amyloidosis. JACC Cardiovasc Imaging 2022;15(1):17–29.
17. Connors LH, Sam F, Skinner M, et al. Heart failure resulting from age-related cardiac amyloid disease associated with wild-type transthyretin: a

prospective, observational cohort study. Circulation 2016;133(3):282–90.

18. Adams D, Koike H, Slama M, et al. Hereditary transthyretin amyloidosis: a model of medical progress for a fatal disease. Nat Rev Neurol 2019;15(7):387–404.

19. Maurer MS, Hanna M, Grogan M, et al. Genotype and phenotype of transthyretin cardiac amyloidosis: THAOS (transthyretin amyloid outcome Survey). J Am Coll Cardiol 2016;68:161–72.

20. Suhr OB, Svendsen IH, Andersson R, et al. Hereditary transthyretin amyloidosis from a Scandinavian perspective. J Intern Med 2003;254(3):225–35.

21. Jacobson DR, Pastore RD, Yaghoubian R, et al. Variant-sequence transthyretin (isoleucine 122) in late-onset cardiac amyloidosis in black Americans. N Engl J Med 1997;336(7):466–73.

22. Booth DR, Booth SE, Persey MR, et al. Three new amyloidogenic TTR mutations: PRO12, GLU18, and VAL33. Neuromuscular Disord. Three new amyloidogenic TTR mutations: PRO12, GLU18, and VAL33 Neuromuscular Disord 1996;6.

23. Reynolds MM, Veverka KK, Gertz MA, et al. Ocular manifestations of familial transthyretin amyloidosis. Am J Ophthalmol 2017;183:156–62.

24. Kittleson MM, Maurer MS, Ambardekar AV, et al. Cardiac amyloidosis: evolving diagnosis and management: a scientific statement from the American heart association. Circulation 2020;142(1):e7–22.

25. Quarta CC, Buxbaum JN, Shah AM, et al. The amyloidogenic V122I transthyretin variant in elderly black Americans. N Engl J Med 2015;372(1):21–9.

26. Grogan M, Scott CG, Kyle RA, et al. Natural history of wild-type transthyretin cardiac amyloidosis and risk stratification using a novel staging system. J Am Coll Cardiol 2016;68(10):1014–20.

27. Gillmore JD, Damy T, Fontana M, et al. A new staging system for cardiac transthyretin amyloidosis. Eur Heart J 2018;39(30):2799–806.

28. Cheng RK, Levy WC, Vasbinder A, et al. Diuretic dose and NYHA functional class are independent predictors of mortality in patients with transthyretin cardiac amyloidosis. JACC Cardiooncol 2020;2(3):414–24.

29. Sperry BW, Reyes BA, Ikram A, et al. Tenosynovial and cardiac amyloidosis inpatients undergoing carpal tunnel release. J Am Coll Cardiol 2018;72(1):2040–50.

30. Geller HI, Singh A, Alexander KM, et al. Association between ruptured distal biceps tendon and wild-type transthyretin cardiac amyloidosis. JAMA 2017;318(10):962.

31. Westermark P, Westermark GT, Suhr OB, et al. Transthyretin-derived amyloidosis: probably a common cause of lumbar spinal stenosis. Ups J Med Sci 2014;119(1):223–8.

32. Castaño A, Narotsky DL, Hamid N, et al. Unveiling transthyretin cardiac amyloidosis and its predictors among elderly patients with severe aortic stenosis undergoing transcatheter aortic valve replacement. Eur Heart J 2017;38(38):2879–87.

33. Scully PR, Treibel TA, Fontana M, et al. Prevalence of cardiac amyloidosis in patients referred for transcatheter aortic valve replacement. J Am Coll Cardiol 2018;71(4):463–4.

34. Ternacle J, Krapf L, Mohty D, et al. Aortic stenosis and cardiac amyloidosis: JACC review topic of the week. J Am Coll Cardiol 2019;74(21):2638–51.

35. Galat A, Guellich A, Bodez D, et al. Aortic stenosis and transthyretin cardiac amyloidosis: the chicken or the egg? Eur Heart J 2016;37(47):3525–31.

36. Longhi S, Lorenzini M, Gagliardi C, et al. Coexistence of degenerative aortic stenosis and wild-type transthyretin-related cardiac amyloidosis. JACC Cardiovasc Imaging 2016;9(3):325–7.

37. Treibel TA, Fontana M, Gilbertson JA, et al. Occult transthyretin cardiac amyloid in severe Calcific aortic stenosis: prevalence and prognosis in patients undergoing Surgical aortic valve replacement. Circ Cardiovasc Imaging 2016;9(8):e005066.

38. Nativi-Nicolau J, Maurer MS. Amyloidosis cardiomyopathy: update in the diagnosis and treatment of the most common types. Curr Opin Cardiol 2018;33(5):571–9.

39. Kyriakou P, Mouselimis D, Tsarouchas A, et al. Diagnosis of cardiac amyloidosis: a systematic review on the role of imaging and biomarkers. BMC Cardiovasc Disord 2018;18(1):221.

40. Cyrille NB, Goldsmith J, Alvarez J, et al. Prevalence and prognostic significance of low QRS voltage among the three main types of cardiac amyloidosis. Am J Cardiol 2014;114(7):1089–93.

41. Kristen AV. Amyloid cardiomyopathy. Herz 2020;45(3):267–71.

42. Di Nunzio D, Recupero A, de Gregorio C, et al. Echocardiographic findings in cardiac amyloidosis: inside two-dimensional, Doppler, and strain imaging. Curr Cardiol Rep 2019;21(2). https://doi.org/10.1007/s11886-019-1094-z.

43. Maurer MS, Elliott P, Comenzo R, et al. Addressing common questions encountered in the diagnosis and management of cardiac amyloidosis. Circulation 2017;135(14):1357–77.

44. Carvalho FP de, Erthal F, Azevedo CF. The role of cardiac MR imaging in the assessment of patients with cardiac amyloidosis. Magn Reson Imaging Clin N Am 2019;27(3):453–63.

45. Fontana M, Banypersad SM, Treibel TA, et al. Native T1 mapping in transthyretin amyloidosis. JACC Cardiovasc Imaging 2014;7(2):157–65.

46. Bokhari S, Castaño A, Pozniakoff T, et al. (99m)Tc-pyrophosphate scintigraphy for differentiating light-chain cardiac amyloidosis from the transthyretin-related familial and senile cardiac amyloidoses. Circ Cardiovasc Imaging 2013;6(2):195–201.

47. Glaudemans AWJM, van Rheenen RWJ, van den Berg MP, et al. Bone scintigraphy with99mtechnetium-hydroxymethylene diphosphonate allows early diagnosis of cardiac involvement in patients with transthyretin-derived systemic amyloidosis. Amyloid 2014;21(1):35–44.

48. Quarta CC, Gonzalez-Lopez E, Gilbertson JA, et al. Diagnostic sensitivity of abdominal fat aspiration in cardiac amyloidosis. Eur Heart J 2017;38(24):1905–8.

49. Ansari-Lari MA, Ali SZ. Fine-needle aspiration of abdominal fat pad for amyloid detection: a clinically useful test? Diagn Cytopathol 2004;30(3):178–81.

50. Fine NM, Arruda-Olson AM, Dispenzieri A, et al. Yield of noncardiac biopsy for the diagnosis of transthyretin cardiac amyloidosis. Am J Cardiol 2014;113(10):1723–7.

51. Bulawa CE, Connelly S, Devit M, et al. Tafamidis, a potent and selective transthyretin kinetic stabilizer that inhibits the amyloid cascade. Proc Natl Acad Sci U S A 2012;109(24):9629–34.

52. Maurer MS, Bokhari S, Damy T, et al. Expert consensus recommendations for the suspicion and diagnosis of transthyretin cardiac amyloidosis. Circ Heart Fail 2019;12(9):e006075.

53. Pollak A, Falk RH. Left ventricular systolic dysfunction precipitated by verapamil in cardiac amyloidosis. Chest 1993;104(2):618–20.

54. Gertz MA, Skinner M, Connors LH, et al. Selective binding of nifedipine to amyloid fibrils. Am J Cardiol 1985;55(13 Pt 1):1646.

55. Bozkurt B, Colvin M, Cook J, et al. Current diagnostic and treatment strategies for specific dilated cardiomyopathies: a scientific statement from the American heart association. Circulation 2016; 134(23). https://doi.org/10.1161/cir. 0000000000000455.

56. Donnelly JP, Sperry BW, Gabrovsek A, et al. Digoxin use in cardiac amyloidosis. Am J Cardiol 2020;133: 134–8.

57. Ritts AJ, Cornell RF, Swiger K, et al. Current concepts of cardiac amyloidosis: diagnosis, clinical management, and the need for collaboration. Heart Fail Clin 2017;13(2):409–16.

58. Sperry BW, Hanna M, Shah SJ, et al. Spironolactone in patients with an echocardiographic HFpEF phenotype suggestive of cardiac amyloidosis: results from TOPCAT. JACC Heart Fail 2021;9(11): 795–802.

59. Mints YY, Doros G, Berk JL, et al. Features of atrial fibrillation in wild-type transthyretin cardiac amyloidosis: a systematic review and clinical experience: atrial fibrillation in wild-type transthyretin amyloidosis. ESC Heart Fail 2018;5(5):772–9.

60. El-Am EA, Dispenzieri A, Melduni RM, et al. Direct current cardioversion of atrial arrhythmias in adults with cardiac amyloidosis. J Am Coll Cardiol 2019; 73(5):589–97.

61. Dli F, Syed IS, Martinez M, et al. Intracardiac thrombosis and embolism in patients with cardiac amyloidosis. Circulation 2009;119(1):2490–7.

62. Barbhaiya CR, Kumar S, Baldinger SH, et al. Electrophysiologic assessment of conduction abnormalities and atrial arrhythmias associated with amyloid cardiomyopathy. Heart Rhythm 2016;13(2):383–90.

63. Longhi S, Quarta CC, Milandri A, et al. Atrial fibrillation in amyloidotic cardiomyopathy: prevalence, incidence, risk factors and prognostic role. Amyloid 2015;22(3):147–55.

64. Towbin JA, McKenna WJ, Abrams DJ, et al. 2019 HRS expert consensus statement on evaluation, risk stratification, and management of arrhythmogenic cardiomyopathy. Heart Rhythm 2019;16(11): e301–72.

65. Donnellan E, Wazni O, Kanj M, et al. Atrial fibrillation ablation in patients with transthyretin cardiac amyloidosis. Europace 2020;22(2):259–64.

66. Kochav SM, Dizon J, Maurer MS. A peak into the pace of cardiac amyloidosis. JACC Clin Electrophysiol 2020;6(9):1155–7.

67. Donnellan E, Wazni OM, Saliba WI, et al. Cardiac devices in patients with transthyretin amyloidosis: impact on functional class, left ventricular function, mitral regurgitation, and mortality. J Cardiovasc Electrophysiol 2019;30(11):2427–32.

68. Giancaterino S, Urey MA, Darden D. Hsu management of arrhythmias in cardiac amyloidosis. J Am Coll Cardiol 2020;6:351–61.

69. Lin G, Dispenzieri A, Kyle R, et al. Implantable cardioverter defibrillators in patients with cardiac amyloidosis: ICD in cardiac amyloidosis. J Cardiovasc Electrophysiol 2013;24(7):793–8.

70. Rehorn MR, Loungani RS, Black-Maier E, et al. Cardiac Implantable Electronic Devices: A Window Into the Evolution of Conduction Disease in Cardiac Amyloidosis. JACC Clin Electrophysiol 2020;6(9): 1144-1154. doi:10.1016/j.jacep.2020.04.020. Epub 2020 Aug 26. PMID: 32972550.

71. Judge DP, Heitner SB, Falk RH, et al. Transthyretin stabilization by AG10 in symptomatic transthyretin amyloid cardiomyopathy. J Am Coll Cardiol 2019; 74(1):285–95.

72. Ibrahim M, Saint Croix GR, Lacy S, et al. The use of diflunisal for transthyretin cardiac amyloidosis: a review. Heart Fail Rev 2021. https://doi.org/10.1007/ s10741-021-10143-4.

73. Benson MD, Waddington-Cruz M, Berk JL, et al. Inotersen treatment for patients with hereditary transthyretin amyloidosis. N Engl J Med 2018;379(1): 22–31.

74. Suhr OB, Coelho T, Buades J, et al. Efficacy and safety of patisiran for familial amyloidotic polyneuropathy: a phase II multi-dose study. Orphanet J Rare Dis 2015;10(1):109.

75. Gillmore JD, Gane E, Taubel J, et al. CRISPR-Cas9 in vivo gene editing for transthyretin amyloidosis. N Engl J Med 2021;385(6):493–502.

76. Griffin JM, Rosenblum H, Maurer MS. Pathophysiology and therapeutic approaches to cardiac amyloidosis. Circ Res 2021;128(10):1554–75.

77. Berk JL, Suhr OB, Obici L, et al. Repurposing diflunisal for familial amyloid polyneuropathy: a randomized clinical trial. JAMA 2013;310(24):2658.

78. Adams D, Gonzalez-Duarte A, O'Riordan WD, et al. Patisiran, an RNAi therapeutic, for hereditary transthyretin amyloidosis. N Engl J Med 2018; 379(1):11–21.

79. Maurer MS, Schwartz JH, Gundapaneni B, et al. Tafamidis treatment for patients with transthyretin amyloid cardiomyopathy. N Engl J Med 2018;379(11): 1007–16.

80. Elliott P, Drachman BM, Gottlieb SS, et al. Long-term survival with tafamidis in patients with transthyretin amyloid cardiomyopathy. Circ Heart Fail 2022; 15(1):e008193.

UNITED STATES POSTAL SERVICE®

Statement of Ownership, Management, and Circulation
(All Periodicals Publications Except Requester Publications)

1. Publication Title	2. Publication Number	3. Filing Date
CARDIOLOGY CLINICS	000 – 701	9/18/2022

4. Issue Frequency	5. Number of Issues Published Annually	6. Annual Subscription Price
FEB, MAY, AUG, NOV	4	$370.00

7. Complete Mailing Address of Known Office of Publication (Not printer) (Street, city, county, state, and ZIP+4®)

ELSEVIER INC.
230 Park Avenue, Suite 800
New York, NY 10169

Contact Person
Malathi Samayan

Telephone (Include area code)
91-44-4299-4507

8. Complete Mailing Address of Headquarters or General Business Office of Publisher (Not printer)

ELSEVIER INC.
230 Park Avenue, Suite 800
New York, NY 10169

9. Full Names and Complete Mailing Addresses of Publisher, Editor, and Managing Editor (Do not leave blank)

Publisher (Name and complete mailing address)

DOLORES MELONI, ELSEVIER INC.
1600 JOHN F KENNEDY BLVD. SUITE 1800
PHILADELPHIA, PA 19103-2899

Editor (Name and complete mailing address)

JOANNA COLLETT, ELSEVIER INC.
1600 JOHN F KENNEDY BLVD. SUITE 1800
PHILADELPHIA, PA 19103-2899

Managing Editor (Name and complete mailing address)

PATRICK MANLEY, ELSEVIER INC.
1600 JOHN F KENNEDY BLVD. SUITE 1800
PHILADELPHIA, PA 19103-2899

10. Owner (Do not leave blank. If the publication is owned by a corporation, give the name and address of the corporation immediately followed by the names and addresses of all stockholders owning or holding 1 percent or more of the total amount of stock. If not owned by a corporation, give the names and addresses of the individual owners. If owned by a partnership or other unincorporated firm, give its name and address as well as those of each individual owner. If the publication is published by a nonprofit organization, give its name and address.)

Full Name	Complete Mailing Address
WHOLLY OWNED SUBSIDIARY OF REED/ELSEVIER, US HOLDINGS	1600 JOHN F KENNEDY BLVD. SUITE 1800 PHILADELPHIA, PA 19103-2899

11. Known Bondholders, Mortgagees, and Other Security Holders Owning or Holding 1 Percent or More of Total Amount of Bonds, Mortgages, or Other Securities. If none, check box ▶ ☐ None

Full Name	Complete Mailing Address
N/A	

12. Tax Status (For completion by nonprofit organizations authorized to mail at nonprofit rates) (Check one)
The purpose, function, and nonprofit status of this organization and the exempt status for federal income tax purposes:
☒ Has Not Changed During Preceding 12 Months
☐ Has Changed During Preceding 12 Months (Publisher must submit explanation of change with this statement)

PS Form **3526**, July 2014 [Page 1 of 4 (see instructions page 4)] PSN: 7530-01-000-9931 PRIVACY NOTICE: See our privacy policy on www.usps.com.

13. Publication Title			14. Issue Date for Circulation Data Below
CARDIOLOGY CLINICS			MAY 2022

15. Extent and Nature of Circulation			Average No. Copies Each Issue During Preceding 12 Months	No. Copies of Single Issue Published Nearest to Filing Date
a. Total Number of Copies (Net press run)			174	156
b. Paid Circulation (By Mail and Outside the Mail)	(1)	Mailed Outside-County Paid Subscriptions Stated on PS Form 3541 (Include paid distribution above nominal rate, advertiser's proof copies, and exchange copies)	85	79
	(2)	Mailed In-County Paid Subscriptions Stated on PS Form 3541 (Include paid distribution above nominal rate, advertiser's proof copies, and exchange copies)	0	0
	(3)	Paid Distribution Outside the Mails Including Sales Through Dealers and Carriers, Street Vendors, Counter Sales, and Other Paid Distribution Outside USPS®	52	43
	(4)	Paid Distribution by Other Classes of Mail Through the USPS (e.g., First-Class Mail®)	0	0
c. Total Paid Distribution (Sum of 15b (1), (2), (3), and (4))		▶	137	122
d. Free or Nominal Rate Distribution (By Mail and Outside the Mail)	(1)	Free or Nominal Rate Outside-County Copies Included on PS Form 3541	21	17
	(2)	Free or Nominal Rate In-County Copies Included on PS Form 3541	0	0
	(3)	Free or Nominal Rate Copies Mailed at Other Classes Through the USPS (e.g., First-Class Mail)	0	0
	(4)	Free or Nominal Rate Distribution Outside the Mail (Carriers or other means)	0	0
e. Total Free or Nominal Rate Distribution (Sum of 15d (1), (2), (3) and (4))		▶	21	17
f. Total Distribution (Sum of 15c and 15e)		▶	158	139
g. Copies not Distributed (See Instructions to Publishers #4 (page #3))		▶	16	17
h. Total (Sum of 15f and g)		▶	174	156
i. Percent Paid (15c divided by 15f times 100)			86.7%	87.86%

*If you are claiming electronic copies, go to line 16 on page 3. If you are not claiming electronic copies, skip to line 17 on page 3.

PS Form **3526**, July 2014 (Page 2 of 4)

16. Electronic Copy Circulation	Average No. Copies Each Issue During Preceding 12 Months	No. Copies of Single Issue Published Nearest to Filing Date
a. Paid Electronic Copies	▶	
b. Total Paid Print Copies (Line 15c) + Paid Electronic Copies (Line 16a)	▶	
c. Total Print Distribution (Line 15f) + Paid Electronic Copies (Line 16a)	▶	
d. Percent Paid (Both Print & Electronic Copies) (16b divided by 16c × 100)	▶	

☒ I certify that 50% of all my distributed copies (electronic and print) are paid above a nominal price.

17. Publication of Statement of Ownership

☒ If the publication is a general publication, publication of this statement is required. Will be printed   ☐ Publication not required.
in the   NOVEMBER 2022   issue of this publication.

18. Signature and Title of Editor, Publisher, Business Manager, or Owner

Malathi Samayan - Distribution Controller   *Malathi Samayan*   Date 9/18/2022

I certify that all information furnished on this form is true and complete. I understand that anyone who furnishes false or misleading information on this form or who omits material or information requested on the form may be subject to criminal sanctions (including fines and imprisonment) and/or civil sanctions (including civil penalties).

PS Form **3526**, July 2014 (Page 3 of 4)   PRIVACY NOTICE: See our privacy policy on www.usps.com.

Moving?

Make sure your subscription moves with you!

To notify us of your new address, find your **Clinics Account Number** (located on your mailing label above your name), and contact customer service at:

Email: journalscustomerservice-usa@elsevier.com

800-654-2452 (subscribers in the U.S. & Canada)
314-447-8871 (subscribers outside of the U.S. & Canada)

Fax number: 314-447-8029

Elsevier Health Sciences Division
Subscription Customer Service
3251 Riverport Lane
Maryland Heights, MO 63043

*To ensure uninterrupted delivery of your subscription, please notify us at least 4 weeks in advance of move.

Printed and bound by CPI Group (UK) Ltd, Croydon, CR0 4YY

03/10/2024

01040363-0016